D1525339

MILITARY PSYCHOLOGY

Also Available

Military Stress Reactions: Rethinking Trauma and PTSD
Carrie H. Kennedy

MILITARY PSYCHOLOGY

CLINICAL AND OPERATIONAL APPLICATIONS

THIRD EDITION

edited by

CARRIE H. KENNEDY
ERIC A. ZILLMER

THE GUILFORD PRESS

New York   London

Copyright © 2022 The Guilford Press
A Division of Guilford Publications, Inc.
370 Seventh Avenue, Suite 1200, New York, NY 10001
www.guilford.com

Printed in the United States of America

This book is printed on acid-free paper.

Last digit is print number: 9 8 7 6 5 4 3 2 1

The authors have checked with sources believed to be reliable in their efforts to
provide information that is complete and generally in accord with the standards
of practice that are accepted at the time of publication. However, in view of the
possibility of human error or changes in behavioral, mental health, or medical
sciences, neither the authors, nor the editors and publisher, nor any other party
who has been involved in the preparation or publication of this work warrants
that the information contained herein is in every respect accurate or complete, and
they are not responsible for any errors or omissions or the results obtained from
the use of such information. Readers are encouraged to confirm the information
contained in this book with other sources.

Library of Congress Cataloging-in-Publication data is available from the
publisher.

ISBN 978-1-4625-4992-4 (hardcover)

The views presented in this book are those of the authors and do not reflect the
official policy or position of the U.S. Air Force, U.S. Army, U. S. Marine Corps,
U.S. Navy, the Department of Defense, the U.S. Government, or any other
institution with which the authors are affiliated.

In memory of my great-uncle,
Boatswain's Mate Third Class (United States Navy)
Heath Ridgeway Harrison,
1931–2021

—C. H. K.

To a patriot, humanitarian, and friend,
Chuck Pennoni,
President Emeritus, Drexel University

—E. A. Z.

In memory of my great-uncle,
Boatswain's Mate Third Class (United States Navy)
Heath Ridgeway Harrison,
1931–2021

—C. H. K.

To a patriot, humanitarian, and friend,
Chuck Pennoni,
President Emeritus, Drexel University

—E. A. Z.

About the Editors

Carrie H. Kennedy, PhD, ABPP, is a Captain in the Medical Service Corps of the U.S. Navy and Assistant Professor of Psychiatry and Neurobehavioral Sciences at the University of Virginia. She is board certified in both clinical and police and public safety psychology and is a Fellow of the National Academy of Neuropsychology and the American Psychological Association (APA). She currently serves as Member-at-Large, American Board of Police and Public Safety Psychology, and as Division 19 (Society for Military Psychology) Representative, APA Council of Representatives. Her awards include the Charles S. Gersoni and Robert S. Nichols Awards from APA Division 19, and she is a two-time Navy Psychologist of the Year winner. Dr. Kennedy has more than 70 publications in the areas of military psychology, aeromedical psychology, and neuropsychology. She is the author or editor of six books, which have been translated into four languages.

Eric A. Zillmer, PsyD, a clinical psychologist, is the Carl R. Pacifico Professor of Neuropsychology at Drexel University in Philadelphia. He is a Fellow of the College of Physicians of Philadelphia, the APA, and the National Academy of Neuropsychology, for which he also served as president. Dr. Zillmer has done extensive work on terrorism as well as the psychology of Nazi Germany, including publications, media, and film. His latest film project was to assist in a Russian documentary entitled *Trawinki: School of Executioners*. He is the author of *The Quest for the Nazi Personality* and the text *Principles of Neuropsychology,* and coauthor of two psychological assessment measures, the d2 Test of Attention and the Tower of London Test. He is a recipient of the Outstanding Faculty Award from the Pennoni Honors College at Drexel.

Contributors

Lieutenant Lyndse S. Anderson, PhD, United States Navy, Assistant Head, Special Psychiatric Rapid Intervention Team (SPRINT) West, Navy Medicine Readiness and Training Command, San Diego, California

Patrick Armistead-Jehle, PhD, ABPP, Chief, Concussion Clinic, Munson Army Health Center, Fort Leavenworth, Kansas

Captain Emmett Arthur, PsyD, United States Army, Brigade Psychologist, Behavioral Health Officer, 75th Field Artillery Brigade, Fort Sill, Oklahoma

Colonel (Ret) L. Morgan Banks, PhD, United States Army; Chief of Operations, Special Psychological Applications, Southern Pines, North Carolina

Heather G. Belanger, PhD, ABPP, Command Surgeon Office, United States Special Operations Command (USSOCOM), MacDill Air Force Base, Florida

Colonel (Ret) Carl Andrew Castro, PhD, United States Army; Professor and Director, USC Center for Innovation and Research on Veterans and Military Families and the Military and Veterans Programs, USC Suzanne Dworak-Peck School of Social Work, University of Southern California, Los Angeles, California

Major Jessica Y. Combs, PsyD, United States Air Force, Spangdahlem Air Base, Germany

Michael J. Craw, PhD, Police Psychologist, Los Angeles Police Department, Los Angeles, California

Major Melisa S. Finley, PsyD, United States Army, Tripler Army Medical Center, Honolulu, Hawaii

Captain Jeffrey L. Goodie, PhD, ABPP, Public Health Service, Director of Clinical Training, Medical and Clinical Psychology Program, Uniformed Services University of the Health Sciences, Bethesda, Maryland

Michael A. Gramlich, PhD, Clinical Psychologist, VA Puget Sound Health Care System, American Lake Division, Tacoma, Washington

Lieutenant Colonel (Ret) Revonda Grayson, PhD, United States Air Force

Colonel (Ret) Sally Harvey, PhD, United States Army

John A. Hodgson, MD, Department of Anesthesiology, Walter Reed National Military Medical Center, Bethesda, Maryland

Tim Hoyt, PhD, MBA, Deputy Director for Force Resiliency, Office of the Under Secretary of Defense for Personnel and Readiness, The Pentagon, Arlington, Virginia

Commander James M. Keener, PsyD, United States Navy, Operational Psychology Subspecialty Leader, Virginia Beach, Virginia

Captain Carrie H. Kennedy, PhD, ABPP, United States Navy, Psychiatry Department, Navy Medicine Operational Training Command Detachment, Naval Aerospace Medical Institute, Pensacola, Florida

Sara Kintzle, PhD, Research Associate Professor, Deputy Director Military and Veterans Programs, USC Suzanne Dworak-Peck School of Social Work, University of Southern California, Los Angeles, California

Jessica M. LaCroix, PhD, Associate Director, Suicide Care, Prevention, and Research Initiative, Henry M. Jackson Foundation; Research Assistant Professor, Uniformed Services University of the Health Sciences, Bethesda, Maryland

Captain Melissa D. Hiller Lauby, PhD, ABPP, United States Navy, Program Director, Warrior Toughness, Naval Service Training Command, Great Lakes, Illinois

Sara M. Lippa, PhD, ABPP, National Intrepid Center of Excellence, Walter Reed National Military Medical Center, Bethesda, Maryland

Commander Robert D. Lippy, PhD, ABPP, United States Navy, Force Psychologist for Commander, Naval Air Forces, U.S. Pacific Fleet, San Diego, California

Lieutenant Commander Stephanie M. Long, PhD, MSCP, ABPP, United States Navy, Suicide Prevention Subject Matter Expert, Office of the Chief of Naval Personnel, 21st Century Sailor Office (OPNAV N17), Arlington, Virginia

Major Carrie L. Lucas, PhD, MSW, MPA, MMOAS, LICSW, United States Air Force, Mental Health Flight Commander, Tinker Air Force Base, Oklahoma City, Oklahoma

Captain Mathew P. McCauley, PsyD, Irish Defence Forces, Consultant Military Clinical Psychologist; Assistant Professor of Clinical Psychology, Trinity College, University of Dublin, Ireland, Dublin, Ireland

Captain (Ret) William A. McDonald, MD, United States Navy, Psychiatry Department, Navy Medicine Operational Training Command Detachment, Naval Aerospace Medical Institute, Pensacola, Florida

Donald D. McGeary, PhD, ABPP, Associate Professor, Department of Psychiatry and Behavioral Sciences, University of Texas Health Science Center at San Antonio, San Antonio, Texas

Lieutenant Colonel Christopher A. Merchant, PsyD, United States Army Reserve, Operational Psychologist, Virginia Beach, Virginia

Charles A. Morgan III, MD, Department of Psychiatry, Yale University School of Medicine and National Center for Posttraumatic Stress Disorder, New Haven, Connecticut

Lieutenant Colonel Chad E. Morrow, PsyD, ABPP, United States Air Force, Command Psychologist, United States Air Force Special Operations Command, Hurlburt Field, Florida

Captain Hannah I. Nordwall, MSW, LCSW, United States Air Force, Clinical Social Worker, United States Air Force Academy, Colorado

Lieutenant Colonel Alan D. Ogle, PhD, United States Air Force, Command Psychologist, 480th Intelligence, Surveillance, and Reconnaisance Wing, Langley Air Force Base, Virginia

Major Stephanie N. Pagano, PsyD, ABPP, United States Army, Chief, Mountain Post Behavioral Health (Multi-D), Fort Carson, Colorado

Russell E. Palarea, PhD, President, Operational Psychology Services, LLC, Alexandria, Virginia

Lieutenant Colonel Jessica Parker, PsyD, ABPP, United States Army, Alexandria, Virginia

Major Thomas J. Patterson, PsyD, United States Army, Director, Clinical Psychology Internship Program, Chief, Behavioral Health Medical Education, Madigan Army Medical Center, Joint Base Lewis-McChord, Washington

Alan L. Peterson, PhD, ABPP, Aaron and Bobbie Elliott Krus Endowed Chair in Psychiatry, Professor and Chief, Division of Behavioral Medicine, Deputy Chair for Military Collaboration, Associate Director of Research, Military Health Institute, University of Texas Health Science Center at San Antonio, San Antonio, Texas; Director, STRONG STAR Consortium

Colonel (Ret) James J. Picano, PhD, United States Army Reserve; Senior Operational Psychologist, NASA Johnson Space Center, Houston, Texas

Commander Mathew B. Rariden, PsyD, ABPP, Department Head, Outpatient Mental Health, U.S. Naval Hospital, Okinawa, Japan

Lieutenant Colonel Patricia J. Razuri, PsyD, ABPP, United States Army, Command Psychologist, 1st Special Forces Group (Airborne), Joint Base Lewis McChord, Washington

Greg M. Reger, PhD, Deputy Associate Chief of Staff, Mental Health Service, VA Puget Sound Healthcare System, Tacoma, Washington; Associate Professor, Department of Psychiatry and Behavioral Sciences, University of Washington School of Medicine, Seattle, Washington

Colonel (Ret) Robert R. Roland, PsyD, United States Army

Ashley C. Schuyler, MPH, College of Public Health and Human Sciences, Oregon State University, Corvallis, Oregon

Nancy A. Skopp, PhD, Psychological Health Center of Excellence, Defense Health Agency (DHA), Joint Base Lewis-McChord, Tacoma, Washington

Christopher J. Spevak, MD, MPH JD, Professor of Clinical Anesthesiology, Georgetown University School of Medicine, Washington, D.C.

Lieutenant Marcus R. VanSickle, PhD, ABPP, United States Navy, Prescribing Psychologist; Forensic Psychology Fellow, Postdoctoral Fellowship Training Program in Forensic Psychology, Walter Reed National Military Medical Center, Bethesda, Maryland

Captain Kelly M. Wails, MSW, LSCW, United States Air Force, Alcohol and Drug Abuse Prevention & Treatment (ADAPT) Program Manager, Moody Air Force Base, Georgia

Captain Aaron D. Werbel, PhD, United States Navy, Executive Officer, Naval Hospital Twentynine Palms, Twentynine Palms, California

Lieutenant Kevin Michael Wilfong, PhD, Department of Medical and Clinical Psychology, Uniformed Services University of the Health Sciences, Bethesda, Maryland

Colonel (Ret) Thomas J. Williams, PhD, United States Army, Senior Operational Psychologist, Houston, Texas

Colonel Eveline F. Yao, MD, MPH, United States Air Force; Command Surgeon Office, United States Special Operations Command (USSOCOM), MacDill Air Force Base, Florida

Eric A. Zillmer, PsyD, Carl R. Pacifico Professor of Neuropsychology, Drexel University, Philadelphia, Pennsylvania

Preface

This volume is an important one to us, since it represents the last edition that we will publish together in our respective professional positions, Carrie in the Navy and Eric at Drexel University. Living with this book over the course of our careers, and in a period where the country was at war, has been formative for both of us.

Initially, the book itself was born of necessity, originally due to Carrie's frustration while on Navy psychology internship that no central repository of information for military mental health providers existed. This realization occurred before September 11, 2001, but once the volume was started, the country went to war, and the volume morphed accordingly in order to meet an even greater need.

At the moment of conception in 1999, however, Carrie had never published a book and needed someone to show her the way. Eric, her dissertation chair, Professor of Psychology at Drexel, and Drexel's Athletics Director, knew the way and he already had a deeply ingrained love of the military. He was the son of Lieutenant Colonel David Zillmer, United States Military Academy, Class of 1944. As an "Army brat," Eric was born in Tokyo and spent 22 years with his family while his father was stationed in Asia, Africa, and Europe. He grew up a child of the Cold War and learned firsthand about life in the military and, by proxy, the policies of détente. Of special impact on Eric was his father's experience in World War II and his role as part of the force that liberated the German concentration camp Dachau at the end of the war. Spending his formative years in Germany and attending Gymnasium in Garmisch-Partenkirchen, Eric became fluent in German and was immersed in German culture. As a result, he later wrote *The Quest for the Nazi Personality* and developed a longstanding interest in terrorism, military issues, and the culture of the military. Needless to say, the idea of a book that would directly benefit military psychologists and service members immediately appealed to him. But arriving at the foundational ideas behind a book and actually seeing that book in print can span a long period. And this book, although conceived in 1999, was mostly written at a time when our country had been thrust into war and it thus took several years to complete. Many things changed along the way, including the practice of military psychology itself. Consequently, the first edition was not published until 2006.

So much has also changed in the military since the first and second (2012) editions were published. After 20 years of war, the stigma of seeking mental health care has declined significantly, evidence-based research supporting specific forms of mental health treatments has grown, military instructions related to mental health have been revised, and the approaches of military mental health providers, as well as the locations in which they practice, have significantly evolved. Many military mental health providers are now engaged in prevention, early intervention, and care within primary-care clinics or military units, as opposed to mental health specialty clinics. Because of these substantial transformations, this volume sees significant updates to the core chapters, in addition to new chapters on military stress reactions; evidence-based treatment of depression, anxiety disorders, and posttraumatic stress disorder; concussion management; the integration of psychological health services within primary-care clinics; embedded psychological practice; sexual assault; and security clearance evaluations.

Of all the ideas we have both realized in our professional careers, we consider this volume our best. It is a practical how-to guide for mental health providers serving the military population and one of the few resources on operational psychology available. It has also sparked our lifelong friendship, and we are grateful for each other.

Finally, we are thankful for the steadfast support we have received from The Guilford Press. It is a significant benefit for authors when there is continuity within a publishing house, and they can work with the same editors across all three editions of a book. Thank you, Seymour Weingarten, Editor in Chief, and Rochelle Serwator, Senior Editor.

Contents

List of Cases

Note. All cases presented in this volume are composites, fictional, or cases in which identifying variables have been changed.

CHAPTER 1

A History of Military Psychology

Mathew P. McCauley, Eric A. Zillmer,
and Carrie H. Kennedy

Military psychology has a rich history. Although military history reaches back thousands of years, the formal establishment of military psychology began as recently as the early 20th century. The scholarly and applied discipline of psychology in the United States and elsewhere has had a similar trajectory as that of military psychology, and it is easy to conclude that their origins and growth are undeniably linked. However, the advancement of military psychology has occurred in spurts, each related to the demands, psychological as well as military, of the conflicts of different nations. Therefore, despite the fact that the history of formalized military psychology is relatively short, its impact pervades the practice of psychology. Military psychology has evolved from that of limited participation in wars of the past to today's conflicts, where it has become an indispensable asset in combat readiness and mission success.

More recently, military engagements and interactions have become increasingly intricate due to the complex geopolitical events evolving around the globe. As a result, the operational demands on the military have expanded accordingly and present the potential to create a novel set of stressors on military personnel and their families. Now more than ever, and related to this newest chapter of the history of military psychology, it would seem appropriate to review and catalog the role of this military specialty across clinical, industrial–organizational, and research domains. This chapter briefly describes the development of the profession of military psychology, including the various functions of the military psychologist through the years.

This chapter is dedicated to Private First Class (United States Army) John Bernard (Ben) McCauley (1934–1997).

THE U.S. CIVIL WAR

During the U.S. Civil War, military medicine was in its infancy, and the discipline of military psychology did not exist in any form. It was throughout the Civil War, however, that the first steps were taken to address overtly the effects of combat and war on servicemen. The concept of nostalgia, a term in use since the 1600s, was first well described (Kennedy, 2020), and military doctors reported treating other psychological concepts, such as phantom pain in amputees (Shorter, 1997), acute and chronic mania, alcoholism, suicidal behavior, and sunstroke (Lande, 1997). Although there is no documentation of the number of nostalgia cases, one anecdote depicts the numbers of psychiatric casualties of the Civil War:

> Both the Union and Confederate Armies attempted to utilize hospital ships to evacuate their wounded situated in areas near the Atlantic coastline. It has been reported that both armies had to abandon the use of such ships because a large number of individuals suffering from what was then called "nostalgia" practically clogged the gangplanks. This precluded such ships' properly caring for the physically sick and wounded. (Allerton, 1969, p. 2)

Following the war, soldiers who presented themselves for mental health care were often diagnosed with "chronic mania." Formal programs to address veterans' problems were limited. These servicemen were mostly cared for at home—although at times housed in the local jail because of the lack of other appropriate means to keep them and others safe—and many were treated in "insane asylums" (Dean, 1997). The United States Government Hospital for the Insane (USGHI; now known as St. Elizabeths Hospital), opened in 1855, was the first federally operated psychiatric hospital in the United States and eventually provided care for all government patients, including those who attempted to assassinate Presidents Andrew Jackson and Ronald Reagan (McGuire, 1990).

The Civil War saw the first documentation of substance use problems related to combat: abuse and addiction to alcohol, chloral hydrate, cocaine, morphine, and opium as well as substance withdrawal (Dean, 1997; Watanabe, Harig, Rock, & Koshes, 1994). Anecdotally, it appears that many of the chronic addiction problems among Civil War veterans were related to medical treatment for pain (Dean, 1997; see Chapter 7, this volume, for more information on substance abuse and the military).

WORLD WAR I

World War I marked the official birth of military psychology. In April 1917, Robert Yerkes, then the head of the American Psychological Association

(APA), convened a group of psychologists, including James McKeen Cattell, G. Stanley Hall, Edward L. Thorndike, and John B. Watson. Their charter was to determine how psychology could help the war effort. The committee recommended that "psychologists volunteer for and be assigned to the work in which their service will be of the greatest use to the nation" (Yerkes, 1917). Committees were developed, ranging from the Committee on the Selection of Men for Tasks Requiring Special Skills to the Committee on Problems of Motivation in Connection with Military Service. On August 17, 1917, Yerkes was commissioned as a Major in the U.S. Army (Uhlaner, 1967; Zeidner & Drucker, 1988), and by January 1918, 132 officers were commissioned for work in the Division of Psychology, Office of the Surgeon General (Zeidner & Drucker, 1988; see Figures 1.1 and 1.2). Their work signified the first concerted efforts to screen military recruits and included such notable statisticians as E. L. Thorndike, Louis Thurstone, and Arthur Otis (Driskell & Olmstead, 1989). World War I had such an impact on psychology that only one paper presented at the 1918 APA annual convention did not have anything to do with the war (Gade & Drucker, 2000), and although there were only 200 members of the APA at the time, 400 psychologists contributed to the war effort.

The Army Alpha Intelligence Test (for those who were literate in English) and Beta (for those who were not literate, who were literate in another language, and/or who failed the Alpha) were developed and administered to 1,750,000 men during the war (Kevles, 1968; see Figure 1.3). Of these men, 7,800 were recommended "for discharge by psychological examiners because of mental inferiority," 10,014 were recommended for assignment "to labor battalions because of low grade intelligence," and 9,487 were recommended for assignment to "development battalions, in order that they might be more carefully observed and given preliminary training to discover, if possible, ways of using them in the Army" (Yerkes, 1921, p. 99).

The Army Alpha evolved into the Wechsler–Bellevue Scale, the precursor to the Wechsler Adult Intelligence Scale, which has become the most frequently used intelligence test today (Boake, 2002). Intelligence testing during World War I marked the first means of testing hundreds of individuals simultaneously and led Lewis Terman (1918) to emphasize the need for standardized administration of psychological tests. Intellectual testing was not the only focus during World War I. The Woodworth Personality Data Sheet, which became the model for subsequent personality assessments, was introduced at that time (Page, 1996), and Yerkes developed procedures to assess and select individuals to become officers and undertake special assignments (Zeidner & Drucker, 1988).

The achievements of psychological testing in World War I were a significant impetus for the earliest recognition of psychology as a respected academic and scientific field. The success of group testing had substantial

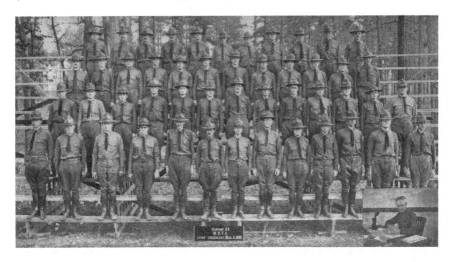

FIGURE 1.1. First company of commissioned psychologists, School for Military Psychology, Camp Greenleaf. (***denotes officer not a psychologist.) From left to right—front row: Wood, Roberts, Brueckner, Stone, Foster (instructor), Tyng (battalion major), Hunter, Hayes, ***, ***, Edwards, Stech, LaRue. Second row: ***, ***, Malmberg, Moore, Norton, Shumway, Arps, ***, ***, Stokes, Jones, Pedrick, Toll. Third row: Manuel, Bates, Miller, Chamberlain, Basset, Estabrook, Poffenberger, Benson, Trabue, Doll, Rowe, Elliott. Top row: Paterson, Dallenbach, Pittenger, Boring, Wylie, Bare, English, Sylvester, Morgan, Anderson, Houser. Major Yerkes is shown in the corner. Reprinted from Yerkes (1921).

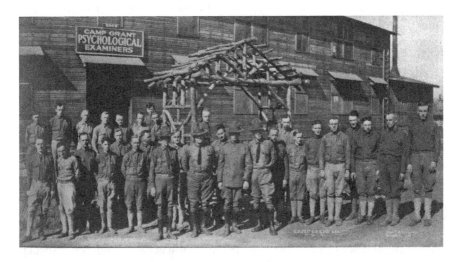

FIGURE 1.2. Supply company barracks assigned to psychological board at Camp Grant, showing typical psychological staff. Of the four officers in front, the captain at the left is the psychiatrist, and the three lieutenants (Sylvester, Benson, Terry) are psychologists. Reprinted from Yerkes (1921).

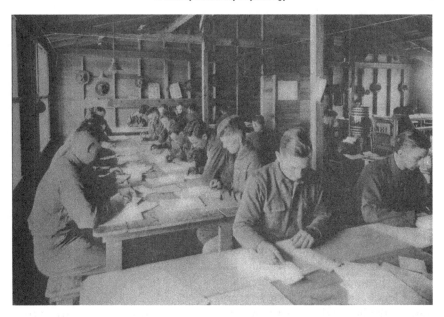

FIGURE 1.3. Scoring examination papers. The scorers are working at mess tables on the alpha examination. Reprinted from Yerkes (1921).

implications for organizations like grade schools, universities, and licensing boards. These tests also kindled the interest of private industry in search of help from psychologists with problems such as employee absenteeism, employee turnover, and ways to increase industrial efficiency (Zeidner & Drucker, 1988).

World War I marked the creation of the specialty of neurosurgery and the means to save the lives of servicemen with head injuries. With these advances arose the field of cognitive rehabilitation, advocated heavily by Shepherd I. Franz, a psychologist at USGHI, whose efforts to create a rehabilitation research institute were unsuccessful. However, Franz went on to publish manuals and books on cognitive assessment and "re-education" (Boake, 1989; Franz, 1923). Most military hospitals did provide rudimentary rehabilitation during World War I but were closed after the war because of lack of need.

Aviation psychology was born during World War I, and its major focus was the psychological screening of pilots in order to select those most likely to successfully complete training and avoid aviation accidents (Driskell & Olmstead, 1989). Early work showed that the best candidates possessed high levels of intelligence, emotional stability (i.e., low levels of excitability), perception of tilt (i.e., proprioception, the perception or awareness of the position and movement of the body), and mental alertness (Koonce,

1984). In addition to widespread intellectual testing, psychological screening, and head injury rehabilitation, the clinical condition of war neurosis was identified (Young, 1999).

During World War I, U.S. military psychiatrists filled the clinical role. In the United Kingdom, however, military psychologists not only provided clinical care but also did so in the combat zone, something U.S. military psychologists would not engage in until the Korean War. With the outbreak of World War I, these medically trained British Army psychologists deployed to wartime France in support of U.K. troops. Operating from field hospitals and casualty clearing stations and, later, not yet diagnosed nervous (NYDN) hospitals, they saw large numbers of personnel suffering from shellshock (Smith & Pear, 1917), disordered action of the heart (DAH), and related syndromes (Jones & Wessely, 2005). British military psychologists also presided over the evacuation, to rear areas or to the United Kingdom, of military personnel who were deemed unfit for further combat, at least in the immediate future.

In Britain, a large number of hospitals were established, including Craiglockhart (made famous in novelist Pat Barker's *Regeneration* trilogy, as the hospital where the writers Siegfried Sassoon and Wilfred Owen were treated together by British Army psychologist W. H. Rivers). Rivers and his colleague C. S. Myers were both medical practitioners who had taken up the new discipline of psychology, and both worked at Sir Frederick Bartlett's Department of Experimental Psychology at the University of Cambridge. Indeed, Rivers held the position of university lecturer in physiological and experimental psychology, while also noted as the founding editor of the *British Journal of Psychology*. He furthermore functioned as cofounder of what later became the British Psychological Society. Both individuals served as commissioned officers in the Royal Army Medical Corps during World War I, with Myers becoming consulting psychologist to the British Expeditionary Force. He established four forward NYDN centers and, later, five forward DAH centers in France, which operated in addition to the hospitals in Britain (Greenberg, Hacker Hughes, Earnshaw, & Wessely, 2011; Shephard, 2000).

World War I also saw the recognition of the first effective intervention for combat stress (i.e., shellshock), and the earliest cognitive restructuring techniques were documented well ahead of the development of formal cognitive theory (Howorth, 2000). Forward psychiatry was implemented, using the concept of assessment and treatment known as PIES (proximity, immediacy, expectancy, and simplicity) and resulted in 40–80% of shellshock cases returning to combat duty (Jones & Wessely, 2003). These early-intervention principles remain the foundation of combat stress intervention today, within the practices of deployed combat stress units (McCauley & Breeze, 2019; Kennedy, 2020).

The conflict of World War I also marked one of the first organized uses of chemical warfare: mustard gas (Harris, 2005). This gave rise to observations of "gas hysteria" and the recognition of a psychological response to threats of this nature. Lessons learned in World War I continue to guide mental health professionals in addressing the response to fears of and current terrorist threats to employ chemical and biological weapons. In short, World War I was a time of major growth for the field of psychology, the successes of which continue to have a profound impact on psychology practice today. G. Stanley Hall (1919) foretold the future when he commented on the work of psychologists in World War I, noting that "only when the history of American psychology is recorded in large terms will we realize the full significance of the work."

WORLD WAR II

Between 1944 and 1946, the APA underwent significant reorganization when it merged with the American Association for Applied Psychology (AAAP). After this merger, the five sections of AAAP became charter divisions in the new APA and included Division 19, Military Psychology (Gade & Drucker, 2000). In addition to stronger organizational foundations, World War II saw an influx of esteemed German and Jewish psychologists to America, which significantly strengthened the field of psychology in the United States.

Psychologists were in high demand during World War II and worked in all branches of the U.S. military, as well as sectors such as the National Research Council, Psychological Warfare Services, Veterans Administration (VA, now known as the United States Department of Veterans Affairs), and Department of Commerce (Gilgen, 1982). Work continued in psychometric testing, but a great diversification of developments and expansion in psychology occurred both during and immediately after the war. Boring (1945) published a comprehensive text on the application of psychology to the military, addressing topics such as adjustment to combat, personnel selection, morale, sexuality, and psychological warfare. He outlined seven fields of the "psychological business of the Army and Navy": observation, performance, selection, training, personal adjustment, social relations, and opinion and propaganda (p. 3). Books were also published for military members about the application of psychological principles to enhance performance (e.g., National Research Council, 1943; Shaffer, 1944) and to develop psychologically informed leadership abilities (Kraines, 1946). The Office of Strategic Services (OSS, now the Central Intelligence Agency) was developed, along with the first psychological selection program for individuals seeking positions as OSS operatives in espionage, counterespionage, and propaganda (Banks, 1995; OSS Assessment Staff, 1948), modeled after the selection procedures used by the German military for officers and others holding leadership positions (Ansbacher, 1949).

Screening for military service was improved, and in 1940 the Army General Classification Test (AGCT), developed by psychologists, was introduced as a means of measuring the aptitude of recruits and also of selecting men for specialist courses (Zeidner & Drucker, 1988) and for officer training (Harrell, 1992). The AGCT was taken by more than 12 million men for classification purposes and was valued over the intellectual testing format because of its minimization of verbal ability and the influence of formal education, its emphasis on spatial and quantitative reasoning, and its efficiency in administration (Harrell, 1992). After World War II, uniform aptitude testing in the military was mandated by the Selective Service Act of 1948, and in 1950 the Armed Forces Qualification Test (AFQT) was born. Although every service branch utilized the AFQT, each also continued to use its own screening procedures and instruments until 1968 (Defense Manpower Data Center, 1999).

Much of the improvement in classification and screening procedures was attributed to military psychologists' opportunity to test large groups of individuals from various geographical and cultural backgrounds. This observation and subsequent recognition that test results must be interpreted differently depending on an individual's background were clearly documented during World War II, marking some of the first succinct reasoning for culturally fair psychological tests. An additional impact was the construction of abbreviated testing techniques, which could easily be applied in the civilian sector (Hunt & Stevenson, 1946). World War II also saw the increased use of personality tests, and in 1943 the Army began using experimentally a newly published test, the Minnesota Multiphasic Personality Inventory, as a screening and selection instrument (Page, 1996; Uhlaner, 1967).

The increased emphasis on screening turned out to be a problem for those experiencing what was then identified as combat fatigue or combat exhaustion. Because the thinking of the time was that screening would exclude those prone to the development of these problems, during World War II, the United States did not initially apply the lessons learned in World War I about combat stress reactions (i.e., the need for timely intervention near the front line). Subsequently, little forward mental health care (i.e., mental health clinicians in the combat zone) was practiced, favoring instead reliance on psychological screening to avoid negative psychological reactions to the war. In fact, in 1943, while the rejection rate based on psychological screening was three to four times that of World War I, the incidence of mental health disorders was three times that seen in World War I (Glass, 1969). General George Marshall, in 1943, observed "that there were more individuals being discharged from the army for psychiatric reasons than the number of individuals being inducted into the army" (Allerton, 1969, p. 3). Between 1943 and 1945, 409,887 U.S. servicemen were hospitalized for combat fatigue in overseas Army hospitals: Of these, 127,660 were aeromedically evacuated to the United States (Tischler, 1969). One unfortunate result of the overemphasis on screening was that 40% of early discharges were attributed to combat fatigue (Neill, 1993), but it solidified the military's recognition of the need for battlefield interventions and preparation for the psychological toll of combat (Department of the Army, 1948). The overwhelming number of psychiatric casualties of World War II also confirmed the notion that combat stress reactions were generally normal responses to the emotional trauma and stressors of war, as opposed to a defect of character (Glass, 1969; see Chapter 3 for a discussion of military stress reactions).

Meanwhile, the U.K. military recruited eight civilian psychologists to produce tests to aid in the selection of candidates for the Royal Navy (RN). As a second filter at the larger naval entry establishments, these psychologists administered short, graded, and easy-to-score tests comprising additional tests of general intelligence, mathematical aptitude, and mechanical aptitude. As noted by Hacker Hughes (2007), the end of 1943 saw the RN retaining a staff of 10 "industrial" psychologists and approximately 300 assistants, mainly from the Women's Royal Naval Service (WRNS), who were involved in the work of personnel selection.

In the British War Office, on the other hand, testers and nontechnical officers and noncommissioned officers (NCOs) were employed within the Army's Directorate of Service Personnel, set up in July 1941 as part of the Adjutant-General's Department. All 19 psychologists—14 men and 5 women—were uniformed officers. Additionally, such work retained 31 officers and NCO testers (26 men and 5 women); along with 584 Nontechnical officers (531 men and 53 women) and a further 697 NCOs (494 men and 203 women). The tests in the standard test battery included assessments of general intelligence, arithmetic, verbal and nonverbal skills, and instructions (comprehension). Tests used for the selection for training in special trades or duties included U.S. Army Morse Aptitude Tests for signalers; spelling, shorthand, and typing tests for Auxiliary Territorial Service (ATS) clerks and signalers; and assembly tests for drivers and mechanical trades (Hacker Hughes, 2007).

More comprehensive testing was involved in British officer selection, in which psychologists collaborated with military officers and psychiatrists in the selection of officer candidates. Their work centered on formal psychological testing as well as the overall selection process. The tests involved not only outdoor selection tasks, in which psychologists and psychiatrists collaborated on test design with the military staff of the War Office selection boards (WOSBs), but also a number of formal psychological tests, including intelligence tests, biographical questionnaires, projective tests, and a more complicated version of the traditional Raven's Progressive Matrices Test; together with tests of verbal intelligence and reasoning. Outside the Adjutant-General's Department, the War Office also employed a small number of men with psychological training at the Directorate of Scientific

Research and the Directorate of Biological Research within the War Office Medical Department (Hacker Hughes, 2007).

Military psychology also achieved advances elsewhere in what was then the British Commonwealth. For example, the Australian military witnessed the establishment of the Australian Army Psychology Service in 1945. This occurred in tandem with Australian developments in psychological test resources for pilot selection, along with advances in cultural sensitivity within the psychological screening and assessment tools for military recruits (Hall & Eaves, 1989).

During the war, multiple psychological articles were published on malingering as a means to avoid military service or discipline, then also referred to as gold-bricking, faking, or malingery. The attitude toward malingerers at this time was summed up by Hulett (1941): "It is indeed devastating to recognize as we must, that all men are not possessed of manhood, and that the yellow streak down the backs of some of our fellows is invisible to the unaided human eye" (p. 138). Common methods of malingering were purported to be the induction of symptoms with substances such as alcohol, epinephrine, sugar, and cathartics; claims of pain or other sensory problems (e.g., blindness); claims of motor dysfunction; feigning of insanity; self-mutilation; exaggeration of real symptoms; or refusing to seek treatment for a curable condition (Campbell, 1943).

During World War II, the top five mental health diagnostic categories were neurosis, personality disorder, alcoholism, epilepsy, and insanity (Stearns & Schwab, 1943). Notably, the inadequacy of the existing mental health diagnostic system (Standard Nomenclature of Diseases and Operations) for military use during World War II was a significant impetus for the development of the *Diagnostic and Statistical Manual of Mental Disorders* (DSM; American Psychiatric Association, 1952). Additionally, head injury rehabilitation reemerged on a large scale (Doherty & Runes, 1943), with many of the leading psychologists later gaining prominence in the field of neuropsychology (Boake, 1989; for further information, see Kennedy, Boake, & Moore, 2010). Unfortunately, once again, many of the rehabilitation centers were closed after the war. The field did not return in a significant way until the late 1960s and early 1970s, in response to the increasing number of survivors of motor vehicle accidents (Boake, 1989).

Aviation psychology continued to evolve during World War II with the development of the U.S. Army Air Forces Aviation Psychology Program in 1941, the focus of which was to assist with the selection of aviation personnel (Driskell & Olmstead, 1989). In addition to the selection for positions such as pilots, navigators, and bombardiers, research was also conducted on the service member–equipment relationship, particularly with regard to the new military technologies of this period (Koonce, 1984). In 1947, the Air Force became a separate branch of the military, and industrial psychological research flourished in the new service (Hendrix, 2003).

As noted by Hacker Hughes (2007), World War II saw the British Air Ministry retain 4 civilian advisors in psychology for training methods; along with 17 Women's Auxiliary Air Force (WAAF) aircrew selection officers, 14 ground crew selection officers, and nearly 100 junior technical assistants. Tests used included measures of general intelligence (including the Royal Air Force [RAF] GVK test of general, verbal, and spatial/practical intelligence) and mathematics (for all RAF and WAAF candidates); Morse aptitude; pilot aptitude and observer (radio) aptitude (for aircrew candidates) and fluency; technical information; Morse reading; and radar (for temperament). In addition to these duties, Air Ministry psychologists also collaborated on a number of research projects from 1937 onward, including tests of reaction time and deftness of speed of hands and feet (the Sensory Motor Apparatus Test to assess flying aptitude and the Angular Perception Test to assess skills in making final approaches and landing aircraft). In addition, the Air Ministry, at the beginning of the war, used two kinds of tests: a group intelligence test prior to the selection board assessment, and experimental preselection aptitude tests to try to determine the sort of flying for which a recruit would be best suited.

Across all three British services, psychologists were involved in the design and interpretation of a variety of questionnaires and interviews, which addressed the layout, arrangement, and display of operational equipment, particularly in RAF operations rooms. Specific contributions were made in regard to the radius and position of turning handles in gunnery controls, along with the design and use of a number of trainers and simulators for pilots, gunners and air gunners, and bomb aimers. Psychologists were integral to work connected with a wide range of visual aspects of operational duties, including the use of goggles, instrument panel lighting, and night flying. Other more operational work involved advising in the special adaptation and modification of a variety of weapon systems. Job analyses and time and motion studies formed another aspect of wartime psychologists' work: for example, the job analyses of WRNS radio mechanics, air mechanics, and torpedo mechanics for the admiralty and the organization of WOSBs for potential ATS officers for the War Ministry; time and motion studies of gun laying and gun drills; and studies of extreme climatic conditions in tropical and Arctic conditions (Hacker Hughes, 2007).

Following World War II, the field of aviation psychology grew dramatically, affecting the practices of civilian airlines and creating new roles for aviation psychologists. Such psychologists are now involved in a wide range of activities, including research and identification of individuals involved in antiterrorism activities, aircraft accident investigations, assessment and selection of flight personnel, performing aeromedical psychological evaluations, and continuing research into human factors issues (Koonce, 1984; Olson, McCauley, & Kennedy, 2013).

World War II was also the first and only time that nuclear weapons were used. Survivors developed both acute and chronic psychological reactions, including withdrawal, severe fear reactions, psychosomatic symptoms, and posttraumatic stress disorder (PTSD; Salter, 2001). Beyond the effect of the bombings on the people of Japan, the images from Hiroshima and Nagasaki in 1945 continue to instill fear into societies threatened with such use today. Concerns mount about the capacity of terrorists to obtain and use these weapons (Knudson, 2001). In a similar vein, World War II was known for Japanese suicide bombers or kamikaze pilots. Kamikaze attacks accounted for a large proportion of the sailors who were wounded in action, second only to attacks that involved multiple weapons (Blood, 1992). The threat of suicide bombers has arisen as a heightened concern in recent decades, and some of the lessons learned in World War II are applicable to this modern-day weapon.

In the United States, military clinical psychology emerged during World War II, with military psychologists assigned to hospitals for the first time (McGuire, 1990; Uhlaner, 1967). Following the war, the growth of clinical psychology in the military continued. With a shortage of physicians and psychiatrists to meet the emotional needs of veterans, psychologists provided both group and individual mental health treatment in VA facilities (Cranston, 1986). In 1946, the first psychology internship programs were established, enrolling 200 interns within the VA system. These efforts resulted in increased acceptance of psychologists, not just as researchers and experts in assessment but also as mental health providers (Phares & Trull, 1997).

As occurred after World War I, psychologists were demobilized following World War II; however, in 1947, they obtained permanent active-duty status (McGuire, 1990; Uhlaner, 1967). Two years later, the first military clinical psychology internship programs were established in the U.S. Army, one of which was at the Walter Reed General Hospital in Washington, D.C. For discussions of military psychologists' current core clinical duties, see Chapters 2 (fitness-for-duty evaluations), 3 (stress reactions), 4 (evidenced-based treatment), 5 (behavioral health in primary care clinics), 7 (substance use), and 9 (suicide), this volume.

The advances of military psychology during World War II cannot be underestimated, and this provided a solid foundation from which the profession of psychology would continue to grow. Indeed, during the war, the Allies' adversary, Germany, deemphasized the study of individual differences and rejected the profession of psychology, replacing, for example, didactic courses in universities in psychology with those of racial theory (Zillmer, Harrower, Ritzler, & Archer, 1995). As such, the United States and United Kingdom became global leaders in the study of human behavior following World War II.

THE KOREAN WAR

During the Korean War, military psychologists served in several new positions: in service overseas, in combat zones, and on hospital ships (McGuire,
1990). The war saw significant use of torture, as well as the execution of
U.S. prisoners of war, and gave rise to the concept of brainwashing (Ursano
& Rundell, 1995). U.S. troops were exposed to forced marches, severe mal-
nutrition, inhumane treatment, and continuous propaganda and "reeduca-
tion" on communism (Ritchie, 2002). The Korean experience prompted
the military to make significant changes in survival schools or training
programs to help service members who are captured as prisoners of war.
Repatriated prisoners of war from the Korean conflict are credited for the
inception of the survival, evasion, resistance, and escape (SERE) model of
training currently provided to U.S. service members whose duties place
them at high risk of enemy capture (e.g., special forces, aviation personnel).
The SERE training paradigm and psychology's role therein are covered in
depth in Chapter 15 (this volume; see also Moore, 2010).

Unfortunately, early in the war, the principle of treating combat stress
near the front line to enable military members to return to duty was not
possible to implement, partly due to the abrupt start of the conflict and the
lack of prepared support units (McGuire, 1990). As a result, 250 troops
per 1,000 were declared psychological casualties. However, the lessons of
World War II regarding the need for mental health providers in the combat zone were not forgotten (Glass, 1969). Later in the war, mental health
providers were deployed, and 80% (Ritchie, 2003) to 90% (Jones, 1995)
of combat fatigue cases returned to duty. After the first year of combat in
Korea, a rotation policy of 9 months in combat was implemented, which
also helped to significantly reduce the number of psychiatric casualties
(Glass, 1969).

Psychology's role in testing did not diminish during the Korean War.
The U.S. Army and Air Force collaborated on a technical manual outlining the roles of the military psychologist and proper use of psychological tests (Departments of the Army and the Air Force, 1951), with such
distinguished contributors as David Wechsler and Paul Meehl (Uhlaner,
1967). Instruments created to select individuals for specific jobs and officer
programs continued to be improved. Additionally, the Korean War saw
advances in military psychology within Australia, one of many nations
involved in the conflict, which achieved enhancements to operational and
organizational structures for military psychology assets. Of note, in 1952,
the Australian Army Psychology Service evolved into its current operationally focused entity as the Australian Army Psychology Corps (Hacker
Hughes, McCauley, & Wilson, 2019).

Following the Korean War, the U.S. Army began to devote significant resources to the study of motivation, leadership, morale, and psychological warfare (Uhlaner, 1967). The study of human systems related to military functioning increased in scope, utility, and popularity (Zeidner & Drucker, 1988). The Air Force and Navy also created research centers for the study of what was then called human engineering. The goal of increasing the performance of military personnel given different equipment, various physical states (e.g., fatigue), and various environments gave rise to increased research in human factors engineering (Roscoe, 1997; Uhlaner, 1967).

THE VIETNAM WAR

After the Korean War, the U.S. Air Force implemented the Airman Qualifying Examination in 1958 for administration to high school students. Shortly thereafter, the Army and Navy developed their own group ability tests, and ultimately in 1968, the Armed Services Vocational Aptitude Battery (ASVAB) was implemented to make a truly uniform aptitude tool (Defense Manpower Data Center, 1999). The ASVAB has become an integral screening and aptitude tool for military recruits, and it is regularly used by military neuropsychologists during the assessment of head-injured service members, as its composite score is a reliable indicator of premorbid intellectual functioning (Kennedy et al., 2000; Welsh, Kucinkas, & Curran, 1990).

As in Korea, psychologists served in combat zones during the Vietnam War. Forward mental health was practiced from the beginning of the conflict, and low levels of traditional combat stress were seen. Compared with the psychiatric casualty rates of World War II (28–101 per 1,000 troops per year) and Korea (37 per 1,000 troops per year), troops in Vietnam exhibited very low rates, 10–12 per 1,000 troops per year (Allerton, 1969). As in no other conflict before or since, however, there was an extraordinary amount of substance abuse (see Chapter 7, this volume).

Also, a higher proportion of character disorders were diagnosed during the war, possibly related to the characteristics of individuals who could not avoid the draft. In other words, those with more resources were able to obtain education deferments or other exemptions to avoid military service (McGuire, 1990). In addition, the spirit of the times in the United States was highly tolerant of drug use, and this probably affected those serving in Vietnam as well. Because of the large numbers of troops who were abusing substances and had to be medically evacuated from the theater, mandatory drug testing was implemented and opportunities for alcohol and drug rehabilitation were increased.

The Vietnam War was a significantly complex conflict, involving the use of weapons technologies not seen before that could inflict substantial destruction, even on the level of the individual soldier (Zeidner & Drucker, 1988). American military members faced a well-trained force and were confronted with challenging jungle warfare as well as horrific prisoner of war experiences (see Moore, 2010). Military rotation policies at the time dictated specific tour lengths for individuals as opposed to rotations of entire units, resulting in poor unit cohesion because of the constant arrivals and departures of personnel (Zeidner & Drucker, 1988). Compounding these problems, the attitude on the home front regarding the utility of the war was largely unsupportive of the troops. The psychological impact of all these factors is hypothesized to have resulted in high rates of PTSD, with some veterans still experiencing symptoms today.

Following Vietnam, the U.S. military recognized the need for a formal response to noncombat critical incidents, including the deaths of service members during training or from suicide. In 1978, the Portsmouth Naval Hospital Psychiatry Department organized a Special Psychiatric Rapid Intervention Team. This multidisciplinary resource comprised psychologists, psychiatrists, chaplains, nurses, and corpsmen (McCaughey, 1987). The team supported psychological casualties arising from critical incidents such as training accidents, suicides, natural disasters, and bombings (for modern disaster response, see Chapter 11, this volume).

OPERATIONS DESERT SHIELD AND DESERT STORM

Military personnel in Operations Desert Shield and Desert Storm were exposed to multiple combat stressors: greater numbers of enemy forces, possible use of chemical and biological weapons, environmental challenges (i.e., desert exposure, sandstorms), lethal animal life, inadequate or insufficient hygiene opportunities, and a culture that did not accept American values (Martin, Sparacino, & Belenky, 1996). Although there was great capacity for significant stress casualties, the limited number of wounded and killed American troops and the availability of forward mental health support resulted in relatively few combat stress casualties; however, rates of PTSD have increased over time in these veterans. In addition to forward mental health support on the ground during the Persian Gulf War, for the first time a psychologist was deployed on a Navy aircraft carrier, the USS *John F. Kennedy*, which subsequently had no incidence of medical evacuation for mental health reasons (Wood, Koffman, & Arita, 2003).

Notwithstanding the contribution of good military mental health support structures, Gulf War syndrome or Gulf War illness, an ambiguous conglomeration of physical and psychological symptoms, emerged uniquely during the Persian Gulf War era. Despite a wealth of research into this phenomenon, there remains uncertainty regarding the characterization of the condition as a specific syndrome (Bieliauskas & Turner, 2000; Everitt, Ismail, David, & Wessely, 2002). Gulf War syndrome was hypothesized to originate from vaccinations, exposure to toxic substances (e.g., smoke from burning oil wells), and psychological trauma. Years of studying Gulf War veterans have largely led to the conclusion that, although risk factors for the syndrome included inoculations and exposures to noxious chemicals and psychological trauma, the persistence of the syndrome is largely the result of previous psychological distress and individual veterans' attribution of their symptoms (i.e., the belief that they were exposed to toxic agents; Hotopf et al., 2004; Stuart, Ursano, Fullerton, Norwood, & Murray, 2003). Despite the lack of a clear definition of Gulf War syndrome, veterans who have unexplained symptoms that began during or after the war are given financial and health benefits (Campion, 1996), and research into this issue continues.

PEACEKEEPING AND HUMANITARIAN OPERATIONS: MILITARY OPERATIONS OTHER THAN WAR

Peacekeeping and humanitarian missions have their own unique characteristics and impact on military personnel. Stress control units have been regularly utilized for those deployed for peacekeeping operations. Such psychological resources have been applied since Operation Restore Hope (ORH) in Somalia in 1992 (Bacon & Staudenmeier, 2003), given that peacekeeping forces often face an unfriendly populace, come under fire, live in unhygienic conditions, and are separated from their families (Hall, Cipriano, & Bicknell, 1997). In addition, peacekeeping missions can put significant strain on individuals who may be vulnerable, have a preexisting mental health condition, are engaging in the abuse of drugs and/or alcohol, or are experiencing relationship problems. These have been deemed risk factors for suicide in peacekeepers specifically (Wong et al., 2001).

Operation Uphold Democracy in Haiti saw significant stress among U.S. troops, including three suicides in the first 30 days of the mission (Hall, 1996). This reinforced the need for frontline mental health providers to administer preventive and early intervention measures for military personnel supporting peacekeeping missions (Hall et al., 1997). With operational stress support, 94% of soldiers presenting with psychological symptoms during Operation Uphold Democracy were returned to full duty without the need for medical evacuation (Hall, 1996).

Operation Joint Endeavor in Bosnia saw an unprecedented number of military mental health professionals on hand for suicide prevention, stress management, critical incident debriefings, and clinical care in-country (Pincus & Benedek, 1998). Mental health providers made advances during this mission in learning to increase awareness of available services and in destigmatizing help-seeking behavior by offering a comprehensive outreach program (Bacon & Staudenmeier, 2003). For more on peacekeeping and humanitarian missions and stress responses, see Kennedy (2020).

IRAQ, AFGHANISTAN, AND BEYOND

Military psychologists continue to make history. During two decades of international conflict in Iraq, Afghanistan, and beyond, there emerged an immediate need for an enhanced understanding of combat stress in the context of modern warfare. Service members have experienced the pervasive use of improvised explosive devices and rocket and mortar attacks causing psychological injuries as well as physical wounds. The frequent blasts and explosions once again brought to the forefront the phenomenon of blast concussion, first examined in World War I. As such, across the services, programs have arisen to educate service members on concussion and combat stress (see Chapter 6, this volume), and significant research has emerged in this area. In addition, prevention, diagnosis, and treatment are increasingly integrated into pre- and postdeployment health readiness programs throughout the military. In particular, military neuropsychologists have made major contributions in establishing guidelines for the assessment and treatment of brain injuries.

Military psychologists continue to expand their roles, including support for conventional and special operations. As early as October 2001, psychologists were deployed to main and forward-staging bases supporting Operation Enduring Freedom (OEF). In addition, psychologists served at forward-fire bases, providing expeditionary support to soldiers and U.S. Marines; along with consultation for commanders in both OEF and Operation Iraqi Freedom (OIF). Psychologists also treated enemy combatants throughout the Global War on Terror, both in theater and in detention facilities such as Guantanamo Bay.

Psychologists provide integral support in repatriation operations (see Chapter 15, this volume), assessment and selection for special operations (see Chapter 13, this volume), hostage negotiation (see Chapter 16, this volume), and human factors research; their roles have also expanded dramatically in counterintelligence, counterterrorism, and interrogation support (Staal & Harvey, 2019; see Chapter 12, this volume, for a discussion of operational psychology, and Chapter 14, this volume, for a discussion of security clearance evaluations).

Furthermore, women now make up an increasing proportion of the U.S. military, and all jobs, including ground combat positions, are open to them. However, women face gender-specific stressors in the military, such as unhealthy stereotypes, lack of female mentors and role models, sexual harassment, and sexual assault. Consequently, there remains much for military psychology to contribute to this emerging area (see Chapter 8, this volume, for more information on sexual assault in the military).

Other recent advances include the expansion of prescription privileges for psychologists. Beginning in 1994, the first cohort of military clinical psychopharmacology fellows graduated from a bespoke postdoctoral training program (Sammons, Levant, & Paige, 2003); followed by the establishment of the psychopharmacology fellowship at the Tripler Army Medical Center in Hawaii in 2005. The military's success in training psychologists as prescribers has served as a model for psychologists in the civilian sector (Dittman, 2003). In addition to the Department of Defense, Public Health Service, and Indian Health Service, five states (New Mexico, Louisiana, Illinois, Iowa, and Idaho) and one U.S. territory (Guam) have since enacted laws granting prescribing privileges to appropriately trained psychologists.

Military psychologists became permanent ship's company on aircraft carriers in 1998. This Psychology at Sea program continues to be highly successful (Wood et al., 2003). Service aboard these ships can be mentally stressful to the crew and is at times referred to as working "on top of a nuclear reactor and under an airport." Each carrier is assigned one psychologist, who serves not only the carrier but also the battle group that accompanies it, comprising a total of approximately 12,000 people. As the sole mental health provider, with assistance from a behavioral health technician and one or two substance abuse counselors, psychologists have had to move away from traditional forms of therapeutic interventions. The success of the carrier psychologists, and the need for mental health providers to be as close to military units as possible, led to an expansion of embedded mental health, to include ground combat units, submarine squadrons, and other operational commands (see Chapter 10, this volume). This mode of care delivery is tackling stigma and shows promise in the arenas of problem prevention and early detection.

In parallel with the long-standing campaigns in Iraq and Afghanistan, military psychology has seen significant expansion in armed forces across international jurisdictions. Many nations now view this specialty as a crucial asset for military health care, research, and organizational systems. In the Irish military, for example, clinical psychologists comprise the largest group of mental health professionals (McCauley & O'Brien, 2017). The Australian Army Psychology Corps remains an integral part of mental health provision throughout that nation's deployment cycles. Additionally, the U.K. Armed Forces now retain over 100 psychologists (i.e., uniformed and Ministry of Defence (MoD) civilian personnel) across military medical, research, and human factors domains (Hacker Hughes et al., 2019). Specifically, the British military has achieved a tenfold increase in their number of clinical psychology personnel during the past 20 years, while also securing the reintroduction of uniformed military psychology officers to the Royal Army Medical Corps. This has resulted in clinical psychologists serving as the U.K. MoD's Deputy Head of Healthcare, with others leading mental health clinical teams across the military (Norris, Renwick, Siddle, & Westlake, 2019).

Additionally, British military psychologists are responsible for delivering specialist neuro- and rehabilitative psychology services, developing new assessment and treatment programs, serving as U.K. representatives to the North American Treaty Organization (NATO) scientific entities, and incorporating psychological resources into both enlisted and officer training courses (Precious & Lindsay, 2019; Rennie, 2019; Sturgeon-Clegg, Hurn, & McCauley, 2019). Such U.K. military psychology personnel have broken new ground in serving as direct assets to special forces units, while also deploying as specialist personnel during the Ebola crisis, and via the provision of expert consultative functions to deployed units in Iraq, Afghanistan, and elsewhere (Norris & McCauley, 2019). These advances in U.K. military psychology had a significant impact on the British Psychological Society (BPS). In 2015, Professor Jamie Hacker Hughes, the former head of the MoD's Clinical Psychology Service, became president of the BPS; and in 2019, the BPS formally established its Defence and Security Psychology Section.

Large-scale international military operations have been reduced over recent years. However, the emergence of COVID-19 in 2020 saw the redeployment of military psychologists to military and civilian medical facilities, where they supported fellow clinicians in responding to the world's largest public health crisis in over 100 years (O'Brien & McCauley, 2020). Psychology served as a key operational asset and force-multiplier. As noted by Shenberger-Hess, Giangrande, and Miletich (2020), military psychologists have faced new and unique behavioral health challenges during the coronavirus pandemic. Serving both military personnel and civilian populations, they continue to apply evidence-based interventions to address the consequences of social distancing, isolation, quarantining, unemployment, and financial difficulties, and fear of direct morbidity and mortality from the virus itself (including the loss of loved ones). In addition, they have adapted to address the challenges in delivering high-quality patient care (e.g., within intensive care units), providing adequate access to care, and administering early intervention for inpatients and outpatients experiencing behavioral health crises (p. 4).

Across the United States and internationally, COVID-19 has seen military psychologists evolve their service delivery models on land and sea. Such duties entail the use of personal protective equipment for in-person clinical care; along with providing their full spectrum of duties via remote and telemedicine platforms (Collins, McCauley, & Norris, 2020; Grant, 2020; Zanov et al., 2020). Such clinical practice innovations hold significant promise for improving access to care during operations, while removing social and cultural barriers to military psychology services (O'Shea, McCauley, & O'Brien, 2019).

SUMMARY

The history of military psychology, although brief, is extensive. Not only has the field of psychology had an extraordinary impact on the military, but also the developments that have grown out of the various wars and the needs of the military have directly affected the practice of psychology across society. Psychologists continue to make history in their support of military missions, in their contributions to national security, and in improving services for active-duty members and their families. The following chapters focus on these efforts, along with military psychologists' increasing roles in clinical, expeditionary, and operational psychology domains. Lessons learned from recent and current campaigns and operations will shape the next chapter in the history of not only military psychology but also the discipline of psychology throughout the world.

REFERENCES

Allerton, W. S. (1969). Army psychiatry in Viet Nam. In P. G. Bourne (Ed.), *The psychology and physiology of stress: With reference to special studies of the Viet Nam War* (pp. 1–17). New York: Academic Press.

American Psychiatric Association. (1952). *Diagnostic and statistical manual of mental disorders*. Washington, DC: Author.

Ansbacher, H. L. (1949). Lasting and passing aspects of German military psychology. *Sociometry, 12*, 301–312.

Bacon, B. L., & Staudenmeier, J. J. (2003). A historical overview of combat stress control units of the U.S. Army. *Military Medicine, 168*, 689–693.

Banks, L. M. (1995). *The Office of Strategic Services psychological selection program*. Unpublished master's thesis, U.S. Army Command and General Staff College.

Bieliauskas, L. A., & Turner, R. S. (2000). What Persian Gulf War syndrome? *The Clinical Neuropsychologist, 14*, 341–343.

Blood, C. G. (1992). Analyses of battle casualties by weapon type aboard U.S. Navy warships. *Military Medicine, 157*, 124–130.

Boake, C. (1989). A history of cognitive rehabilitation of head-injured patients, 1915–1980. *Journal of Head Trauma Rehabilitation, 4*, 1–8.

Boake, C. (2002). From the Binet–Simon to the Wechsler–Bellevue: Tracing the history of intelligence testing. *Journal of Clinical and Experimental Neuropsychology, 24*, 383–405.

Boring, E. G. (1945). *Psychology for the armed forces*. Washington, DC: National Research Council.

Campbell, M. M. (1943). Malingery in relation to psychopathy in military psychiatry. *Northwest Medicine, 42*, 349–354.

Campion, E. (1996). Disease and suspicion after the Persian Gulf War. *New England Journal of Medicine, 335*, 1525–1527.

Collins, R., McCauley, M., & Norris, R. (2020). UK military clinical psychology during Covid19. *The Military Psychologist, 35*(2), 18–21.

Cranston, A. (1986). Psychology in the Veterans Administration: A storied history, a vital future. *American Psychologist, 41*, 990–995.

Dean, E. T., Jr. (1997). *Shook over hell: Post-traumatic stress, Vietnam, and the Civil War*. Cambridge, MA: Harvard University Press.

Defense Manpower Data Center. (1999). *Technical manual for the ASVAB 18/19 career exploration program* (rev. ed.). North Chicago: HQ USMEPCOM.

Department of the Army. (1948). *Military leadership psychology and personnel management* (an extract from the *Senior ROTC Manual*, Vol. II). Washington, DC: Author.

Departments of the Army and the Air Force. (1951). *Military clinical psychology, technical manual, TM 8–242, Air Force manual, 1600–45.* Washington, DC: Author.

Dittman, M. (2003). Psychology's first prescribers. *Monitor on Psychology, 34,* 36.

Doherty, W. B., & Runes, D. D. (1943). *Rehabilitation of the war injured: A symposium.* New York: Philosophical Library.

Driskell, J. E., & Olmstead, B. (1989). Psychology and the military: Research applications and trends. *American Psychologist, 44,* 43–54.

Everitt, B., Ismail, K., David, A. S., & Wessely, S. (2002). Searching for a Gulf War syndrome using cluster analysis. *Psychological Medicine, 32,* 1371–1378.

Franz, S. I. (1923). *Nervous and mental re-education.* New York: Macmillan.

Gade, P. A., & Drucker, A. J. (2000). A history of Division 19 (Military Psychology). In D. A. Dewsbury (Ed.), *Unification through division: Histories of the divisions of the American Psychological Association* (Vol. V, pp. 9–32). Washington, DC: American Psychological Association.

Gilgen, A. R. (1982). *American psychology since World War II.* Westport, CT: Greenwood Press.

Glass, A. J. (1969). Introduction. In P. G. Bourne (Ed.), *The psychology and physiology of stress: With reference to special studies of the Viet Nam War* (pp. xiii–xxx). New York: Academic Press.

Grant, N. (2020). Steaming to assist Los Angeles with COVID-19. *The Military Psychologist, 35*(2), 21–22.

Greenberg, N., Hacker Hughes, J. G. H., Earnshaw, N. M., & Wessely, S. (2011). Mental healthcare in the United Kingdom Armed Forces. In E. C Ritchie (Ed.), *Textbook of military medicine* (pp. 657–665). Washington, DC: Department of the Army, Office of the Surgeon General, Borden Institute.

Hacker Hughes, J. G. H. (2007). *British naval psychology 1937–1947: Round pegs into square holes.* Unpublished master's thesis, University of London.

Hacker Hughes, J. G. H., McCauley, M., & Wilson, L. (2019). History of military psychology. *Journal of the Royal Army Medical Corps: International Journal of Military Health; Military Psychology Special Issue, 165,* 68–70.

Hall, D. P. (1996). Stress, suicide, and military service during Operation Uphold Democracy. *Military Medicine, 161,* 159–162.

Hall, D. P., Cipriano, E. D., & Bicknell, G. (1997). Preventive mental health interventions in peacekeeping missions to Somalia and Haiti. *Military Medicine, 162,* 41–43.

Hall, G. S. (1919). Some relations between the war and psychology. *American Journal of Psychology, 30,* 211–223.

Hall, W. H., & Eaves, J. L. (1989). *Military psychology: Its role in the growth of psychology in Australia* (1st ed.) Psychological Research Unit, Directorate of Psychology Publication, Australian Defence Force. Retrieved February 25, 2020, from *https://apps.dtic.mil/dtic/tr/fulltext/u2/a217966.pdf.*

Harrell, T. W. (1992). Some history of the Army General Classification Test. *Journal of Applied Psychology, 77,* 875–878.

Harris, J. C. (2005). Gassed. *Archives of General Psychiatry, 62,* 15–17.

Hendrix, W. H. (2003). Psychological fly-by: A brief history of industrial psychology in the U.S. Air Force. *American Psychological Society Observer, 16.* Retrieved May 20, 2012, from *www.psychologicalscience.org/observer/getArticle.cfm?id=1451.*

Hotopf, M., David, A., Hull, L., Nikalaou, V., Unwin, C., & Wessely, S. (2004). Risk factors for continued illness among Gulf War veterans: A cohort study. *Psychological Medicine, 34,* 747–754.

Howorth, P. (2000). The treatment of shell-shock: Cognitive theory before its time. *Psychiatric Bulletin, 24,* 225–227.

Hulett, A. G. (1941). Malingering—A study. *The Military Surgeon, 89,* 129–139.

Hunt, W. A., & Stevenson, I. (1946). Psychological testing in military clinical psychology: I. Intelligence testing. *Psychological Review, 53,* 25–35.

Johnson, R. D. (1997). *Seeds of victory: Psychological warfare and propaganda.* Atglen, PA: Schiffer.

Joint Chiefs of Staff. (2003). *Doctrine for joint psychological operations.* Washington, DC: Author.

Jones, E., & Wessely, S. (2003). "Forward psychiatry" in the military: Its origins and effectiveness. *Journal of Traumatic Stress, 16,* 411–419.

Jones, E., & Wessely, S. (2005). *Shell shock to PTSD: Military psychiatry from 1900 to the Gulf War.* New York: Psychology Press.

Jones, F. D. (1995). Psychiatric lessons of war. In R. Zattchuk & R. F. Bellamy (Eds.), *Textbook of military medicine: War psychiatry* (pp. 1–33). Washington, DC: Office of the Surgeon General, U.S. Department of the Army.

Kennedy, C. H. (2020). *Military stress reactions: Rethinking trauma and PTSD.* New York: Guilford Press.

Kennedy, C. H., Boake, C., & Moore, J. L. (2010). A history and introduction to military neuropsychology. In C. H. Kennedy & J. L. Moore (Eds.), *Military neuropsychology* (pp. 1–28). New York: Springer.

Kennedy, C. H., Kupke, T., & Smith, R. (2000). A neuropsychological investigation of the Armed Service Vocational Aptitude Battery (ASVAB). *Archives of Clinical Neuropsychology, 15,* 696–697.

Kevles, D. J. (1968). Testing the Army's intelligence: Psychologists and the military in World War I. *Journal of American History, 55,* 565–581.

Knudson, G. B. (2001). Nuclear, biological, and chemical training in the U.S. Army Reserves: Mitigating psychological consequences of weapons of mass destruction. *Military Medicine, 166,* 63–65.

Koonce, J. M. (1984). A brief history of aviation psychology. *Human Factors, 26,* 499–508.

Kraines, S. H. (1946). *Managing men: Preventive psychiatry.* Denver: Hirschfeld Press.

Lande, R. G. (1997). The history of forensic psychiatry in the U.S. military. In R. G. Lande & D. T. Armitage (Eds.), *Principles and practice of military forensic psychiatry* (pp. 3–27). Springfield, IL: Charles C. Thomas.

Martin, J. A., Sparacino, L. R., & Belenky, G. (1996). *The Gulf War and mental health.* Westport, CT: Praeger.

McCaughey, B. G. (1987). U.S. Navy Special Psychiatric Rapid Intervention Team (SPRINT). *Military Medicine, 152,* 133–135.

McCauley, M., & Breeze, J. (2019) Dispatches from the editor: Military psychology, a force multiplier. *Journal of the Royal Army Medical Corps: International Journal of Military Health; Military Psychology Special Issue, 165,* 63–64.

McCauley, M., Hacker Hughes, J. G. H., & Liebling-Kalifani, H. (2008). Ethical considerations for military clinical psychologists: A review of selected literature. *Military Psychology, 20,* 7–20.

McCauley, M., & O'Brien, D. (2017). Military clinical psychology in the Irish Defence Forces. *The Irish Psychologist, 44,* 10–15.

McGuire, F. L. (1990). *Psychology aweigh! A history of clinical psychology in the United States Navy, 1900–1988.* Washington, DC: American Psychological Association.

Moore, J. L. (2010). The neuropsychological functioning of prisoners of war following repatriation. In C. H. Kennedy & J. L. Moore (Eds.), *Military neuropsychology* (pp. 267–295). New York: Springer.

National Research Council. (1943). *Psychology for the fighting man.* Washington, DC: Penguin.

Neill, J. R. (1993). How psychiatric symptoms varied in World War I and II. *Military Medicine, 158,* 149–151.

Nguyen, D. S. (1969). Psychiatry in the army of the republic of Viet Nam. In P. G. Bourne (Ed.), *The psychology and physiology of stress: With reference to special studies of the Viet Nam War* (pp. 45–73). New York: Academic Press.

Norris, R., & McCauley, M. (2019). Defence Clinical Psychology Service: An overview of clinical psychology in the UK Ministry of Defence. *Journal of the Royal Army Medical Corps: International Journal of Military Health; Military Psychology Special Issue, 165,* 71–73.

Norris, R., Renwick, S., Siddle, R., & Westlake, P. (2019). Leadership in 21st century military healthcare: What did clinical psychologists ever do for us? *Journal of the Royal Army Medical Corps: International Journal of Military Health; Military Psychology Special Issue, 165,* 74–79.

O'Brien, D., & McCauley, M. (2020). Covid-19 and defence mental health: The journey of the military clinical psychologist. *The Irish Psychologist, 46*(6), 152–156.

Olson, T., McCauley, M., & Kennedy, C. H. (2013). *History of aeromedical psychology.* In C. H. Kennedy & G. Kay (Eds.), *Aeromedical psychology* (pp. 1–17). Aldershot, UK: Ashgate.

O'Shea, E., McCauley, M., & O'Brien, D. (2019). Tele-mental health and psychosocial support: A case for implementation with Irish Defence Forces personnel. *Defence Forces Review,* pp. 85–92

OSS Assessment Staff. (1948). *Assessment of men.* New York: Rinehart.

Page, G. D. (1996). Clinical psychology in the military: Developments and issues. *Clinical Psychology Review, 16,* 383–396.

Phares, E. J., & Trull, T. J. (1997). *Clinical psychology: Concepts, methods, and profession* (5th ed.). Pacific Grove, CA: Brooks/Cole.

Pincus, S. H., & Benedek, D. M. (1998). Operational stress control in the former Yugoslavia: A joint endeavor. *Military Medicine, 163,* 358–362.

Precious, D., & Lindsay, A. (2019). Mental resilience training. *Journal of the Royal*

Army Medical Corps: International Journal of Military Health; Military Psychology Special Issue, 165, 106–108.

Rennie, A. M. (2019). Here, there, and everywhere: Psychologists and the training of British Army officers at the Royal Military Academy Sandhurst. *Journal of the Royal Army Medical Corps: International Journal of Military Health; Military Psychology Special Issue, 165,* 109–112.

Ritchie, E. C. (2002). Psychiatry in the Korean War: Perils, PIES, and prisoners of war. *Military Medicine, 167,* 898–903.

Ritchie, E. C. (2003). Psychiatric evaluation and treatment central to medicine in the U.S. military. *Psychiatric Annals, 33,* 710–715.

Roscoe, S. N. (1997). *The adolescence of engineering psychology.* Human Factors History Monograph Series 1. Retrieved September 14, 2005, from *www.hfes.org/PublicationMaintenance/FeaturedDocuments/27/adolescencehtml.html.*

Salter, C. A. (2001). Psychological effects of nuclear and radiological warfare. *Military Medicine, 166,* 17–18.

Sammons, M. T., Levant, R. F., & Paige, R. U. (2003). *Prescriptive authority for psychologists: A history and guide.* Washington, DC: American Psychological Association.

Shaffer, L. F. (1944). *The psychology of adjustment: An objective approach to mental hygiene.* Washington, DC: Houghton Mifflin, for the United States Armed Forces Institute.

Shenberger-Hess, A., Giangrande, S., & Miletich, D. (2020). COVID-19's impact on mental health. *The Military Psychologist, 35*(2), 4–6.

Shephard, B. (2000). *A war of nerves: Soldiers and psychiatrists 1914–1994.* London: Jonathan Cape.

Shorter, E. (1997). *A history of psychiatry.* New York: Wiley.

Smith, G. E., & Pear, T. H. (1917). *Shell shock and its lessons.* Manchester, UK: Manchester at the University Press.

Staal, M., & Harvey, S. (2019). *Operational psychology: A new field to support national security and public safety.* Westport, CT: Praeger.

Stearns, A. W., & Schwab, R. S. (1943). Five hundred neuro-psychiatric casualties at a naval hospital. *Journal of the Maine Medical Association, 34,* 81–89.

Stuart, J. A., Ursano, R. J., Fullerton, C. S., Norwood, A. E., & Murray, K. (2003). Belief in exposure to terrorist agents: Reported exposure to nerve or mustard gas by Gulf War veterans. *Journal of Nervous and Mental Disease, 191,* 431–436.

Sturgeon-Clegg, J., Hurn, H., & McCauley, M. (2019). Neuropsychology and clinical health psychology in the UK Ministry of Defence. *Journal of the Royal Army Medical Corps: International Journal of Military Health; Military Psychology Special Issue, 165,* 87–89.

Terman, L. M. (1918). The use of intelligence tests in the Army. *Psychological Bulletin, 15,* 177–187.

Tischler, G. L. (1969). Patterns of psychiatric attrition and of behavior in a combat zone. In P. G. Bourne (Ed.), *The psychology and physiology of stress: With reference to special studies of the Viet Nam War* (pp. 19–44). New York: Academic Press.

Uhlaner, J. E. (1967, September). *Chronology of military psychology in the Army.*

Paper presented at the 75th Annual Convention of the American Psychological Association, Washington, DC.

Ursano, R. J., & Rundell, J. R. (1995). The prisoner of war. In R. Zajtchuk & R. F. Bellamy (Eds.), *Textbook of military medicine: War psychiatry* (pp. 431–455). Washington, DC: Office of the Surgeon General, U.S. Department of the Army.

Walters, H. C. (1968). *Military psychology: Its use in modern war and indirect conflict.* Dubuque, IA: Wm. C. Brown.

Watanabe, H. K., Harig, P. T., Rock, N. L., & Koshes, R. J. (1994). Alcohol and drug abuse and dependence. In R. Zajtchuk & R. F. Bellamy (Eds.), *Textbook of military medicine: Military psychiatry: Preparing in peace for war* (pp. 61–90). Washington, DC: Office of the Surgeon General, U.S. Department of the Army.

Welsh, J. R., Kucinkas, S. K., & Curran, L. T. (1990). *Armed Services Vocational Aptitude Battery (ASVAB): Integrative review of reliability studies.* Brooks Air Force Base, TX: Air Force Systems Command.

Wong, A., Escobar, M., Lesage, A., Loyer, M., Vanier, C., & Sakinofsky, I. (2001). Are UN peacekeepers at risk for suicide? *Suicide and Life-Threatening Behavior, 31,* 103–112.

Wood, D. P., Koffman, R. L., & Arita, A. A. (2003). Psychiatric medevacs during a 6-month aircraft carrier battle group deployment to the Persian Gulf: A Navy force health protection preliminary report. *Military Medicine, 168,* 43–47.

Yerkes, R. M. (1917). Psychology and national service. *Journal of Applied Psychology, 1,* 301–304.

Yerkes, R. M. (Ed.). (1921). *Memoirs of the National Academy of Sciences: Psychological examining in the United States Army* (Vol. XV). Washington, DC: U.S. Government Printing Office.

Young, A. (1999). W. H. R. Rivers and the war neuroses. *Journal of the History of the Behavioral Sciences, 35,* 359–378.

Zanov, M., Genkov, K., Taylor, D., Hein, C., Crittenden, B., & Eklund, K. (2020). Madigan fight with COVID-19: Department of Behavioral Health response to the pandemic. *The Military Psychologist, 35*(2), 6–9.

Zeidner, J., & Drucker, A. J. (1988). *Behavioral science in the Army: A corporate history of the Army Research Institute.* Washington, DC: Army Research Institute for the Behavioral and Social Sciences.

Zillmer, E. A., Harrower, M., Ritzler, B., & Archer, R. P. (1995). *The quest for the Nazi personality: A psychological investigation of Nazi war criminals.* New York: Routledge.

CHAPTER 2

Military Fitness-for-Duty Evaluations

James M. Keener, Christopher A. Merchant,
and Chad E. Morrow

Clinical military psychologists assess a service member's fitness for duty each time they conduct a psychological evaluation, whether in a deployed or an expeditionary setting, at a stateside military treatment facility (MTF), in an overseas hospital, or in an outpatient clinic. Based on Department of Defense (DoD) terminology, fitness for duty is defined as a service member's ability to perform the duties of his or her office, grade, rank, or rating.

When meeting with a service member for the first time, military psychologists make an initial assessment of the member's fitness for duty and write a narrative report. On the basis of this evaluation, they determine whether the service member is fit and suitable for full duty or whether further review is needed. In some services, such as the Army, more specific policy requires that military psychologists document whether a service member is fit for duty during every encounter (U.S. Army Medical Command, 2017). To find a service member unfit for duty, the military uses a formal review process that involves a Medical Evaluation Board (MEB) and a Physical Evaluation Board (PEB). Suitability for further service is determined at the command level and refers to issues of development and personality. In addition to this form of medical evaluation, commanders also have service-specific regulations to administratively separate service members due to psychological fitness for duty concerns that do not rise to the level, or meet requirements of, the MEB process. This chapter guides the reader through the military fitness and suitability-for-duty evaluation process.

CONDUCTING A FITNESS-FOR-DUTY EVALUATION

Fitness-for-duty evaluations can arise from one of three sources: self-referral, referral from other medical providers, or command referral. Initially, we discuss a non-emergent fitness-for-duty evaluation (self-referral and voluntary medical referral) and then focus on the special requirements of a command-directed evaluation (CDE). It should be noted that the different branches of service have somewhat differing administrative requirements and language; however, the components of the fitness-for-duty evaluation are very similar across all branches.

It is generally accepted that a service member rarely presents to a military mental health provider as a first response in coping with psychological problems. Friends, family members, other service members, members of the chain of command, and chaplains are often the first-line resources for emotional support. Most often then, other self-help approaches have been tried without adequate success before mental health professionals are approached. Therefore, when a service member comes to a mental health clinic, he or she usually presents with problems that significantly affect quality of life. Most often, the individual is experiencing problems in relationships, self-image, and performance of duties. Although it is usually the individual who decides to seek help, this decision is often influenced by the advice of friends, family members, coworkers, or supervisors; it may be generally recognized that the individual's level of functioning has declined. Therefore, it is necessary for the military psychologist to determine whether the decline in functioning has reached a level at which the service member can no longer adequately perform his or her assigned military duties (i.e., determine fitness for duty). While the military psychologist is thoughtful about fitness for duty, he or she is also focused on treating the service member with the ultimate goal of returning that individual to full functioning.

MILITARY OCCUPATION

To determine whether the service member can adequately perform his or her assigned duties, the military psychologist must first understand what the person's job responsibilities involve.

There are hundreds of distinct military occupations within each branch of service throughout a vast network of bases around the globe. Each of these occupations requires specific education, training, and experience that can offer a unique challenge to understanding a service member's fitness for duty. To understand whether a service member is fit or not fit for duty, military psychologists initially need to understand the unique occupational skills involved in the service member's day-to day-activities and how his or her symptoms impact his or her ability to function in a specific job.

The U.S. Navy and U.S. Coast Guard have a system of ratings or "rates" such as Hospital Corpsman (HM); the U.S. Army uses Military Occupational Specialties such as Infantryman (11B); the U.S. Marine Corps uses Military Occupational Specialties such as Infantry Rifleman (0311); the U.S. Air Force uses a system of Air Force Specialty Codes (AFSC) such as Aircraft Loadmaster (1A2X1); and the U.S. Space Force uses specialty codes such as Space Systems Operations (1C6). The duty requirements of each of these occupations can vary widely; for example, the day-to-day requirements of a Coast Guard HM will be very different from those of an aircraft loadmaster serving in the Air Force. For this reason, certain military occupational specialties and special duty assignments require specialized assessments and consideration when determining fitness or suitability. An explanation of special screenings for several specialized communities is provided later in this chapter. Also see Chapter 13 (this volume) for information on assessing and selecting personnel for high-risk jobs.

SOURCES OF COLLATERAL INFORMATION

The process for assessing a service member's fitness for duty requires a comprehensive evaluation of his or her situation. The primary instruments for this evaluation are the clinical interview, a review of pertinent history and collateral information. In addition to the careful history obtained by interviewing the patient, the military psychologist will also need to conduct a thorough review of the service member's service and medical records and, if necessary, obtain a history from his or her collateral sources to include military service record, supervisors, family members, and embedded medical professionals.

The military service record contains details about the service member's training, performance of duties, educational history, military award history, enlistment waivers, disciplinary issues, and Armed Services Vocational Aptitude Battery (ASVAB) scores. The ASVAB is an entry-level screening tool, and the scores can be useful for understanding baseline intellectual functioning (DoD, 1984; Kennedy, 2020). The service member's hard copy and electronic medical record details medical issues beginning with the service member's entry into the military and all subsequent contacts in the military health care system, including mental health. Importantly, medical records originating in deployed and operational settings are increasingly becoming available for review.

Understanding the service member's occupation and work setting will likely be more straightforward for embedded psychologists who serve in the same units as their patients. For psychologists attached to military treatment facilities, responsible for the treatment of a variety of service members with a multitude of occupations, they will need to rely heavily on consultation with the embedded medical providers who provide routine medical care for expeditionary units. These embedded medical providers offer a key source of collateral information and a critical resource to better understand the often complex and multifaceted day-to-day responsibilities that their service members must meet. Examples of valuable collateral sources include an independent duty corpsman attached to a Navy submarine, a flight surgeon attached to an Air Force air wing, or brigade surgeon attached to an Army infantry brigade.

If given permission to contact family members, the psychologist is able to gain a better understanding of the service member's preservice personality, developmental history, the family's perception of any changes, and general functioning, contrasting information to verify the accuracy of the interview data and gathering details regarding developmental and preservice influences and behaviors. Consider the following example in which collateral information was key is assisting with the case conceptualization and intervention plan.

Case 2.1. The Struggling Sailor

A 21-year-old BM3 (boatswain's mate petty officer third class) with 2 years of active service returned from a 9-month deployment at sea with limited opportunities for liberty off the ship. During the deployment, his wife gave birth to their first child. After returning from postdeployment leave, the BM3 presented for an intake to the ship's psychologist with a chief complaint of feeling disconnected from his wife and child. During the evaluation, the BM3 indicated that his wife had convinced him to see the ship's psychologist because she was worried about him being distant, lacking joy when interacting with the baby, and sleeping too much. The psychologist learned that the sailor was having challenges reintegrating with his wife, guilty thoughts about missing the birth of his son, and concerns about his abilities as a new father. During the evaluation, the BM3 agreed to allow the psychologist to contact his wife to gather collateral information about predeployment and postdeployment functioning. The psychologist learned from the BM3's wife that she was primarily concerned about her husband's unwillingness and inability to effectively interact with their son. The collateral information from the spouse validated the BM3's concerns and the psychologist's suspicions that the sailor was having difficulty with postdeployment reintegration and with his confidence in his own abilities as a new father. Using this information, the psychologist was able to develop an individual treatment plan that focused on behavioral strategies to help the BM3 engage with his son and communicate more effectively with his wife. The collateral information gained from his wife also helped to guide a referral for the sailor to a new parent support program that helped him gain confidence in his parenting abilities.

Furthermore, in routine behavioral health evaluations, if given permission to contact supervisors in the chain of command, the military psychologist is better able to assess how the individual's mental health problems are affecting his or her ability to perform assigned duties. The military branches recognize the importance of maintaining privacy and confidentiality while carefully balancing a commanding officer's (CO) right/need to know to ensure that he or she can manage operational risk. According to the Code of Federal Regulations, "A covered entity may use and disclose the protected health information of individuals who are U.S. Armed Forces personnel for activities deemed necessary by appropriate military command authorities to assure the proper execution of the military mission" (Public Welfare, Security & Privacy 45 C.F.R. § 164, 2020). By DoD Instruction (DoDI) 6490.08, "Healthcare providers shall follow the presumption that they are not to notify a Service member's commander when the Service member obtains mental healthcare" (DoD, 2011). The presumption of privacy is overcome in specific instances, including concern about harm to self, harm to others, harm to mission, inpatient care, and acute medical conditions interfering with duty, if the member has entered into a substance abuse treatment program, for specialized personnel, and CDEs.

Routine evaluations will usually find the service member fit for full duty. However, when the psychologist finds the individual unable to adequately perform assigned duties, the psychologist must determine whether a course of treatment is likely to return the individual to full-duty status within a reasonable period (e.g., 6–12 months). As an example, each branch of service has the ability to utilize a temporary period whereby a change in the service member's duty status is permitted. This brief period is called limited duty (LIMDU) in the Navy and Marine Corps and temporary limited duty (TLD) in the Coast Guard. LIMDU is an official documented period of restricted duty during which the service member receives ongoing treatment. The Army and Air Force use a physical profile serial report in place of a LIMDU board. Profiles and LIMDU are time limited and allow the service member to have his or her duty temporarily restricted (e.g., no overseas deployments, no overnight watch standing), so he or she can receive adequate treatment with limited interruptions. However, these profiles or LIMDU boards are usually designed for a specific period of time. For example, military psychologists evaluating an Army soldier can assign a temporary profile for up to 90 days without restriction, but the process must involve a physician if a profile extends beyond that time (Department of the Army, 2019c). Due to these time limitations, it is incumbent on the mental health professional to closely monitor the member's progress during LIMDU and facilitate return to full duty as soon as he or she is ready. If

LIMDU does not return the service member to full duty within the allowed time frame or the illness is sufficiently severe and chronic such that the member is not expected to return to unrestricted duty, then he or she is typically referred to an MEB.

The Army and Air Force are guided in the fitness for duty process by their own instructions on how to evaluate and communicate potential issues. Although similar to Navy guidelines, there are subtle differences to address mission-specific requirements. Military psychologists working with Army soldiers frequently communicate with commanders through the Report of Mental Status Evaluation (Department of the Army Form 3822) to record the results of an evaluation that may include temporary duty restrictions, safety concerns, or brief profile recommendations. An example of a common duty-limiting recommendation is the restriction of a service member's ability to carry a weapon (Department of the Army, 2019d). Once these recommendations are made, the temporary profiles are also documented in a Physical Profile Record (Department of the Army Form 3349), which is defined as the single source for communicating a soldier's comprehensive medical fitness for duty to commanders and medical professionals (Department of the Army, 2019c). These formal tools help maintain the balance between service member privacy and the commander's need to maintain the readiness and safety of the force. Regardless of service, military psychologists must be skilled in how to effectively and appropriately communicate the psychological needs and risk factors of service members to commanders. The reader is invited to review the branch-specific instructions for MEBs referenced in Table 2.1.

DISABILITY EVALUATION SYSTEM

The military Disability Evaluation System (DES), often referred to as the medical board system, has undergone considerable changes in the past decade. DoD Instruction (DoDI) 1332.18 defines the DES as the "mechanism for determining fitness for duty, separation, or retirement of service members because of disability" (DoD, 2018b). Notable aspects of the DES are the MEB, PEB, and nonmedical assessment.

Medical Evaluation Board

An MEB "reviews all available medical evidence, to include any examinations completed as a part of DES processing, and documents the medical status and duty limitations of Service members who meet referral eligibility criteria." For an example of a thorough MEB narrative summary, see Appendix 2.1 at the end of this chapter. The role of the MEB is to document whether the service member "has medical conditions whether singularly,

TABLE 2.1. Regulations and Instructions by Branch of Service

Organization	Title	Regulation or Instruction
Air Force	Medical examinations and standards (Secretary of the Air Force, 2013)	USAF Instruction 48-123
	Physical evaluation for retention, retirement, and separation (Secretary of the Air Force, 2019)	USAF Instruction 36-3212
	Nuclear Weapons Personnel Reliability Program	USAF Guidance Memorandum
Army	Medical record administration and health care documentation	AR 40-66
	Patient administration (Department of the Army, 2014)	AR 40-400
	Active duty enlisted administrative separations	AR 635-200
	Assignment of enlisted personnel to Army Recruiting Command	AR 601-1
	Disability evaluation for retention, retirement, and separation	AR 635-40
	Enlisted assignments and utilization management	AR 614-200
	Medical readiness procedures (U.S. Department of the Army, 2019b)	AR 40-502
	Standards of medical fitness (U.S. Department of the Army, 2019e)	AR 40-501
Navy	Manual of the medical department (Secretary of the Navy, 2005)	NAVMED P-117 and Change 164
	Separation by reason of convenience of the government—medical conditions not amounting to a disability	Article 1900-120
DoD	Manual for courts-martial	Military Rules of Evidence 706
	Command notification requirements to dispel stigma in providing mental health care to service members	DODI 6490.08
	Mental health evaluations of members of the armed forces	DODI 6490.04
	Medical standards for appointment, enlistment, or induction in the military services	DODI 6130.03
	Physical disability evaluation	DODI 1332.18
	Enlisted administrative separations	DODI 1332.14

Note. Full reference entries for the specific publications noted in this table are listed in the end-of-chapter References.

collectively or through combined effect, that will prevent them from reasonably performing the duties of their office, grade, rank, or rating." If the service member cannot perform these duties, he or she is referred to a PEB. An MEB is made up of two or more physicians, and any MEB that includes a mental health diagnosis "must contain a thorough behavioral health evaluation and include the signature of at least one psychiatrist or psychologist" (DoD, 2018b). The MEB does not make the final determination on fitness for duty; this is determined by the PEB, later in the process. Of note, under the provisions of Title 10, U.S.C., Chapter 61, branch secretaries of the military are given the authority to separate members found unfit for duty.

The MEB considers several sources when making a determination, including the provider's narrative summary, line-of-duty (LOD) determination, and a statement from the CO describing the impact of the condition on the service member's military duties. An LOD determination is necessary if there is a question about the member's duty status at the time of an injury or disease, or if the condition was caused by other factors. A nonmedical assessment provides the MEB with critical information regarding the member's performance of assigned duties at the work site, supervisors' behavioral observations, and possible psychosocial factors. The MEB makes its determinations based on the diagnosis, prognosis for return to full duty, need for further treatment, and medical recommendations. If the MEB determines that the service member is unable to adequately perform his or her duties, it will refer the case to a PEB. The member can file an appeal if he or she does not agree with the findings of the MEB.

Physical Evaluation Board

By DOD Instruction (DoDI) 1332.18, the PEB includes three formal processes: the Informal Physical Evaluation Board (IPEB), the Formal Physical Evaluation Board (FPEB), and a review of PEB results. The IPEB includes at least two military officers or the civilian equivalent. In the event of a split opinion, a third officer will be brought in. The IPEB reviews all the documents from the MEB and issues initial findings. When the service member is presented with the findings from the IPEB, he or she may decide to accept or rebut the findings. At this time, the service member can request a formal hearing (FPEB), which he or she can personally attend, and offer witnesses who may testify, challenging the IPEB's conclusions. The FPEB consists of at least three members: a 0–6 president of the board (or the civilian equivalent), a medical officer who is not the service member's treating physician or the physician who originated the MEB, and a line officer or E-9 staff noncommissioned officer (NCO) for enlisted cases who is familiar with duty assignments. At the conclusion of the FPEB, a determination of fitness for duty is made (fit vs. unfit) and a disability rating is assigned if applicable.

ADMINISTRATIVE SEPARATIONS

Certain diagnoses lead to an administrative separation rather than initiation of the PEB process, including, but not limited to, personality disorders and conditions that existed prior to service (EPTS) and that were not exacerbated by military service. When a service member is deemed unable to perform assigned duties because of one of these conditions, he or she is considered for an administrative separation rather than a medical separation (PEB). These conditions typically lead to discharge only if they affect the service member to the degree that he or she cannot adequately perform assigned duties. Guidance for administrative separations is extensive and can be found in DoDI 1332.14 (DoD, 2019). Services may require mental health evaluations for administrative separations. The Army provides service-specific guidance through Army Regulation 635–200 for administrative separations. Military psychologists working with Army soldiers should be aware that this regulation requires verification that mental health conditions that qualify for the MEB process did not contribute to the reason for administrative separation. If a condition that qualifies for MEB is present, commanders are required to use the MEB process for separation (Department of the Army, 2016a). This is to protect soldiers who are experiencing disabling conditions from being administratively separated for misconduct. For example, a soldier with schizophrenia may miss work or display bizarre conduct due to psychosis, which the command may misinterpret as misconduct. Mental health evaluations are also required for separation for conditions not rising to the level of MEB, such as claustrophobia or personality disorder, in the case of the absence of other conditions that qualify for MEB (Department of the Army, 2016a). Personality disorders are addressed in detail in the "Suitability Evaluations" section later in this chapter.

COMPETENCY EVALUATIONS

Competency evaluations, commonly referred to as 706 boards, are completed in accordance with the guidelines established by the *Manual for Courts-Martial* (2019). A 706 board is ordered by a military judge if "it appears to any commander who considers the disposition of charges, or to any preliminary hearing officer, trial counsel, defense counsel, military judge, or member that there is reason to believe that the accused lacked mental responsibility for any offense charged or lacks capacity to stand trial" (*Manual for Courts-Martial*, 2019, p. II-86). This formal inquiry into mental capacity or responsibility is conducted by a physician or clinical psychologist and serves to answer a number of questions posed by the court. These questions include an understanding of the state of mind of the

accused service member at the time of the alleged crime, the diagnosis of the service member, and if the accused service member was able to "appreciate the nature and quality or wrongfulness of his or her conduct" at the time of the alleged crime (*Manual for Courts-Martial,* 2019, p. II-86). Furthermore, the court seeks to understand from the 706 board if the service member is "presently suffering from a mental disease or defect rendering the accused unable to understand the nature of the proceedings against the accused or to conduct or cooperate intelligently in the defense" (*Manual for Courts-Martial,* 2019, p. II-86). For a comprehensive review of military forensic psychology, the military justice system, and psychologists' roles in courts-martial, see Stein and Younggren (2019).

COMMAND-DIRECTED EVALUATIONS

CDEs are performed when a CO becomes concerned about the emotional state and subsequent fitness for duty of a service member under his or her command. It should be noted that pre- and postdeployment mental health assessments, special duty evaluations, evaluations arising as a result of family advocacy involvement (e.g., domestic violence), and evaluations related to substance abuse rehabilitation programs, are covered under different instructions and are not considered CDEs. Moreover, the process for conducting both nonemergency and emergency CDEs has changed considerably in the past decade, and the DoD has streamlined the process to ensure that service members receive the treatment they need.

The responsibility for ordering a mental health evaluation rests with the CO or supervisor. When an enlisted service member is the subject of an emergency command-directed mental health evaluation, the CO or supervisor can delegate the order to a senior enlisted member. If a commissioned officer is the subject of a command-directed mental health evaluation, the order for the CDE may be delegated to a commissioned officer senior to the officer being referred. The steps involved in a CDE have been simplified in the past decade and are described in DOD Instruction 6490.04 (2013). When a commander believes that a service member requires a nonemergent evaluation, the commander will:

- *Step 1:* Advise the service member that there is no stigma associated with obtaining mental health services.
- *Step 2:* Refer the service member to a mental health provider utilizing the provider's name and contact information. Precoordination with the mental health professional is recommended as the CO will need to inform the provider and de-conflict scheduling to ensure a smooth appointment. Mental health providers authorized to conduct CDEs are clinical psychologists, psychiatrists, psychiatric nurse

practitioners, and doctorate-level social workers. In outpatient settings, LCSWs who hold a master's degree in social work will be
considered to conduct CDEs.
- *Step 3:* Inform the service member of the necessary details of the
appointment, including its date, time, and location.

When a commander or supervisor is concerned about potential suicidal or homicidal behavior, he or she will take steps to ensure that the
safety of the service member and others is protected and transportation is
obtained for the emergency CDE. Finally, the commander or supervisor
will inform the receiving mental health provider that the service member is
arriving to his or her treatment facility and what prompted the referral for
the emergency CDE. Consider the following example.

Case 2.2. The Concerned Command

An embedded psychologist with an Army infantry unit was contacted by
the battalion commander who reported that he recently learned a previously high-performing specialist (SPC) had shown up to work smelling
of alcohol, missed important meetings, had recently given away prized
photographs, and had commented to a friend that "the world would be
better if I was gone." Many of the SPCs friends had tried to convince him
to speak with the embedded psychologist, but he refused, stating, "I won't
do it, I don't need any help." Due to the SPCs behaviors, concerning statement, and unwillingness to voluntarily meet with the psychologist, the
battalion commander requested a CDE. During the course of the evaluation, it became clear to the psychologist that the SPC had become increasingly depressed after a divorce and a lengthy custody dispute. Through
the CDE, the psychologist discovered that he began binge-drinking and
was contemplating suicide as a result of his stressors. He was subsequently
hospitalized for 3 days and, upon discharge, was connected with follow-
up care to begin treatment for his symptoms of depression and alcohol
use, and to set up a consultation for legal assistance for his divorce. The
battalion commander's swift and deliberate actions through a referral for
a CDE were critical in understanding the SPCs circumstances and condition as well as providing him with time-sensitive treatment and support.

Post-CDE, follow-up communication with COs is critical, so they can
better care for their service member and ensure safe and effective execution of the military mission. Mental health providers are instructed to limit
their communications to "the minimum necessary disclosure" that often
includes diagnosis, prognosis, discharge, and duty limitations. The Army
(2008) specifies the use of the Report of Mental Status Evaluation (Department of the Army Form 3822) to further structure feedback to commanders from military psychologists. This form is a tool for the above-minimum

necessary disclosers when used for a CDE, though it is also used to communicate with commanders for other types of psychological evaluations as well. Of note, the other services meet the same post-CDE communication standards utilizing official memorandums or other documentation. Regardless of service, military mental health providers can, if necessary, inform the referring CO or supervisor of how they can assist the service member with future treatment.

SUITABILITY EVALUATIONS

Mental health separations from the military based on unsuitability are often due to personality disorders. For a service member to be found unsuitable, the personality disorder must impair his or her ability to perform assigned duties and to work with and take guidance from others. Being unable to do so can result in adjustment difficulties, disciplinary issues, and inadequate performance of assigned duties. When the personality disorder is severe, the individual may become a threat to his or her own safety or the safety of others. Before a service member can be separated as unsuitable because of inadequate performance of assigned duties, his or her command must have counseled the member about his or her deficiencies and given reasonable time for the service member to correct the deficiencies "unless an appropriate medical provider finds that the condition precludes the member from overcoming the deficiencies" (MILPERSMAN 1900–120; Department of the Navy, 2018a). Moreover, extensive documentation from multiple sources will need to be obtained, including supervisors and coworkers to "establish that the behavior is persistent, interferes with assignment to or performance of duty and has continued after the member was counseled and afforded an opportunity to overcome the deficiencies" (MILPERSMAN 1900–120; Department of the Navy, 2018a). As in fitness-for-duty evaluations, the military psychologist must make the determination that mental health treatment will not adequately change the service member's suitability status. In other words, when finding a member unsuitable, the psychologist is saying that the service member and the military would be best served if the service member left the service.

When a military psychologist finds a service member unsuitable for military service because of a personality disorder, an administrative separation is recommended. This is only a recommendation made by the mental health professional and does not constitute a final decision. In most cases, the separation authority that makes the ultimate retention decision is the service member's service headquarters. Moreover, if the service member has been diagnosed with a personality disorder and has more than 4 years of service, has deployed to an imminent danger pay area in the past 24 months, or has ever completed a postdeployment health assessment, a flag medical officer will need to review the record. Military psychologists must also be aware of service-specific policy and guidance. The Army (2016a) has further restrictions, stating the service member must have served less than 24 months on active duty at the time the recommendation for separation is initiated and must not have comorbid diagnoses of posttraumatic stress disorder (PTSD), traumatic brain injury, or another mental health disorder that significantly contribute to the diagnosis of personality disorder. If these criteria are not met, the service member will be recommended for separation through the MEB process rather than administrative separation. These policies were instituted to protect combat veterans from the possibility of being misdiagnosed with a personality disorder when they exhibit behavioral problems secondary to combat stress or concussive injuries.

FITNESS FOR ENLISTMENT AND ENTRY INTO MILITARY SERVICE

Fitness for military service is assessed for every person who desires enlistment or commissioning. The DoD sets common physical and psychological standards that are assessed prior to taking the oath of enlistment or oath of office. Once prospective applicants have consulted with a recruiter and then choose to join the service, they are taken to a local Military Entrance Processing Station (MEPS), where they undergo a variety of assessments, including an intensive physical exam. At MEPS, prospective service members are medically screened and a comprehensive review of their past record is completed. Candidates who have a history of a mental health condition may be referred to a psychologist or psychiatrist by MEPS personnel who will consider past treatment records and current presentation to assist in determining their fitness for military service. The DoD (2020) has established a policy that clearly identifies medical standards for appointment, enlistment, or induction in the military service. These medical and mental health standards are comprehensive. Prospective service members are found fit for enlistment or commissioning once they have met these medical standards. While a condition may be disqualifying according to the DoD, it is important to note that service-specific waivers can be requested in some cases where the prospective service member does not meet the minimum standards of enlistment.

These medical standards are important points of reference for military mental health professionals working at MEPS; civilian mental health professionals utilized by MEPS; and at mental health clinics attached to a recruit training command, such as the Navy Recruit Training Command outside Chicago, the Marine Corps Recruit Depot at Parris Island, Army Basic Training in Fort Jackson, South Carolina, or Air Force Basic Military Training (BMT) at Joint Base San Antonio Lackland. At these recruit training commands, mental health professionals perform fitness-for-duty evaluations on a regular basis. It is possible that during training a recruit will disclose a history of a psychological condition that was not previously disclosed and that is not consistent with military service. Based on a comprehensive clinical interview and a review of available records, a decision will need to be made regarding whether the recruit's condition existed prior to enlistment (EPTE) and whether the recruit can continue to train. If the recruit is found not fit for continued training, a recommendation is made to the recruit's command for an entry-level separation (ELS) for an EPTE condition. A service member is eligible for an ELS if he or she has been in the service for less than 180 days. Consider the following example.

Case 2.3. The Recruit with a History of Inattention

During medical in-processing at the local MEPS, a prospective Marine recruit reported to the medical staff that he had been prescribed a stimulant for attention-deficit/hyperactivity disorder (ADHD) from the ages of 9 to 13 years old. The prospective recruit was concerned that the history of a diagnosis and subsequent treatment for ADHD would disqualify him from service. During his physical exam, the prospective recruit denied symptoms of ADHD, but he had difficulty remembering the circumstances that led to his diagnosis and subsequent treatment. The HM attached to MEPS worked with the prospective Marine recruit to gather the necessary records from his former psychiatrist, but she had retired and the records were not available. Thus, MEPS referred him for a one-time diagnostic evaluation with a local psychologist who periodically conducted such evaluations for MEPS. During the evaluation, the psychologist gathered an extensive history, ranging from childhood until the present, to better understand past symptoms of inattention and hyperactivity. In addition to the interview, the psychologist utilized self-report measures of ADHD and gathered collateral information from the prospective recruit's parents. After the evaluation, it was determined that he did not meet the criteria for ADHD and he was subsequently granted a waiver.

These standards do not offer fitness-for-duty guidance on the numerous special or arduous duties that are available to some service members (e.g., aviation, special operations, or submarine duty). There are myriad specialized duties within the military in which initial or ongoing psychological evaluations are conducted. Knowledge of the specific rules and regulations impacting service members is crucial for mental health professionals who are routinely called on to consult, evaluate, and treat service members from a variety of communities.

OVERSEAS SCREENINGS

In 2018, the DoD released its annual base structure report that indicated the DoD manages "a worldwide real property portfolio that spans all 50 states, 8 U.S. territories with outlying areas, and 45 foreign countries" (DoD, 2018a). The bases that are outside of the continental United States (OCONUS) are often occupied by uniformed service members who, in some cases, are accompanied by their families. The size, structure, and mission of these bases vary considerably, as do the medical and mental health resources available. At some of the smaller locations, treatment options are limited. To determine medical and psychological fitness for overseas duty, the service member and accompanying family members must complete an overseas screening (OSS). While each service varies slightly in how they complete an OSS, the general process and structure are similar across branches. A suitability screening is designed to determine appropriateness for service in overseas or remote duty assignments. This screening is conducted by a medical provider at the service member's current command, whose goal is to identify medical, psychological, dental, and educational needs that may be duty limiting due to the available resources at the gaining command.

Mental health professionals may be asked to complete a supplemental evaluation as part of the screening to determine whether a psychological condition or educational need (e.g., Individualized Education Plan) is present and what treatment or services are required. If a need for ongoing mental health services is identified, information from the evaluation is sent to the gaining command, which determines whether the necessary treatment options are available at that location. If the recommended treatment options are not available, it may be determined that the service member or family member cannot have his or her health care needs met at the overseas duty station, and new orders are issued.

SUBMARINE DUTY

The environment and mission of a submarine are unique: Serving on a submarine can be an extremely difficult and arduous duty, marked by long periods of limited contact with family and friends, a high operational tempo, and intense cognitive demands. While onboard care is available for many physical complaints and illnesses through a dedicated independent duty corpsman (IDC), mental health professionals are not assigned to individual submarines, but provide care pier-side when the submarine is in port. Due to the limited availability of mental health resources and the demanding nature of submarine duty, rigorous psychological standards must be met before a sailor can serve aboard a submarine.

Once sailors complete recruit training, their path to service aboard a submarine is voluntary and varies depending on their chosen rate. If their rate will require them to perform a support function aboard the submarine, such as in the case of a Culinary Specialist (CS) or Yeoman (YN), they will first learn about the technical aspects of their rate at "A" School. Once they complete their technical training at A School, they will attend Basic Enlisted Submarine School (BESS), where they will learn about the basic operations of the submarine. If their rate will require them to perform more technical duties, such as machinist's mate (MM), electronics technician (ET), or electrician's mate (EM), then they will attend BESS shortly after completing recruit training. After completing BESS, they will attend A School, where they will gain the technical knowledge of their rate. Prospective submariner candidates are assessed during training at BESS for psychiatric suitability using screening tools and, if necessary, a follow-up evaluation with a psychologist or psychiatrist.

Once a submariner has completed the required training, and been found physically and psychologically fit for submarine duty, there are strict regulations that determine continued fitness for duty. According to the Department of the Navy (2018b), "Psychological fitness for submarine duty must be carefully and continuously evaluated in all submarine designated personnel. It is imperative that individuals working in this program have a very high degree of reliability, alertness, and good judgment" (p. 15-93a). There are a litany of psychiatric conditions that are disqualifying for submarine service, given that no care is available during frequent deployments, including psychotic disorders, anxiety and mood disorders, somatoform disorders, dissociative disorders, eating disorders, impulse control disorders, and severe personality disorders. Some psychiatric conditions are not disqualifying from service, including adjustment disorders and bereavement, after the service member is evaluated by their undersea medical officer (UMO) and a psychologist or psychiatrist. For some psychiatric conditions, a waiver can be requested by the submariner's UMO in consultation with the treating psychologist or psychiatrist. Mental health professionals who have contact with submariners should closely consult with UMOs and IDCs because they can provide further guidance on fitness-for-duty issues arising with this unique population.

NUCLEAR FIELD DUTY

Nuclear field duty is a specialized Navy program open to officers and certain enlisted ratings and involves work in the Naval Nuclear Propulsion Program. Enlisted sailors who work in the nuclear field perform a variety of highly skilled duties. Nuclear field duty is highly competitive and requires a great deal of motivation, a clean service record, and a strong academic background. Upon completion of a unique and academically rigorous training program, sailors are sent to Nuclear Prototype School, where their education continues in an environment similar to that of their work in the fleet.

Mental health professionals may encounter service members who are qualified to work in nuclear field duty after a self-referral, a CDE, or a referral from the service member's medical provider related to a periodic medical exam. Service members who are qualified for nuclear field duty receive periodic medical exams, during which, according to the Department of the Navy (2018b), the medical provider "will pay special attention to the mental status, psychiatric, and neurological components of the examination, and will review the entire health record for evidence of past impairment. Specifically, the individual will be questioned about anxiety related to working with nuclear power, difficulty getting along with other personnel, and history of suicidal or homicidal behavior" (p. 15-79). Mental health professionals who encounter nuclear field–qualified personnel should work closely with these service members' radiation health officer (RHO), UMO, or IDC, because there are numerous psychological and neurological conditions that are disqualifying from duty. A fitness-for-duty evaluation should be comprehensive, and evaluators should pay special attention to current mental health symptoms and a history of impulsivity, evidence of poor judgment, poor interpersonal skills, and anxiety or mood symptoms impacting ability to function in a high-stress environment.

PERSONNEL RELIABILITY PROGRAM

The Air Force has a program and evaluation processes for those working with nuclear materials. The Air Force's Personnel Reliability Program (PRP) is an extensive and continuous process, and an airman who is in PRP requires substantial medical and psychological oversight that is managed by certifying officials. Certifying officials typically are commanders, and they ensure PRP airmen are constantly assessed, monitored, and cared for throughout their time in the PRP. If any airman in the PRP receives any type of treatment (e.g., medical or psychological) or experiences any significant personal life events (e.g., foreclosure on a house or a divorce), that individual is obligated to report such changes to his or her certifying official. At that time, the certifying official determines if the airman needs to be placed on alternate duties or can continue to work in his or her designated field. In recent years, the PRP program has been implementing changes to create objective versus subjective standards. The PRP manual (Secretary of the Air Force, 2020) has been streamlined and has standardized the guidance and policies from the Headquarters Air Force (HAF) level.

POSITIONS OF TRUST AND AUTHORITY

The secretary of the Army defined certain assignments as positions of trust and authority (Department of the Army, 2019a). By Army regulation, the commander of any soldier pending assignment to become a drill sergeant, Advance Individual Training (AIT) platoon sergeant, recruiter, sexual assault response coordinator (SARC), or sexual assault prevention and response victims' advocate (SAPR-VA) must review the behavioral health record of the soldier prior to authorizing his or her assignment. This review is conducted through the Report of Mental Status Evaluation (DA 3822) form mentioned previously in this chapter; such an evaluation is mandated by an administrative requirement for a fitness-for-duty evaluation and because commanders do not have direct access to a soldier's behavioral health records, he or she must rely on evaluations communicated by military psychologists (Department of the Army, 2008). The Air Force conducts similar evaluations for a military training instructor (MTI), a military training leader (MTL), and service members with recruiting duties. The Marine Corps has a process for conducting psychological assessments and subsequent monitoring of drill instructors, whereas the Navy developed a process for conducting psychological assessments and follow-up skills training for recruit division commanders (RDCs).

The criteria for fitness for duty differ by position, but rely on the judgment of military psychologists who understand the unique requirements of all positions. In general, these positions involve contact with potentially vulnerable populations, authority over others, or positions with limited oversight. For drill instructors and AIT platoon sergeants, the language determining their fitness for duty to proceed to their assignment is similar and broad. The regulation requires a licensed, doctoral-level mental health provider to verify that the soldier has no record of emotional instability. If a soldier is found fit for duty and successfully assigned to the position and then removed from the position for a mental health reason, the soldier is not eligible to return to the assignment. The criteria for a SARC or SAPR-VA are more stringent and require the evaluation of the applicant for domestic violence, substance abuse, financial instability, and any history of removal from previous positions of trust.

Army recruiters also serve in positions of trust with specific fitness-for-duty requirements defined by a separate regulation from the other positions (Department of the Army, 2016b). These recruiters often serve in remote locations with less access to care and under much different chain of command oversight than other active-duty soldiers. They also routinely interact with high school students and their families as the face of the military. As a result, there is increased scrutiny of their behavior and stability. This is mirrored in the depth of the fitness-for-duty evaluations conducted by military psychologists. Objective testing is recommended, and treatment for any significant mental health condition is disqualifying for 12 months. In addition, any evidence of current emotional instability or distress related to a temporary condition is disqualifying and requires the evaluating psychologist to provide the expected duration of the instability and when the soldier can be reevaluated for recruiting duty. Chronic or recurrent conditions are disqualifying without exception.

MENTAL HEALTH EVALUATIONS IN A COMBAT ENVIRONMENT

Mental health professionals working in combat zones will often find themselves assisting service members with managing the challenges of separation from family and friends while simultaneously managing the day-to-day operational demands unique to a combat environment. While providing care and evaluations in the combat zone is challenging, the process of assessing a service member's fitness for a combat zone deployment begins prior to the service member traveling to that environment. The DoD requires a Pre-Deployment Health Assessment (Department of Defense Form 2795) that includes mental health screening questions (Department of Defense, 2015). This assessment is evaluated by medical professionals who refer to mental health professionals when that is indicated. Mental health professionals then perform evaluations, as required, to determine the service member's fitness for deployment. In 2013, the Office of the Assistant Secretary of Defense for Health Affairs published further guidance with specific mental health requirements for a service member to be considered fit for combat deployment. One notable takeaway from this guidance is the requirement of 3 months of stability without significant impairments for any service member diagnosed with a mental health disorder. These requirements are more stringent due to the unique stressors and limited resources available in combat zones. Combat troops are exposed to experiences difficult for those outside the combat zone to fully grasp. Service members' safety is of the utmost importance, and safety is paramount in an environment where all service members, including the psychologist, have access to one or multiple weapons.

Despite the obvious challenges of serving in an operational setting, the fitness-for-duty process remains essentially the same. Over the past decade, military mental health personnel, both officers and enlisted, from all branches of service have been routinely deployed to combat zones to support combat troops during Operation Iraqi Freedom, Operation Enduring Freedom, and Operation Inherent Resolve. Fitness-for-duty evaluations in a combat zone must take into consideration the specific duty requirements of the service member and the challenges of the combat environment. Some combat troops go on daily combat missions, while others remain mostly "within the wire" in combat support positions. From a mental health perspective, deployed military psychologists must help make a determination regarding the service member's ability to function within this unique environment while taking into account the unique stressors that the service member faces. They will work closely with the service member and his or her command unit to ensure the member can safely remain on full duty. Requirements for CDEs remain the same. Recommendations to the service member's commander may include keeping the service member behind the wire for a specified period so he or she can get consistent sleep, hot food, and a chance to receive mental health services. The goal is to return the service member to normal operations as soon as possible. Depending on the mission of the service member's command, the specified period away from combat operations may be extended for days or even weeks. However, based on our experience, if the service member does not benefit significantly from a brief mental health intervention, then he or she will typically be evacuated from theater to the continental United States (CONUS), where there are greater resources for further evaluation and treatment. In cases where the service member is considered a danger to self or others, the evacuation is expedited.

SUMMARY

Psychologists working with service members regularly evaluate and make recommendations related to fitness for duty at the initial point of enlistment into the service, during recruit training, during selection for special communities, at any time when a CO becomes concerned for a service member's welfare, and at additional points throughout a service member's career. Fitness-for-duty evaluations are a critical responsibility that active-duty and civilian psychologists are routinely asked to perform. Psychologists working within military institutions should be well versed and knowledgeable about the various occupational settings and specialties, the service-specific requirements for these specialties, and the instructions that guide the evaluations they must perform. Conducting these multifaceted and at times complex evaluations allows psychologists to make an impact on the lives of individual service members and the fighting force as a whole by identifying those members who are fit and suitable for various occupations, evaluating when psychological interventions may be beneficial, and helping them return to productive service whenever possible.

REFERENCES

Assistant Secretary of Defense for Health Affairs. (2013). *Clinical practice guidance for deployment-limiting mental disorders and psychotropic medications* (memorandum for Assistant Secretary of the Army [Manpower and Reserve Affairs], Assistant Secretary of the Navy [Manpower and Reserve Affairs], Assistant Secretary of the Air Force [Manpower and Reserve Affairs], Joint Staff Surgeon, Vice Commandant of the Coast Guard). Washington, DC: Author.

Department of the Army. (2008). *Medical record administration and healthcare documentation* (Army Regulation 40–66). Arlington, VA: Author.

Department of the Army. (2014). *Patient administration* (Army Regulation 40–400). Arlington, VA: Author.

Department of the Army. (2016a). *Active duty enlisted administrative separations* (Army Regulation 635–200). Arlington, VA: Author.

Department of the Army. (2016b). *Assignment of enlisted personnel to U.S. Army Recruiting Command* (Army Regulation 601–1). Arlington, VA: Author.

Department of the Army. (2017). *Disability evaluation for retention, retirement, and separation* (Army Regulation 635–40). Arlington, VA: Author.

Department of the Army. (2019a). *Enlisted assignments and utilization management* (Army Regulation 614–200). Arlington, VA: Author.

Department of the Army. (2019b). *Medical readiness* (Army Regulation 40–502). Arlington, VA: Author.

Department of the Army. (2019c). *Medical readiness procedures* (Department of the Army Pamphlet 40–502). Arlington, VA: Author.

Department of the Army. (2019d). *Report of mental status evaluation* (Department of the Army Form 3822). Arlington, VA: Author.

Department of the Army. (2019e). *Standards of medical fitness* (Army Regulation 40–501). Arlington, VA: Author.

Department of Defense. (1984). *Test manual for the Armed Services Vocational Aptitude Battery.* North Chicago: U.S. Military Entrance Processing Command.

Department of Defense. (2011). *Command notification requirements to dispel stigma in providing mental health care to service members* (Department of Defense Instruction 6490.08). Arlington, VA: Author.

Department of Defense. (2013). *Mental health evaluations of members of the armed forces* (Department of Defense Instruction 6490.04). Arlington, VA: Author.

Department of Defense. (2015). *Pre-deployment health assessment* (Department of Defense Form 2795). Arlington, VA: Author.

Department of Defense. (2018a). *Base structure report: Fiscal year 2018 baseline.* Retrieved March 6, 2020, from *www.acq.osd.mil/eie/Downloads/BSI/Base%20Structure%20Report%20FY18.pdf.*

Department of Defense. (2018b). *Physical disability evaluation* (Department of Defense Instruction 1332.18). Arlington, VA: Author.

Department of Defense. (2019). *Enlisted administrative separations* (Department of Defense Instruction 1332.14). Arlington, VA: Author.

Department of Defense. (2020). *Medical standards for appointment, enlistment, or induction in the military services* (Department of Defense Instruction 6130.03). Arlington, VA: Author.

Department of the Navy. (2018a). *Naval military personnel manual. Article 1900–120: Separation by reason of convenience of the government—medical conditions not amounting to a disability.* Arlington, VA: Author.

Department of the Navy. (2018b). *Change 164: Manual of the medical department* (NAVMED P-117). Arlington, VA: Author.

Manual for courts-martial. (2019). Military Rules of Evidence 706. Washington, DC: U.S. Government Printing Office.

Public Welfare, Security and Privacy, 45 C.F.R. § 164 (2020).

Secretary of the Air Force. (2013). *Medical examinations and standards* (Air Force Instruction 48–123). Washington, DC: Author.

Secretary of the Air Force. (2019). *Physical evaluation for retention, retirement and separation* (Air Force Instruction 36–3212). Washington, DC: Author.

Secretary of the Air Force. (2020). *Nuclear Weapons Personnel Reliability Program* (Air Force Guidance Memorandum to DODM5210.42_AFMAN 13–501). Washington, DC: Author.

Secretary of the Navy. (2005). *Manual of the Medical Department U.S. Navy* (NAVMED P-117). Washington, DC: Author.

Stein, C. T., & Younggren, J. N. (2019). *Forensic psychology in military courts.* Washington, DC: American Psychological Association.

U.S. Army Medical Command. (2017). *Behavioral health eProfiling standardization policy* (Medical Command Policy Memorandum 17–079). Joint Base San Antonio Fort Sam Houston: Author.

APPENDIX 2.1. REPORT TO MEDICAL EVALUATION BOARD

Date and Time: 23 March 2020 1200 to 1330

Service Member's Name: Sergeant First Class (SFC) Joe Example

Reason for Convening of the MEB: SFC Joe Example is being recommended for a Medical Evaluation Board by Dr. Zelda Q. Williams because of a history of posttraumatic stress disorder (PTSD).

Nature of the Evaluation (*voluntary or command-directed mental health evaluation*):
SFC Example self-referred to treatment. He was initially evaluated on 14 July 2019 by Dr. Williams.

Sources of Information (*initial assessment; number of follow-up sessions; review of inpatient and outpatient treatment records; interview with collateral sources; interview with command sources; psychological assessments*): The information for the current report was received from SFC Example and from a review of his outpatient medical records (both hard copy and electronic).

Identifying Information (*age; marital status; ethnicity*): SFC Example is a 32-year-old, married, Caucasian and Hispanic male with 15 years of continuous active duty service. SFC Example's military occupational specialty (MOS) is military police (MP, 31B), and his current home duty station is Any Base, USA. SFC Example reported that he has deployed three times to an imminent-danger pay area.

Military Status and Military History (*date of first and most recent entry into service; estimated termination of service [i.e., EAOS/EAS]; duty status: active duty or reservist; time in service; military occupational specialty [MOS]; dates and locations of deployments; pertinent history of improvised explosive device [IED] or other blast exposure; motor vehicle accidents; vehicle rollovers; significant mortar fire; or rocket attacks that landed close to the service member; taking small-arms fire; seeing fellow service members who were injured or killed; treating wounded; attending to service members who were killed in action [KIA]; being injured in combat; awards received; pending disciplinary action and punishments; past disciplinary actions and punishments*): SFC Example reported that he enlisted in the Army in 2005 because he wanted to serve his country and learn a valuable skill. He has served on three combat deployments including deployments in support of Operation Iraqi Freedom (OIF; 2006–2007 and 2009–2010) and Operation Enduring Freedom (OEF; 2011). He endorsed numerous examples of small-arms engagements, seeing fellow service members who were injured and killed, treating wounded, and attending to service members KIA during each of his deployments. He denied a history of IED blast exposure, motor vehicle accidents in theater, tactical vehicle rollovers, significant mortar or rocket attacks that landed close to him, or being injured in combat. SFC Example stated that he has performed well in his military career thus far, has never received a nonjudicial punishment or other disciplinary action, and until recently has typically gotten along well with peers and superiors. He has been awarded three Army Commendation Medals, one Army Achievement Medal, the Combat Infantryman Badge, an Iraqi Campaign Medal, and a Global War on Terror Service Medal. SFC Example is pending end of obligated service in 2014, and per his report he hopes to attend college and study international finance.

Chief Complaint at Intake (*chief complaint at time of initial outpatient visit or inpatient hospitalization in the service member's own words*): "Deployment stress"

History of Present Illness (*circumstances surrounding initial presentation of symptoms/stressors; current and past symptoms; frequency of symptoms; duration of symptoms*):

SFC Example was initially evaluated on 14 July 2010 when he presented on a walk-in basis to the Behavioral Health Clinic. His chief complaint during that evaluation was "deployment stress" and he described numerous symptoms of anxiety and depression. During the initial evaluation, SFC Example stated that he had been feeling increasingly anxious and depressed since returning from a 12-month deployment in support of OIF in early 2010. He stated that his wife complained that he was "jumpy," on guard, and irritable, and that members of his extended family were concerned about his visible change in mood and behaviors. He stated that he was often on guard and fearful that he would be attacked. SFC Example also stated that he felt distant and detached from his wife and two young sons. He described trouble connecting with his wife and children and noted that he would often feel guilty for wanting to isolate himself from his family. Other symptoms endorsed included trouble falling asleep, nightmares (three to four per week), experiencing moments in which he would "zone out" and remember his deployment experiences, difficulties concentrating, avoidance of large crowds (including busy restaurants, classrooms, amusement parks, and church), avoidance of talking about his deployment experiences, and avoidance of driving on busy streets. He also noted periods of depressed mood, never lasting more than 2 days at a time. He denied symptoms consistent with a mood disorder, mania, or psychosis during his initial presentation.

Present Condition/Review of Symptoms and Current Functional Status (*current psychiatric symptoms; required treatment; service member's ability to perform required duties; compliance with treatment*): SFC Example completed a course of outpatient individual psychotherapy targeting symptoms of PTSD, monthly medication management appointments, and an intensive outpatient treatment program specifically for PTSD. A significant improvement was seen in his ability to manage his irritable moods and connect with family. However, he continues to complain of difficulties falling and staying asleep, nightmares, increased anxiety, increased arousal, difficulties with sustained attention and concentration, avoidance of thinking and speaking about his deployment experiences, avoidance of large crowds, and feeling fearful and on guard. These symptoms have impacted his occupational functioning, because he cannot perform the typical duties of an MP or standard administrative duties without extreme difficulties. His symptoms have also greatly impacted his social functioning; he has noted declines in his relationships with his extended family and friends, mainly attributed to his fearfulness and symptoms of avoidance. He has been compliant thus far with his treatment regimen, although avoidance of initial treatment was seen, and he has stated multiple times that he does want to continue with treatment. Future treatment recommendations include continued outpatient psychotherapy and medication management.

Mental Health History (*history of mental health diagnoses; history of mental health treatment; past hospital course; history of suicidal and/or homicidal ideations, intentions, urges, or plans; past disability rating; supporting data*): SFC Example denied a significant history of diagnoses or treatment for mental health illnesses prior to presenting to the Behavioral Health Clinic. SFC Example reported that he has never participated in individual psychotherapy as an adult but at age 7 he saw a child psychologist for three sessions. SFC Example reported that his mother wanted him to see a child psychologist to process some of his feelings following his parents' divorce. Records from this psychologist were unavailable. SFC Example stated that he has never had a mental health hospitalization. He went on to deny a history of suicidal ideations, intentions, plans, urges, or attempts. He further denied a history of homicidal ideations, intentions, urges, or plans.

Family Psychiatric History (*family history of mental health diagnoses; family history of mental health treatment; family history of suicidal behaviors*): SFC Example stated that his biological grandmother drank excessively throughout her adult years, and he described memories of seeing her intoxicated at family functions. He was unclear whether she ever received treatment for substance abuse. SFC Example denied any further history of mental illness or treatment for mental illness in his family. SFC Example also denied a family history of suicide and a family history of hospitalizations for mental health reasons.

Psychosocial History (*information related to birth and childhood; relevant childhood events [including abuse]; current relationships with parents and siblings; current sources of social support; current living arrangements, current information related to functioning in relationships*): SFC Example was born in Europe and raised throughout the northeastern United States. He is the youngest of five children. He described his childhood as "wonderful" until his parents divorced when he was 7 years old. He denied a history of physical, verbal, or sexual abuse as a child; however, he noted that he was often exposed to verbal arguments between his parents centered on their difficult financial situation. SFC Example described his father as a successful international salesman who often spent money on expensive cars, and his mother was a Spanish teacher who tutored middle school children. He noted that his parents had joint physical custody after their divorce; however, he spent most of his time with his mother because of his father's busy travel schedule. He noted that he performed well throughout grade school and into high school with the exception of the year that his parents divorced. SFC Example noted that his grades slipped and his teachers complained that he was preoccupied, which prompted his mother to consult with his pediatrician, who subsequently referred him to a child psychologist. SFC Example graduated from high school on time with a 3.65 grade point average (GPA), and he participated in band, drama club, and lacrosse. He denied any behavioral difficulties during high school and noted that he got along well with classmates, teachers, and coaches. After high school graduation, he applied to three local universities and decided to enroll in Any Town University to study finance and play lacrosse. He met his future wife during his first year of college and was married 8 months later. He completed 1½ years of college, obtaining a 3.0 GPA and making the lacrosse team, before he was forced to leave school because his father could no longer afford the high tuition. At the urging of his lacrosse coach, he spoke with an Army recruiter. He is currently married and has twin sons (6 years of age). His social support network includes his wife, Army buddies, siblings, and mother. He noted that during the past year he has been withdrawing from others and now only speaks with his friends and family when they stop by his home unannounced. He stated that he has 16 voicemails from friends and family on his cell phone that he has not yet returned. He also noted that his young sons complain that he no longer plays with them and his wife complains that he will not attend social functions with other families.

Legal History (*history of police contact and arrests*): SFC Example stated that he has never been arrested. He did report that 2 months ago he received a ticket for failing to stop at a stop sign while driving home from work. He stated that he was distracted and wasn't paying attention when he ran the stop sign. He denied any other police contact, which is consistent with his command's report.

Substance Use/Abuse (*alcohol: include age of first use, past heavy use, current frequency and duration of use, and symptoms consistent with abuse or dependence; illicit drugs: include age of first use, past heavy use, current frequency and duration of use, and symptoms consistent with abuse or dependence; supplements, including workout supplements and energy drinks; caffeine; nicotine; misuse of over-the-counter [OTC] medications*):

- *Alcohol:* SFC Example noted that he first drank alcohol at the age of 18 while at a school party. He reportedly drinks two alcoholic beverages one to two times per week. He denied a history of heavy alcohol use and stated that seeing his grandmother's drinking was influential. He denied ever experiencing symptoms consistent with alcohol withdrawal or symptoms consistent with an alcohol use disorder.
- *Illicit drugs:* SFC Example stated that he smoked marijuana approximately six times with members of his lacrosse team during his sophomore year of high school. He denied any further history of illicit drug use.
- *Supplements:* He denied current supplement use.
- *Caffeine:* He reported that he currently drinks six to seven cups of coffee per day. He stated that he drinks coffee because he believes that it will help him stay awake and "get through the day" without dozing off. He noted that he has also tried various energy drinks to help him stay awake throughout the day.
- *Nicotine:* SFC Example reported that he currently does not smoke cigarettes; however, he has tried chewing tobacco and uses one can of chewing tobacco per month.

Current Medications: SFC Example is currently prescribed fluoxetine hydrochloride, 40 mg per day. He has previously been prescribed citalopram and zolpidem in the past, both of which have been discontinued.

Medical History (*current treatment for significant medical illnesses; history of major medical illnesses or treatment; history of head traumas or injuries; past disability rating*): SFC Example is currently not receiving any treatment for significant medical illnesses. He has a history of tonsillectomy at the age of 13. He denied a history of head traumas and concussion, seizures and hospitalizations.

Pain Assessment (*current pain*): SFC Example denied current pain (0/10).

Mental Status Exam (*current*): SFC Example arrived to his last appointment 15 minutes late, complaining that he overslept. He had dark circles under his eyes, was unshaven, and was dressed in the uniform of the day. He appeared his stated age, with multiple tattoos on his right arm. He walked without assistance and presented with some psychomotor agitation (leg tapping). He was awake, alert, and oriented to person, place, time, and situation. His speech was of normal rate, rhythm, prosody, and volume. He described his mood as "nervous" and his affect was mood congruent. His thoughts were logical, linear, and goal directed and focused on his current symptoms. There was no evidence of psychosis, and auditory, visual, olfactory, and tactile hallucinations were denied. Insight was fair. Judgment was fair and impulse control appeared intact during the session. Memory for past events appeared normal, and attention and concentration waned at times; however, he was responsive to redirection. Suicidal ideations, intentions, urges, or plans were consistently denied. Homicidal ideations, intentions, urges, or plans were also denied.

Suicidal/Homicidal Ideation Behavioral Review: SFC Example denied current suicidal or homicidal ideations, intentions, urges, or plans in our last session. During the initial evaluation, he also denied a history of suicidal or homicidal ideations, intentions, urges, or plans and described numerous deterrents to suicide, including a desire to see his children grow up, personal beliefs against suicide, and religious beliefs against suicide. He does not have a family history of suicide and does not have weapons at home. He was agreeable to following a clear safety plan should suicidal or homicidal ideations arise in the future.

Psychological Testing Results: SFC Example was administered a battery of psychological assessment measures on 23 August 2019 that included the Minnesota Multiphasic Personality Inventory–2-RF (MMPI-2RF) and PTSD Checklist for DSM-5 (PCL-5). A full copy of these results is available in his electronic medical record. Results of the MMPI-2RF were valid and consistent. Results of the MMPI-2RF indicated that SFC Example endorsed increased negative emotions, including pervasive anxiety, sleep disturbances, and guilt (RC7; $T = 71$ and ANX; $T = 70$). Responses on the PCL-5 indicate a total severity score of 52 with moderately or higher on criterion B, C, D, and E. Both measures are consistent with SFC Example's self-reported symptomology.

DSM-5 Diagnosis: Posttraumatic Stress Disorder, Chronic (309.81)

- *Military Impairment* (*clearly state how these symptoms impact the service member's occupational functioning and how current symptoms will likely impact the military mission; describe how the service member's symptoms impact ability to work in his or her MOS and whether impairment would be evident if he or she were moved to a new MOS*): SFC Example is unable to function fully in his current position as an MP. He will likely not be able to safely perform his role as an MP in a combat zone and has experienced continued difficulties with his duties in a garrison environment. He has trouble sleeping through the night, does not awake feeling rested, is easily distracted, has trouble focusing and concentrating when speaking to others and when writing reports, is often irritable, and experiences anxiety, which results in his leaving situations where more than three people are in attendance. He has been moved to an administrative position within his unit where he has fewer responsibilities and a more flexible schedule; however, he continues to have difficulties with interpersonal interactions and with writing. It is unlikely that another change in job responsibilities or change in MOS will be beneficial.

• *Social Impairment* (*clearly state how these symptoms impact the service member's family life, ability to attend school, ability to establish and maintain relationships*): SFC Example's family life has been greatly impacted by his current symptoms of PTSD. He noted that he has withdrawn from his wife, children, extended family, and friends. He stated that he loves his family very much and feels guilty that he has "cut off" others; however, he believes that he can no longer connect with those who were previously close with him. His interactions with his wife and children have improved while at home, but he continues to avoid social activities outside of the home, including his son's soccer games, the theater, and going out to a restaurant to eat. He enrolled in a course at the local community college, but dropped out because of the increased anxiety he felt around others in the classroom. He was able to successfully complete one online business course. Although his avoidant symptoms have been a target of treatment throughout the past year, he continues to struggle.

• *Treatment Plan:* It is recommended that SFC Example continue in weekly Prolonged Exposure therapy with a psychologist and continue to follow up for medication reviews on a monthly basis. His spouse has been given information regarding couples therapy and further resources for the family.

• *Barriers to Care:* SFC Example has avoided treatment in the past, and his ambivalence about attending psychotherapy was an impediment to treatment for the first month. His command has been flexible with his schedule and allowed him to attend all appointments as scheduled. When he transitions to a new provider in the VA system, his avoidance will likely need to be targeted.

Administrative Recommendations: Physical Evaluation Board

Recommendation for Medical Evaluation Board:

1. Is the service member considered fully competent to be discharged to his or her own custody? YES
2. Are there past findings of incompetence or incapacitation? NO
3. Is there pending disciplinary action, investigation, or administrative discharge pending? NO
4. Is the service member considered fit to administer to his or her own financial and legal affairs? YES
5. Is continued mental health treatment recommended during the processing of the board? YES—see treatment plan

SIGNATURE OF WRITER   CO-SIGNATURE
Specialty of Writer   Specialty of Co-Signer
Originating Department   Department

CHAPTER 3

Military Stress Reactions

Marcus R. VanSickle, Emmett Arthur,
and Jessica M. LaCroix

Service in the United States military is both an honor and a privilege for those who volunteer, many out of a sense of patriotism in addition to multiple career, academic, and travel opportunities. Service also develops multiple character benefits for members, such as resilience, grit, and determination. However, service is not without challenges. In this chapter, we provide a brief overview of military service-related stressors, types of stress reactions, impact of stress on service members, and stress mitigation and support resources. Although an exhaustive review of military stress and stress reactions is beyond the scope of this chapter (see Kennedy, 2020, for a comprehensive review), our aim is to provide an introduction to the risks and predictors for maladaptive military stress reactions paired with available support options to support military service members. It is our hope that this chapter, and the remainder of this volume, will increase awareness and cultural competence when working with the U.S. military, while providing realistic and relevant examples of courses of action to support military service members.

OPERATIONAL DEFINITIONS

The term *stress* has been defined in multiple ways and can relate to an action synonymous with emphasize (e.g., to stress a point) or an experience, a state, or a response. For the purposes of this chapter, we consider stress as the physical or psychological experience subsequent to external forces exceeding the mind's and/or body's ability to respond in an adaptive way. The term *reaction* refers specifically to one's response to a stimulus, without reference to valence. Thus, reactions to stress can be either adaptive or maladaptive, depending on outcome, and valence exists on a continuum. Accepting these definitions permits the interpretation of stress as both inevitable and preventable. Additionally, Yerkes and Dodson (1908) posited an association between stress and performance, whereby moderate levels of stress enhance performance, but low and high levels of stress are detrimental to performance. From this framework, we can further delineate stress into categories of eustress and distress, where the former refers to positive stress that can contribute to feelings of fulfillment and well-being, and the latter refers to negative stress that can contribute to anxiety and mental health problems. Indeed, stress is inevitable. Chronic stressors may exist across times within a life span, and acute stressors often present without sufficient warning. Overcoming chronic and acute distress, while capitalizing on eustress, is critical to optimal performance expected within military settings, punctuating the need to prepare minds, bodies, and lifestyles to survive and thrive despite many types of stressors.

Military-specific training addresses stress reactions along a continuum of colored zones, each with increasing severity. *Green* is adaptive and indicative of resilience, the ability to (1) withstand adversity without becoming significantly affected, and (2) recover quickly and fully from any impairment that has occurred (Department of the Navy, U.S. Marine Corps, 2010). In contrast, *yellow, orange,* and *red* are maladaptive, ranging in severity from mild and transient distress, to more severe and persistent distress, to disabling illness. Adverse reactions to stress requiring traditional mental health treatment are addressed by other chapters within this volume. The following chapter focuses primarily on reactions within the *yellow* zone, those that are maladaptive, but temporary, and lack the severity associated with injury and illness. Notably, recent research indicates that resilience in the face of major life stressors (e.g., spousal loss, divorce, unemployment) is not as common as previously thought and there is substantial variability in how people respond to adverse life events (Infurna & Luthar, 2016). Resolution of reactions within the yellow zone may require involvement of multiple parties, including unit leadership, individuals, peers, family members, as well as community-based and clinical caregivers.

MILITARY SERVICE-RELATED PROTECTIVE FACTORS

Military service offers multiple protective benefits, including pride, confidence, discipline, independence, respect, openness, leadership and job skill development, and friendship (Gade, Lakhani, & Kimmel, 1991). In particular, group cohesion, defined as the "inclination to forge social bonds, resulting in members sticking together and remaining united" (Carron, 1982,

p. 124), is built via dedication of effort under a specified mission, syntonic with a person's values, and shared goals among members (Yukelson, 1997). Group cohesion is associated with mutual support, cooperation, and shared commitment (Consortium for Health and Military Performance [CHAMP], 2020), and the proximity inherent in military settings can enhance cohesiveness (Festinger, Schachter, & Back, 1950). Many military service-related protective factors are associated with both performance as well as mental health (e.g., Ahronson & Cameron, 2007; Rugo et al., 2020; Zalta et al., 2021).

In addition to the protective factors described above, military-specific stress may also be beneficial. Consistent with the Yerkes-Dodson law (1908), veterans with low combat exposure reported greater perceived wisdom years later than those with no or high combat exposure (Jennings, Aldwin, Levenson, Spiro, & Mroczek, 2006). Perceived benefits of military service and coping were also associated with greater perceived wisdom later in life, indicating that appraisal and coping strategies, rather than experiences with stress alone, may facilitate eustress. Additionally, experiencing stress, anxiety, and fear motivates social affiliation (Sarnoff & Zimbardo, 1961), and ambiguous situations in particular promote a desire to be with other people as a means of social evaluation and determination of appropriate responses (Schachter, 1959). Thus, stress reactions such as fear and anxiety are common and, in general, dissipate over time. However, in situations where fear and anxiety do not dissipate, and individuals isolate instead of affiliate, stress reactions may become more severe, debilitating, and persistent over time, ultimately contributing to injury or illness.

MILITARY SERVICE-RELATED STRESSORS

Service members, while experiencing similar stressors to civilian peers, are also subject to stressors unique to military service. Most notable to military service is the stress associated with military deployment and service in combat environments. However, it is a misconception to consider these as the only or primary contributors to stress reactions for service members. While stressors related to a military career vary significantly by branch of service, military occupation, age, sex, and other demographic factors, some commonalities exist across a "typical" career life cycle and are experienced by the majority of service members.

Accession/Entry-Level Training

Upon entry to the military, all members are required to complete some form of military-specific training designed to screen, evaluate, and prepare applicants for service in the U.S. Armed Forces. First, this process typically requires a geographic shift away from family and friends, a separation from common comforts, and a rapid introduction to military culture delivered in environments designed to generate stress. The second stage of the accession process generally focuses on occupation-specific training, preparing new members to function in their new specialty. Common stressors within this stage include performance-related demands (e.g., time pressure, performing in physically demanding situations), interpersonal stress (e.g., being yelled at by instructors), and challenges associated with adjusting to the military environment (e.g., lack of sleep, lack of privacy, feeling homesick) (Adler et al., 2013). Additional stressors can include adjustment to military service, introduction to new and diverse groups, physical and academic demands, and for many—their first step toward independence and adulthood (Gade et al., 1991).

Duty Station/Permanent Change of Station

After completion of initial training, service members report to their initial assigned duty station. For many, this time period may closely resemble civilian occupations and lifestyle with the added stress of military-specific demands. Depending on branch of service, paygrade, location, and marital status, members may reside in dormitory-style barracks, on board ships, or in apartments or houses within the local community. In this setting, service members endure common stressors associated with maintaining a home, family, and social network (e.g., finances, physical separation, communication). Military-specific stressors of frequent moves, unpredictable training and operational schedules, limited privacy, and the impact of high physical demands coupled with irregular sleep and dietary changes are also commonly experienced by members. Previously utilized stress management strategies may be unavailable for service members, driving the need for rapid adaptation. For many, this includes establishing community within their unit, installation, or surrounding areas.

Service members receive permanent change of station (PCS) orders frequently, such that the word *permanent* is not to be taken literally. With every new PCS, service members and their families may experience loss of community and are faced with the task of reestablishing new social networks at their new command. Geographic separation from supportive social systems, frequently utilized as a powerful coping mechanism, is one of the most ubiquitous military stressors. As described above, this separation occurs immediately upon entry into military service for many service members, and may recur every 2 to 4 years throughout one's military career. Separation from support systems further occurs during temporary duty assignments, readiness training, underway periods, and deployment.

Deployment

Depending on branch of service and type of unit, deployment can be operationalized in multiple ways. In general, deployment refers to movement as either an individual or unit, away from an assigned geographic location for the purpose of completing a specific combat, combat support, or humanitarian mission within the range of military operations other than war. As such, the range of specific stressors associated with deployment can include boredom, moral conflict, interruption of routines, separation from family, exposure to new environments, isolation, combat, and fear of loss of life. Intensity of deployment-related stressors can also vary based on military occupational specialty; for instance, combat medics are exposed not only to combat, but also to trauma care on the battlefield (Russell, Russell, Chen, Cacioppo, & Cacioppo, 2019).

Post-deployment Reintegration

Returning home from deployment is often viewed as a positive end to a challenging tour; however, multiple stressors are inherent within the process of returning. Reintegration challenges including intimate relationship stress, parenting challenges, financial stress, and the difficulties of shifting between one mind-set on deployment and then another after service members return home can generate significant levels of individual and social stress. For example, in a deployed setting, aggression, lack of emotional expression, assertive driving, and the need to account for subordinates' whereabouts may all be considered adaptive; on return from deployment, these behaviors may be viewed as anger, detachment, recklessness, and efforts to obtain excessive control (Danish & Antonides, 2013). As such, in many cases, service members may have to unlearn much of what was necessary during deployment in order to reintegrate successfully. Additional stress may result from a perceived decrease in comradery, intensity, and sense of purpose in garrison environments. Finally, another common reintegration challenge is role conflict; service members and their partners must navigate changes and uncertainty regarding gender roles, routines, and joint decision making that may have been well established prior to the deployment (Jeschke, LaCroix, Fox, Novak, & Ghahramanlou-Holloway, 2020; Knobloch & Theiss, 2012).

TYPES OF STRESS REACTIONS

The biopsychosocial model (Engel, 1977) provides a framework for understanding the interactions between biological, psychological, and social factors on the development of illness and understanding the etiology of disease. Stress reactions manifest in each of these domains in unique ways; awareness and recognition of these reactions coupled with targeted interventions can help prevent distress from being amplified to disease, reducing the likelihood that service members will fall below the green and yellow ranges of the stress continuum.

Biological

Acute physiological stress reactions in the military are commonly associated with operational stress in a deployed or combat setting; however, these occur throughout military service (at varying levels) in response to the stressors associated with service described above. These reactions include the neurobiological response of the autonomic nervous system (ANS) during the actual threat of death during combat and perceived threats of harm during high-stress interactions. Specifically, within the ANS, the sympathetic nervous system (SNS) reaction to danger (i.e., fight or flight response) includes deficits or impairment in fine motor coordination, vision, hearing, attention, processing speed, memory encoding and retrieval, and anxiety. Service members are likely to perceive their own physiological symptoms as increased heart rate and respiration, muscle tension and abnormal movement (e.g., shaking), headache, nausea, and perspiration. The subsequent inhibitory response of the parasympathetic nervous system (PNS) allows the brain to restore primary frontal lobe functioning and regulate physiological responses. Many components of military training aim for stress inoculation, with goals to decrease the PNS response and/or enhance PNS regulation during periods of elevated stress through habituation to stress (Meichenbaum, 1985).

Psychological

Innate to military service are persistent stressors that may overburden or deplete typically available supportive psychological resources. Military-specific stressors include unexpected changes in mission demands, frequent PCS moves, geographic distance from protective support systems (e.g., family, community), high-demand operational schedules, and typical daily stressors. Given that the military is a microcosm of society within the United States, service members do not enter with a "blank slate." The stressors associated with military service are additive to the common stressors and histories these members share with the civilian population, often generating a greater than average demand for resilience, with higher risk of adverse outcomes when depleted. Decreased resilience may contribute to sustained anxiety, restlessness, insomnia, poor attention, and mood challenges, increasing the likelihood of a future stress injury.

Social

Military service may fundamentally change one's social environment. The systems a service member engages within can both create stress (frequent moves, performance demands) and buffer stress while encouraging growth (team focus, engaged leadership, access to medical care). Social environment changes alone may limit one's ability to participate in previously enjoyable or stress management activities due to geographic or logistic changes in resources. Social behavior changes within these environments may also parallel physiological and psychological responses to stress, worsening with each stage of change. Decreased engagement means that individuals who previously exercised regularly, socialized with friends and family, or spent their free time participating in hobbies are likely to experience higher levels of stress with worsening mood symptoms, with only the return of prior behaviors predicting improvement (Grippo, Beltz, & Johnson, 2003). Synergistic impacts also occur within the social domain. For example, service members who experience impulsive, disruptive, and antisocial behavior in their stress response can engage in misconduct, resulting in judicial or nonjudicial punishment, demotion, or bad conduct discharges, further restricting available resources within their environment (Booth-Kewley, Highfill-McRoy, Larson, & Garland, 2010).

IMPACT OF STRESS ON SERVICE MEMBERS

Chronicity, accumulation, and/or acuity of a stress reaction can cross the threshold to a level of impairment consistent with a clinical disorder (e.g., major depressive disorder), to be addressed in depth in later chapters. Notably, subclinical stress reactions are some of the most common causes of impairment associated with military service. For example, the most prevalent and costly mental health problem within the U.S. Armed Forces is adjustment disorder (Armed Forces Health Surveillance Branch [AFHSB], 2020; Morgan & Kelber, 2018). In 2019, adjustment disorders affected 91,571 active-duty service members and accounted for a total of 472,436 medical encounters (AFHSB, 2020). Adjustment disorder directly reduces readiness in multiple ways: (1) time required to attend medical appointments (AFHSB, 2020), (2) logistically challenging medical evacuations from theater (AFHSB, 2020), (3) health care costs that exceed posttraumatic stress disorder (PTSD) or anxiety disorders (Morgan & Kelber, 2018), (4) reduced retention (Maby et al., 2017), and (5) a link with more severe mental health issues, including suicide ideation and attempts (George et al., 2019). Additional subclinical stress reactions include combat or operational exhaustion, episodic and cumulative combat stress reaction, and episodic and cumulative operational stress reaction (Kennedy, 2020). Table 3.1 provides an overview of these reactions.

TABLE 3.1. Conceptual Framework of Military Stress Reactions

Type of military stress reaction	Definition	Immediate	Acute	Chronic
Adjustment problems	Stress reaction related to adjusting to a military event or any aspect of life in the military.	Adjustment problems are not conceptualized as immediate or acute in the same way as the stress reactions. Adjustment problems tend to resolve on their own or with mentorship over the course of several weeks to several months.		This is reserved only for those who are unable to adjust to the stressor at hand. Clinically, this is conceptualized as a persisting adjustment disorder, which is still expected to resolve within 6 months of removal of the stressor.
Combat or operational exhaustion	Exhaustion that develops over several weeks or more of combat or other prolonged operations, arduous conditions, and/ or physical, environmental, and mission stressors.	Exhaustion is not conceptualized as immediate or acute as it takes several weeks to develop.		Exhaustion becomes a chronic, clinically diagnosable problem only when early intervention is unsuccessful in reregulating mood and sleep symptoms.
Episodic combat stress reaction	Stress response that results from a discrete event that occurs in the course of a combat situation.	Presentation lasts several hours to days.	Presentation lasts from a week to months.	Presentation lasts several months or arises/is exacerbated months or years later; a traditional clinical diagnosis is likely appropriate.
Cumulative combat stress reaction	Stress response that results from prolonged and repetitive combat experiences; this is a combined stress and exhaustion response.	Presentation lasts several hours to days.	Presentation lasts from a week to months.	Presentation lasts several months or arises/is exacerbated months or years later; a traditional clinical diagnosis is likely appropriate.
Episodic operational stress reaction	Stress response that results from a specific event that occurs in the course of military duties and is unrelated to combat.	Presentation lasts several hours to days.	Presentation lasts from a week to months.	Presentation lasts several months or arises/is exacerbated months or years later; a traditional clinical diagnosis is likely appropriate.

(continued)

TABLE 3.1. (*continued*)

Type of military stress reaction	Definition	Immediate	Acute	Chronic
Cumulative operational stress reaction	Stress response that results from prolonged operations, arduous conditions, and/or physical, environmental, and mission stressors that are unrelated to combat; this comprises a combined stressor and exhaustion response.	Presentation lasts several hours to days.	Presentation lasts from a week to months.	Presentation lasts several months or arises/is exacerbated months or years later; a traditional clinical diagnosis is likely appropriate.

Note. Reprinted with permission from Kennedy (2020).

The value of recognizing subclinical stress reactions, and subsequently intervening at the preclinical level, cannot be overstated. The PIES (proximity, immediacy, expectancy, and simplicity) model provides an example of the benefits of targeting challenges early, close to the source of a problem, with an expectation of rapid return to wellness (Artiss, 1963). The risk of failing to recognize these states is also significant. Stress can have a deleterious effect on performance and mission accomplishment and can also contribute to more severe personal consequences (e.g., excessive alcohol use). Indeed, only 30 percent of military suicide decedents in 2018 were identified to have been treated by mental health or recognized as having a clinical disorder (Tucker, Smolenski, & Kennedy, 2019), and the most commonly identified stressors among military suicide decedents included failing relationships, administrative or legal problems, and workplace difficulties. Case 3.1 below is one example of a common stress reaction and PIES-consistent response, highlighting the roles of leadership and other nonclinical helping services in supporting the service member.

Case 3.1. The Soldier Who Was Never Home

The specialist (SPC) was a Blackhawk crew chief. He was described as a stellar soldier by his chain of command. Unfortunately, the time he was deployed and high operational demands required him to spend significant time away from family. His leadership noticed significant changes in his behavior shortly after he and his wife separated, but attributed these to normal stress. After presenting to work intoxicated, however, his leadership became concerned, grounded him (i.e., removed his flight status), and had the flight surgeon check in with him after he shared that he was having difficulty sleeping, was feeling "angry all the time," and thinking "things would be better for everyone if I were dead." He identified his primary stressors as financial challenges related to his recent separation and inability to engage in marital counseling due to his work schedule. In support, the flight surgeon and the SPC's leadership collaborated to connect him with Army Community Services (ACS) and the Army Substance Abuse Program, to provide financial counseling, marital counseling, and substance use education. ACS also helped him establish budgeting and billing management for future deployments and trainings to help manage his schedule to allow more time with his family. Unfortunately, despite implementing these changes, the specialist was unable to save his marriage. However, he was able to learn to manage the stress related to the divorce in healthy and adaptive ways, and was able to regain his flight status.

STRESS MITIGATION AND SUPPORT

Efforts to mitigate the adverse impacts of stress in service members, individually and through support services, serve to keep members in the *green* and decrease the likelihood of stress injuries. Multiple nonmedical efforts have been undertaken to reach service members with these tools "left of bang" (prior to injury), including the use of Military Family Life Counselors, deployed resiliency counselors, the U.S. Army's Master Resilience Trainer program, and the mental fitness-focused Rational Thinking, Emotion Regulation, and Problem Solving (REPS) program currently being piloted within the U.S. Navy. Each of these programs shares some foundation in cognitive, behavioral, and/or social restructuring—all with the primary foci of stress mitigation, resilience development, and performance enhancement. While a summary of all psychological stress mitigation strategies is outside the scope of this chapter and text, the following highlights of stress mitigation, coping skills, and social support are discussed as a demonstration of effective tools within these domains.

Cognitive Stress Mitigation

Psychological approaches derived from cognitive-behavioral therapy with a focus on the cognitive components of aversive emotional responses have been demonstrated to mitigate these responses in a variety of psychological disorders, limiting further exacerbation and injury (Butler, Chapman, Forman, & Beck, 2006). Furthermore, additional efforts may be focused on identifying maladaptive thoughts, challenging dysfunctional thinking styles, and encouraging thought stopping (recognition of a maladaptive thought, followed by a service member telling him- or herself to stop fixating on the thought once it emerges) (Chesney et al., 2006). Alternatively, service members may use a range of additional strategies designed to reduce cognitive rigidity and enhance cognitive flexibility. For example, service members may practice exploring evidence for and against a particular thought, rather than accepting thoughts as true facts. They may also practice reframing their thoughts in order to introduce shades of gray into all-or-nothing cognitions. Over time, the goal is to replace maladaptive thoughts with more balanced and realistic thoughts that can help individuals adapt to acute and chronic stressors. As service members practice these strategies, their self-confidence and beliefs about stress may change. Notably, recent research found that confidence in one's ability to stop unpleasant thoughts was uniquely associated with lower prevalence of lifetime suicide-related behavior among an outpatient sample of military service members (Cunningham, Cramer, Cacace, Franks, & Desmarais, 2020).

Problem-Focused Coping

Research has highlighted the role of appraisal and effective coping as key to stress-related growth (Jennings et al., 2006). Coping consists of both emotion-focused coping and problem-focused coping; the former refers to regulation of emotional responses to stress, and the latter to efforts to change the characteristics of stressful conditions (Lazarus & Folkman, 1984). Coping self-efficacy may be particularly important to managing stress reactions and minimizing the amount of time one spends in the *yellow* zone, as self-efficacy, or confidence in one's abilities (Bandura, 1997), is an important component of behavior change. There are three main components of coping self-efficacy: (1) belief in one's abilities to stop maladaptive thoughts, (2) belief in one's abilities to find solutions to problems, and (3) belief in one's ability to get social support (Chesney et al., 2006).

Having a positive problem orientation means appraising problems as challenges or opportunities, rather than as insurmountable setbacks. People with a positive problem orientation recognize negative emotions, understand that experiencing negative emotions is part of the problem-solving process, and feel confident that they can overcome problems (e.g., planful problem solving; D'Zurilla & Nezu, 1982). Enhancing effective problem-solving strategies may therefore be an added component in the approach to stress mitigation.

Social Support

Service members, like civilians, who have established a community of social support may be better equipped when faced with acute stress. For example, the presence of social support among veterans is negatively correlated with suicidal ideations (Wilks et al., 2019). Furthermore, service members who perceive cohesive relationships among their unit are also at lower risk for suicide (Rugo et al., 2020). Establishing strong interpersonal relationships within a unit may also influence a service member's job satisfaction (Ahronson & Cameron, 2007).

In addition to peer support, multiple support services exist that may be useful for stress mitigation (see Table 3.2). Examples of these services include the Military OneSource and Military Family Life Counseling programs, service-specific support centers, and service-specific financial relief organizations. Military OneSource offers nonmedical individual and couples counseling for military personnel and their families in the community, in addition to financial consulting, tax filing services, and a multitude of other support services at no cost to service members. Nonmedical counseling is also available on multiple military installations through Military Family Life Counselors (MFLCs). MFLCs are licensed clinicians contracted to provide mobile and confidential supportive nonmedical counseling to service members and their families. These organizations each function to help mitigate psychosocial stress and improve service member well-being. Military branch-specific organizations such as the Army's Community Services and the Navy's Fleet and Family Support Center provide similar resources and recreational activities for active-duty personnel and families. Branch-specific financial support organizations exist to help during significant financial crises (e.g., Navy and Marine Corps Relief Society, Army Emergency Relief) through no interest loans or grants, when needed. Notably, each of these services will also connect service members with higher levels of care, if indicated, conducting warm hand-offs to embedded mental/behavioral health assets or military treatment facilities to ensure safety.

Case 3.2 offers an example of the use of these resources, in partnership with medical and mental health services, in addressing stress reactions.

Case 3.2. *The Sailor Who Had a Difficult Adjustment to the Navy*

A seaman (SN) presented to the emergency room (ER) shortly after arrival at her first duty station, a naval destroyer, after a report of suicide ideation while at sea for a brief training period. She experienced immediate resolution of symptoms upon removal from her ship and expressed fears that she could not handle the stress of the operational schedule, describing multiple upcoming brief underway periods to prepare for a longer, shipboard deployment. The ER connected the sailor with her local mental health clinic for further support and evaluation of suitability for continued service. Clinically, the SN did not meet the criteria for any psychiatric condition that would preclude further service, but rather she presented with the common challenge of difficulty adjusting to a new and stressful environment. She reported feeling overwhelmed at work, with subsequent physiological arousal, then seeking private spaces to calm down. She stated this pattern repeats daily and described feeling embarrassed to ask for help in understanding work expectations ("They will think I'm stupid") or support in adjusting to naval service ("They will think I can't hack it"). Working with MFLC, she learned ways to challenge negative thinking ("Everybody starts somewhere"), diaphragmatic breathing to reduce arousal, social skills to connect with her peers, and goal setting to help her prepare for the upcoming deployment. After six sessions, she noted increased self-confidence for "sticking it out" and reported she had begun to help other new sailors learn how to adjust to shipboard life.

TABLE 3.2. Support Services Available to Military Personnel

Resource	Mental health services	Financial services	Family support services	Spiritual services	Website
Army morale, welfare, and recreation/Army community services		✓	✓		www.armymwr.com
Military OneSource	✓	✓	✓		www.militaryonesource.mil
Fleet and Family Support Center	✓	✓	✓		www.cnic.navy.mil/ffr/family_readiness/fleet_and_family_support_program.html
Navy–Marine Relief Society	✓	✓	✓		www.nmcrs.org
Marine Corps community services	✓	✓	✓		www.usmc-mccs.org/services
Airman and Family Readiness Center	✓	✓	✓		www.afpc.af.mil/Airman-and-Family
Military Family Life Counselors	✓		✓		www.militaryonesource.mil/confidential-help/non-medical-counseling/military-and-family-life-counseling
Embedded mental health	✓		✓		Installation dependent. Check installation directories for resources.
Chaplains				✓	Installation dependent. Check installation directories for resources.
Military medical centers	✓		✓		www.tricare.mil

SUMMARY

Throughout this chapter, we have attempted to detail the sources of military stress, impacts of adverse stress reactions, and methods and resources to mitigate the impacts of stress to prevent further injury. Attempting to summarize military stress and stress reactions within the confines of a single chapter is not possible (for a comprehensive review, see Kennedy, 2020). It is our intent, however, to leave you with some critical takeaways to carry with you through the remainder of this volume:

• Stress, whether eustress or distress, can generate significant change (adaptive or maladaptive) within the person experiencing it, and this change can vary in both intensity and reach depending on the acuity and/or chronicity of the stressor(s); a stress reaction can transition to a stress injury or illness if ignored.

• Military service is associated with multiple unique stressors in both deployed and garrison environments, and these stressors may impact both the service member and their support system synergistically, thus increasing the effect of the stressor; service members are not a blank slate such that the stressors associated with military service are in addition to the shared stressors experienced by civilian and military alike.

• Despite increased risk of exposure to stressors, military service is also associated with multiple protective and psychologically strengthening factors including a sense of purpose, social support, and access to abundant resources to support personal and family stress, mental and physical health, and financial well-being.

• Adverse reactions to military-specific stressors may have clinical and nonclinical interventions that may improve service member functioning. Clinicians, military leaders, and/or other influential personnel working with service members under such conditions should take an integrative approach in their conceptualization of the issues, which includes biological, cognitive, behavioral, social, and environmental factors. When a whole person approach such as this is used, improved abilities to identify pathology and formulate and provide interventions may be achieved.

• This chapter is not meant to serve as an exhaustive description of stress, military service, how one many react to it, or how best to prevent these reactions from escalation to injuries, but rather as an overview for those unfamiliar with military populations or as an overlay for those with hopes of encouraging further engagement in the understanding of service members and actions to support those who serve. The risk of adverse outcomes following unaddressed stress reactions cannot be overstated.

REFERENCES

Adler, A. B., Delahaij, R., Bailey, S. M., Van den Berge, C., Parmak, M., van Tussenbroek, B., et al. (2013). NATO survey of mental health training in Army recruits. *Military Medicine, 178,* 760–766.

Ahronson, A., & Cameron, J. E. (2007). The nature and consequences of group cohesion in a military sample. *Military Psychology, 19*(1), 9–25.

Armed Forces Health Surveillance Branch. (2020). Hospitalizations, active component, U.S. Armed Forces, 2019. *Medical Surveillance Monthly Report, 27*(5), 10–17.

Artiss, K. L. (1963). Human behavior under stress: From combat to social psychiatry. *Military Medicine, 128,* 1011–1015.

Bandura, A. (1997). *Self-efficacy: The exercise of control.* New York: Freeman.

Booth-Kewley, S., Highfill-McRoy, R. M., Larson, G. E., & Garland, C. F. (2010). Psycosocial predictors of military misconduct. *Journal of Nervous and Mental Disorders, 198*(2), 91–98.

Butler, A. C., Chapman, J. E., Forman, E. M., & Beck, A. T. (2006). The empirical status of cognitive-behavioral therapy: A review of meta-analyses. *Clinical Psychology Review, 26*(1), 17–31.

Carron, A. V. (1982). Cohesiveness in sport groups: Interpretations and considerations. *Journal of Sport Psychology, 4*(2), 123–138.

Chesney, M. A., Neilands, T. B., Chambers, D. B., Taylor, J. M., & Folkman, S. (2006). A validity and reliability study of the coping self-efficacy scale. *British Journal of Health Psychology, 11*(3), 421–437.

Consortium for Health and Military Performance (CHAMP). (2020). *Building team cohesion in military units.* Retrieved March 23, 2021, from *www.hprc-online.org/social-fitness/teams-leadership/building-team-cohesion-military-units.*

Cunningham, C. A., Cramer, R. J., Cacace, S., Franks, M., & Desmarais, S. L. (2020). The Coping Self-Efficacy Scale: Psychometric properties in an outpatient sample of active duty military personnel. *Military Psychology, 32*(3), 261–272.

Danish, S. J., & Antonides, B. J. (2013). The challenges of reintegration for service members and their families. *American Journal of Orthopsychiatry, 83*(4), 550–558.

Department of the Navy and U.S. Marine Corps. (2010). *Combat and operational stress control.* Retrieved March 23, 2021, from *www.med.navy.mil/sites/nmcphc/Documents/LGuide/pdf/COSC_MRCP_NTTP_Doctrine.pdf.*

D'Zurilla, T. J., & Nezu, A. M. (1982). Social problem solving in adults. In P. C. Kendall (Ed.), *Advances in cognitive-behavioral research and therapy* (Vol. 1, pp. 201–274). New York: Academic Press.

Engel, G. (1977). The need for a new medical model: A challenge for biomedicine. *Science, 196,* 129–136.

Festinger, L., Schachter, S., & Back, K. (1950). *Social pressures in informal groups: A study of human factors in housing.* New York: Harper.

Gade, P., Lakhani, H., & Kimmel, M. (1991). Military service: A good place to start? *Military Psychology, 3,* 251–267.

George, B. J., Ribeiro, S., Lee-Tauler, S. Y., Bond, A. E., Perera, K. U., Grammer,

G., et al. (2019). Demographic and clinical characteristics of military service members hospitalized following a suicide attempt versus suicide ideation. *International Journal of Environmental Research and Public Health, 16,* 3774.

Grippo, A., Geltz, T., & Johnson, A. (2003). Behavioral and cardiovascular changes in the chronic mild stress model of depression. *Physiology and Behavior, 78*(4–5), 703–710.

Infurna, F. J., & Luthar, S. S. (2016). Resilience to major life stressors is not as common as thought. *Perspectives on Psychological Science, 11*(2), 175–194.

Jennings, P. A., Aldwin, C. M., Levenson M. R., Spiro, A., & Mroczek, D. K. (2006). Combat exposure, perceived benefits of military service, and wisdom in later life. *Research on Aging, 28*(1), 115–134.

Jeschke, E. A., LaCroix, J. M., Fox, A. M., Novak, L. A., & Ghahramanlou-Holloway, M. (2019). Military training and its relationship to post-deployment role conflict in intimate partner relationships. In U. Kumar (Ed.), *The Routledge international handbook of military psychology and mental health* (pp. 232–248). New York: Routledge.

Kennedy, C. (2020). *Military stress reactions: Rethinking trauma and PTSD.* New York: Guilford Press.

Knobloch, L. K., & Theiss, J. A. (2012). Experiences of U.S. military couples during the post-deployment transition: Applying the relational turbulence model. *Journal of Social and Personal Relationships, 29*(4), 423–450.

Lazarus, R. S., & Folkman, S. (1984). *Stress, appraisal, and coping.* New York: Springer.

Maby, J. I., Kwon, P. O., Washington, W., Pearce, T. D., Cowan, D. N., Kelley, A. L., et al. (2017). *Disability evaluation system analysis and research annual report.* Silver Spring, MD: Walter Reed Army Institute of Research.

Meichenbaum, D. (1985). *Stress inoculation training.* Oxford, UK: Pergamon Press.

Rugo, K. F., Leifker, F. R., Drake-Brooks, M. M., Snell, M. B., Bryan, C. J., & Bryan, A. O. (2020). Unit cohesion and social support as protective factors against suicide risk and depression among National Guard service members. *Journal of Social and Clinical Psychology, 39*(3), 214–228.

Russell, D. W., Russell, C. A., Chen, H. Y., Cacioppo, S., & Cacioppo, J. T. (2019). To what extent is psychological resilience protective or ameliorative: Exploring the effects of deployment on the mental health of combat medics. *Psychological Services, 18*(1), 51–63.

Sarnoff, I., & Zimbardo, P. G. (1961). Anxiety, fear, and social isolation. *The Journal of Abnormal and Social Psychology, 62*(2), 356–363.

Schachter, S. (1959). *The psychology of affiliation: Experimental studies of the sources of gregariousness.* Stanford, CA: Stanford University Press.

Tucker, J., Smolenski, D. J., & Kennedy, C. H. (2019). *Department of Defense Suicide Event Report (DoDSER) calendar year 2018 annual report.* Falls Church, VA: Psychological Health Center of Excellence (PHCoE), Defense Health Agency (DHA).

Wilks, C. R., Morland, L. A., Dillon, K. H., Mackintosh, M., Blakey, S. M, Wagner, H. R., et al. (2019). Anger, social support, and suicide risk in U.S. military veterans. *Journal of Psychiatric Research, 109,* 139–144.

Yerkes, R. & Dodson, J. The relation of strength of stimulus to rapidity of habit formation. *Journal of Comparative Neurology and Psychology, 18,* 459–482.

Yukelson, D. (1997). Principles of effective team building interventions in sport: A direct services approach at Penn State University. *Journal of Applied Sport Psychology, 9*(1), 73–96.

Zalta, A. K., Tirone, V., Orlowska, D., Blais, R. K., Lofgreen, A., Klassen, B., et al. (2021). Examining moderators of the relationship between social support and self-reported PTSD symptoms: A meta-analysis. *Psychological Bulletin, 147*(1), 33–54.

CHAPTER 4

Evidence-Based Treatments of Common Psychological Health Disorders in the Military

Michael A. Gramlich, Nancy A. Skopp,
and Greg M. Reger

$\mathbf{M}$ilitary service members are subject to constant change, and the anticipation of an uncertain future is a way of life. Leadership during combat and other operations requires the use of decision making that is adaptable. Plans can change with little notice, based on ever-changing situations and circumstances. Deployment requirements evolve based on world/political events and military personnel may not know when an operation will occur, or whether they will be involved. The duration of some deployments can change, and in some instances, service members may only have partial information on where they will be located. Furthermore, the experience of combat is characterized by threats that are, to a large degree, difficult to predict. Exposure to potentially traumatic events is common. Stress and anxiety are also present simply in the preparations for combat and other military operations. Because the military aims to always be ready to fight and win America's wars, service members train as they fight, and military training calendars are littered with intentionally stressful and demanding events. All of this occurs in the context of young adulthood, a period during which baseline onset of behavioral health conditions occurs among some, regardless of military service.

In this context, it is self-evident that all service members experience stress and anxiety as a result of combat and military operations. In most cases, combat and operational stress results in reactions that can be managed by simple interventions adopted by the service member and aided by their leaders (Department of Army, 2016; see also Chapter 3, this volume). However, in other cases, military personnel may experience more significant effects. These can include trauma-reactions, depression, apprehension, worry, and fear about perceived threats, or future events, that negatively impact their functioning. In these instances, the service member may meet the criteria for a psychological disorder. This chapter reviews three common psychological health disorders among military personnel—namely, posttraumatic stress disorder (PTSD), depression, and generalized anxiety disorder (GAD)—and discusses the evidence-based treatments available for effective treatment.

POSTTRAUMATIC STRESS DISORDER

Military service is associated with exposure to traumatic stressors including war zone dangers, accidents, and other occupational hazards that may place military personnel at elevated risk for the development of PTSD (Joellenbeck, Russell, & Guze, 1999). In this section, we provide guidance on recommended assessment and treatment procedures in conformance with the Department of Veterans Affairs (VA) and the Department of Defense (DoD) Clinical Practice Guideline for the Management of PTSD (VA/DoD, 2017) and also incorporate other evidence-based sources of information.

Diagnostic Criteria for PTSD

PTSD is a highly debilitating and potentially chronic mental health condition that may occur following trauma exposure. PTSD was formerly classified as an anxiety disorder in the fourth edition of the *Diagnostic and Statistical Manual of Mental Disorders* (DSM-IV; American Psychiatric Association, 1994); however, the fifth edition (DSM-5; American Psychiatric Association, 2013) now classifies PTSD in a separate category denoted as Trauma and Stressor-Related Disorders. DSM-5 describes PTSD as a disorder resulting from trauma exposure involving actual or threatened death, serious injury, or sexual violence either through direct experience or witnessing of the event; learning that a close family member or friend experienced the event; or experiencing repeated or extreme exposure to aversive details of the traumatic event (e.g., police officers repeated exposure to child abuse; American Psychiatric Association, 2013). Diagnostic criteria from each of four distinct symptom clusters must be met for PTSD to be diagnosed: (1) reexperiencing symptoms (e.g., recurrent dreams, involuntary distressing memories [Criterion B]); (2) persistent avoidance of stimuli related to the event (Criterion C); (3) symptoms of negative alternation of cognitions or mood (Criterion D); and (4) alterations in arousal and reactivity associated with the event (Criterion E). The duration of the symptoms must be a month or more and cause significant distress or impairment in social, occupational, or other important domains of functioning. When PTSD onset occurs 6 or more months after the traumatic event, this is designated with the specifier "with delayed expression."

DSM-5 introduced a dissociative subtype of PTSD that is characterized by symptoms of derealization (i.e., sense of detachment from the world or a perception of unreality) and depersonalization (i.e., feeling that one's body is detached from oneself; Dutra & Wolf, 2017). This subtype is given when a patient meets all PTSD criteria plus derealization and/or depersonalization symptoms; it appears to be characteristic of a clinical population with unique neurobiological and epidemiological features, which may confer greater severity and comorbidity (see Schiavone, Frewen, McKinnon, & Lanius, 2018, for a discussion). Although there has been some controversy about whether this subtype requires a specialized form of treatment, the majority of research indicates that current evidence-based PTSD treatments are effective for this subtype (Dutra & Wolf, 2017).

Course of PTSD

Empirical data show that the course of PTSD is not linear but rather may wax and wane across time (Bryant, 2019). A 20-year prospective study examined combat-related PTSD symptoms among Israeli war veterans, comparing those with and without a history of a combat stress reaction (CSR). This study defined CSR as a diagnosis that reflected a psychological breakdown on the battlefield characterized by cognitive, behavioral, and affective responses and the inability to function as a combatant (Karstoft, Armour, Elklit, & Solomon, 2013). Accordingly, this study compared the course of PTSD among soldiers from the same units who were and were not diagnosed with an acute stress reaction, similar in some respects to acute stress disorder. Four trajectories were identified for both groups: (1) resilient, (2) recovering, (3) delayed, and (4) chronic; however, 76.5% of non-CSR cases were classified as resilient compared to 34.4% of the CSR cases. A 10-year study involving combat- and non-combat-exposed U.S. veterans similarly identified four trajectories, described as resilient, preexisting, new-onset, and moderate-stable (Donoho, Bonanno, Porter, & Kearney, 2017). Persistence of PTSD in active-duty service members (ADSMs) and veterans appears to be strongly associated with combat and PTSD symptom severity; additional risk factors include comorbidity, illness/injury, physical symptoms, and sleep problems (Armenta et al., 2018).

Acute Stress Disorder

Acute stress disorder (ASD) may be conceptualized as existing on the same spectrum as PTSD. It differs from PTSD in its duration (less than 1 month) and lower symptom threshold. Instead of requiring symptoms from multiple clusters, 9 out of 14 symptoms must be present. Individuals with subthreshold PTSD symptoms may still experience significant impairment and distress, including suicidal ideation (Marshall et al., 2001). ASD is responsive to trauma-focused psychotherapies containing exposure and/or cognitive restructuring components; thus, such treatments are recommended for the prevention of PTSD among patients diagnosed with ASD (VA/DoD, 2017).

Prevalence of PTSD

Epidemiological studies conducted with the general population report overall lifetime PTSD prevalence rates of 10.0–11.3% for women and 5.0–6.0% for men (Breslau, Davis, Andreski, & Peterson, 1991; Kessler, Sonnega, Bromet, Hughes, & Nelson, 1995). Among veterans, lifetime PTSD prevalence has been estimated to be 13.4% and 7.7%, for women and men, respectively (Lehavot, Katon, Chen, Fortney, & Simpson, 2018). These findings are consistent with a large-scale civilian meta-analysis that reported a twofold greater risk for PTSD among women compared to men (Tolin & Foa, 2006). In contrast, a more recent meta-analysis of PTSD prevalence rates among 4,945,897 Operation Enduring Freedom and Operation Iraqi Freedom (OEF/OIF) veterans yielded an overall PTSD prevalence rate of 23% and indicated that PTSD was more prevalent in men compared to women (Fulton et al., 2015). Although some debate about sex differences occurs in PTSD prevalence, in general, rate estimates indicate that PTSD is more common among women compared to men in both civilian and military populations.

Etiology of PTSD

Individuals vary in their risk for exposure to various types of traumatic events as well as in their responses (Breslau et al., 1991). Although many people experience traumatic events, the majority do not develop PTSD (Breslau et al., 1991). Differences in biological, psychological, and cognitive vulnerabilities (i.e., diatheses), as well as features of the event itself, influence the development and course of PTSD after traumatic exposure (e.g., Bryant, 2019; Elwood, Hahn, Olatungi, & Williams, 2009; Keane, Marshall, & Taft, 2006). Psychiatric history, childhood abuse, and family history, for example, have been shown to consistently relate to PTSD vulnerability (Brewin, Andrews, & Valentine, 2000; see McLaughlin & Lambert, 2017, for a discussion of developmental pathways). In addition, some types of traumatic experiences appear to be more strongly related to PTSD than others. Exposure to natural disasters appears to be considerably less likely to result in PTSD compared to sexual assault and other forms of interpersonal violence (Creamer, Burgess, & Mclaughlin, 2001; Forbes et al., 2014). Although roughly equal proportions of men and women report exposure to various forms of interpersonal violence (Iverson, Mercado, Carpenter, & Street, 2013), men are more likely to experience nonsexual assault, whereas women are more likely to experience sexual assault (Tolin & Foa, 2006; Iverson et al., 2013; Kessler et al., 1995).

Risk and Protective Factors

Certain distal and proximal factors influence susceptibility to PTSD. Such factors can be conceptualized temporally as preexisting factors (e.g., sex, psychiatric history, genetics); factors relating to the trauma (e.g., severity, pain, peritraumatic dissociation, alcohol use); and posttrauma factors (e.g., social support, financial stress; Keane et al., 2006; see Sareen, 2014, for a review). For example, peritraumatic intoxication during sexual assault has been shown to relate to more severe PTSD symptoms, intrusive thoughts, self-blame, and use of alcohol for coping (Jaffe et al., 2017; Littleton, Grills-Taquechel, & Axsom, 2009). Several pretrauma risk factors for combat-related PTSD have been identified among military personnel, including female sex, ethnic minority status, U.S. Army service, enlisted rank, low educational attainment, combat specialization, adverse life events, length of deployment, and prior trauma and psychological problems (Xue et al., 2015). Aspects of the trauma that confer elevated PTSD risk include increased combat exposures, discharge of a weapon, witnessing injury or killing, severe trauma, and deployment-related stressors (Xue et al., 2015). Female ADSMs exposed to combat are significantly more likely than nondeploying women to experience sexual assault (LeardMann et al., 2013), potentially placing them at especially high risk for PTSD. Postdeployment risk factors for PTSD include unemployment, alcohol misuse, stressful events, and poor social support (Possemato, McKenzie, McDevitt-Murphy, Williams, & Ouimette, 2014). In the aftermath of a traumatic experience, increased social support may help mitigate the development of PTSD (Sareen, 2014).

VA/DoD PTSD Treatment Recommendations

The VA/DoD Clinical Practice Guideline for the Management of PTSD recommends diagnostic evaluation and assessment that include the following components: determination of DSM criteria, acute risk of harm to self or others, functional status including duty and work responsibilities, risk and protective factors, treatment history, medical history, and pertinent family history. Given that PTSD is strongly associated with risk for suicidal behavior (Panagioti, Gooding, & Tarrier, 2012), it is especially important to assess for suicidal ideation and prior engagement in suicidal behaviors. PTSD is also often associated with relationship discord and social isolation; thus, it is necessary to evaluate functioning in these domains as well.

Shared decision making (SDM) is the recommended approach to PTSD patient care. SDM involves the incorporation of the patient's preferences to inform treatment and to increase patient involvement, quality decision making, and outcomes. Patient and collateral education on psychological trauma and PTSD, as well as a review of the pros and cons of available treatment options, are key components of SDM in the treatment of PTSD.

Evidence-Based Treatments

The VA/DoD PTSD Clinical Practice Guideline strongly recommends the use of individual and manualized trauma-focused psychotherapeutic treatments containing exposure and/or cognitive restructuring as a principal focus. Treatments that meet these criteria include prolonged exposure (PE; Foa, Hembree, Rothbaum, & Rauch, 2019), cognitive processing therapy (CPT; Resick, Monson, & Chard, 2016), cognitive-behavioral PTSD therapies (e.g., Ehlers et al., 2003), brief eclectic psychotherapy (Gersons, Carlier, Lamberts, & van der Kolk, 2000), narrative exposure therapy (Neuner, Elbert, & Schauer, 2020), eye movement desensitization and reprocessing (EMDR; Shapiro, 1989), and written exposure therapy (WET; Sloan & Marx, 2019).

An estimated third of patients, however, may not respond to trauma-focused cognitive-behavioral therapies (Bradley, Greene, Russ, Dutra, & Westen, 2005), and PE and CPT have been associated with unfavorable rates of attrition (Najavits, 2015). WET may be particularly useful in such cases, as it has demonstrated noninferiority to CPT and significantly lower treatment dropout rates than CPT (6.4% vs. 39.7%), and involves fewer treatment sessions and less in-session provider time (Sloan, Marx, Lee, & Resick, 2018).

Pharmacotherapy or manualized non-trauma-focused psychotherapies including stress inoculation training (Meichenbaum & Deffenbacher, 1988), present-centered therapy (Resick et al., 2015), and interpersonal psychotherapy (Markowitz et al., 2015) are recommended in situations where providers are not trained in trauma-focused psychotherapies or when patients decline to engage in first-line treatments. Although limited empirical data guiding the use of these treatment options exist, meta-analytic findings indicate that pharmacological and individual non-trauma-focused therapies can help alleviate PTSD symptoms.

Additional PTSD Diagnostic and Treatment Considerations

Trauma History

There is a robust dose–response relationship between exposure to traumatic events and risk for PTSD (Dohrenwend et al., 2006). Individuals presenting with PTSD symptomatology may have been exposed to multiple traumatic experiences; thus, the event associated with the clinical presentation may be tied to exposures to several earlier or chronic trauma exposures that may exert a cumulative negative effect (Sareen, 2014). It is therefore recommended that clinicians conduct a thorough assessment of patient trauma history and the trauma's significance to the patient's sense of self and future to inform treatment planning (Coyle et al., 2019; Sareen, 2014).

Complex PTSD

The World Health Organization (WHO) in the *International Classification of Diseases, 11th Revision for Mortality and Morbidity Statistics* (ICD-11; WHO, 2018) describes complex PTSD (CPTSD) as a condition characterized by core PTSD symptoms (i.e., reexperiencing, avoidance, sense of threat) and disturbances in self-organization, including emotion dysregulation, negative self-concept, and interpersonal problems. CPTSD is not included in the DSM-5 (American Psychiatric Association, 2013); however, a considerable volume of research has emerged since the publication of the DSM-5 in support of the validity of this syndrome among both civilians and military personnel (e.g., Folke, Nielsen, Anderson, Karatzias, & Karstoft, 2019; Knefel et al., 2020). CPTSD can result from a single traumatic exposure, although multiple and/or prolonged traumatic exposures may be stronger risk factors for the development of CPTSD (Cloitre, Garvert, Brewin, Bryant, & Maercker, 2013). Sexual assault in childhood and adulthood is a particularly salient predictor of CPTSD (e.g., Villalta et al., 2020). Because of the association of CPTSD with multiple traumatic exposures, ADSMs may be at elevated risk for CPTSD due to deployment-related trauma such as combat and sexual assault as well as other traumatic exposures during and/or predating military service (LeardMann et al., 2013; Letica-Crepulja et al., 2020; Surís, Lind, Kashner, Borman, & Petty, 2004; Zinzow, Grubaugh, Monnier, Suffoletta-Maierle, & Frueh, 2007).

Given the multidimensional symptom profile associated with CPTSD, some have suggested that the efficacy of frontline trauma-focused cognitive-behavioral treatments may be significantly downgraded among CPTSD patients (Corrigan, Fitzpatrick, Hanna, & Dyer, 2020; Ferdinand, Kelly, Skelton, Stephens, & Bradley, 2011; Najavits, 2015). As an alternative, phase-oriented CPTSD treatment approaches target several aspects of treatment in stages (Ford, Courtois, Steele, Hart, & Nijenhuis, 2005). The initial phase is oriented toward stabilization via coping and emotion regulation skill building, followed by a second phase in which trauma-focused exposure treatment is delivered (Ford et al., 2005). The final phase typically focuses on patient aspirations and the restoration of social connections (Ferdinand et al., 2011; Ford et al., 2005). A recent meta-analysis of phase-oriented treatments for CPTSD demonstrated a large effect size (Corrigan et al., 2020), and a few initial studies conducted with veterans and ADSMs also support the model (Ferdinand et al., 2011; Held et al., 2020; Zalta et al., 2018).

Comorbidity

PTSD commonly co-occurs with other mental health conditions. According to the National Comorbidity Survey, 16% of patients diagnosed with PTSD have one coexisting psychiatric disorder, 17% have two psychiatric disorders, and 50% have three or more (Kessler et al., 1995). A large military cohort study that examined medical encounter data over 7 years reported that 83% of PTSD patients had one comorbid diagnosis, and 62.2% had three (Walter, Levine, Highfill-McRoy, Navarro, & Thomsen, 2018). Depressive, anxiety, and substance abuse disorders are two to four times more prevalent among patients with PTSD, and the use of substances for self-medication is common (Leeies, Pagura, Sareen, & Bolton, 2010). There has been controversy about whether or not patients with comorbid PTSD and substance abuse should be treated sequentially or concurrently; the available evidence indicates that concurrent treatment is feasible and efficacious for military veterans (e.g., Back et al., 2019). Significant comorbidity can greatly complicate treatment and may require a broader scope of intervention and adjunct treatment.

In addition to the aforementioned PTSD comorbidities, traumatic brain injury (TBI) and obsessive–compulsive disorder (OCD) are two problems that are particularly difficult to identify, and the failure to do so is likely to substantially prolong distress and negatively impact treatment outcome and quality of life.

Traumatic Brain Injury

PTSD is often comorbid with mild and moderate TBI but can be difficult to identify because of delayed-onset PTSD (Bryant, O'Donnell, Creamer, McFarlane, & Silove, 2013). When both problems are present and only one is identified, however, treatment is adversely affected (see Rosen & Ayers, 2020, for a discussion). Fortunately, frontline treatments for PTSD can be readily adapted to patients with TBIs (Rosen & Ayers, 2020). Thus, careful assessment and monitoring are required of patients who have experienced traumatic experiences and injuries.

Obsessive–Compulsive Disorder

PTSD and OCD are both trauma-related and often co-occur (Badour, Bown, Adams, Bunaciu, & Feldner, 2012; Gershuny et al., 2008). An estimated 24–40% of patients with PTSD have comorbid OCD (Brown, Campbell, Lehman, Grisham, & Mancill, 2001; Gershuny et al., 2008). Thirty-six percent of veterans seeking PTSD treatment exhibited elevated obsessive–compulsive (OC) symptoms and more severe PTSD compared to PTSD patients without OC symptoms (Aldea, Michael, Alexander, & Kison, 2019). It is therefore recommended that clinicians assess OC symptoms in PTSD patients. Although PTSD screening and treatment are routine in the DoD and VA health care systems, OCD is very frequently unrecognized and undiagnosed, with few patients completing a full course of treatment (Aldea, Michael, Alexander, & Kison, 2019). For example, ruminative tendencies for self-blame and guilt found among PTSD patients may be, in part, attributable to coexisting OCD.

Individually, OC and PTSD symptoms may severely impair functioning; however, their co-occurrence is likely to greatly intensify distress, particularly if only one disorder is recognized and treated. Even when both disorders are identified, treatment can be problematic. One study found that behavioral interventions for OCD may increase and intensify PTSD symptoms (Gershuny, Baer, Jenike, Minichiello, & Wilhelm, 2002). Moreover, awareness of potential OCD and PTSD co-occurrence and how it may influence treatment is essential. Although no guidelines or integrated treatment approaches exist for treating comorbid PTSD and OCD, exposure and response prevention (Foa, Yadin, & Leichner, 2012) is the psychotherapeutic treatment of choice for OCD, and trauma-focused exposure-based therapies are recommended by VA/DoD for PTSD. A dual-focus simultaneous approach would appear to be a prudent approach. Both conditions also have been shown to respond to selective serotonin uptake inhibitors (SSRIs).

Case 4.1. The Marine Who Was Sexually Assaulted

The lance corporal (LCpl) sought treatment because she felt "exiled from life," after a sexual assault while deployed 4 months ago. She experienced multiple stressors during the deployment, including poor social support, financial burdens, adaptation to an environment that occasionally exposed her to combat, and sexual harassment by her assailant. After the rape, she experienced emotional disconnection, irritability, and difficulty executing her duties, as well as intrusive thoughts and a strong sense of self-blame. She was sleeping poorly and starting misusing alcohol and sleep medication to cope. She expressed reluctance to report the assault because she had consumed alcohol at the time. The assessment procedure included a diagnostic interview and an assessment battery comprising screening tools for both PTSD and other comorbidities. She was diagnosed with PTSD and opted to engage in PE. Additionally, she was referred to substance abuse counseling to address medication and alcohol misuse, sleep hygiene, and emotion regulation difficulties. She was also provided with a referral to a Sexual Assault Response Prevention Victim's Advocate (SAPR-VA).[1] Over the course of her PE sessions, her self-blame and intrusive thoughts subsided, she reframed the assault as an event that she could not have foreseen occurring, and her work performance returned to normal. She also increased engagement in social activities, and her problematic use of substances improved.

DEPRESSIVE DISORDERS

Depressive disorders were introduced as a new chapter in DSM-5 (American Psychiatric Association, 2013) and include major depressive disorder (MDD), persistent depressive disorder, disruptive mood dysregulation disorder, substance/medication-induced depressive disorder, depressive disorder due to another medical condition, and premenstrual dysphoric disorder. The disorders share the presence of sadness, irritable mood, or feeling hopeless; however, they are differentiated based on the onset, duration, or presumed etiology (American Psychiatric Association, 2013). This section focuses on MDD due to its prevalence among ADSM and veteran populations (Liu et al., 2019; Mustillo et al., 2015) and relevance to the VA/DoD Clinical Practice Guideline for the Management of MDD (VA/DoD, 2016).

Major Depressive Disorder

MDD is the most studied among the depressive disorders. It is defined by experiencing a *major depressive episode* (MDE) without a history of a manic episode or hypomanic episode (characterized by an acute period of intense energy, euphoria, or irritable mood, pressured speech, or behavioral excesses). The classification of an MDE involves experiencing five out of the nine following symptoms for most of the day, nearly every day, for at least 2 weeks, and the symptoms must occur during that same period: depressed mood, little interest or pleasure in activities (anhedonia), change in appetite, change in sleep, psychomotor agitation or slowing, loss of energy, decreased concentration or trouble making decisions, feeling guilty or worthless, and thoughts of death or suicide. Furthermore, an individual must experience at least depressed mood or anhedonia to qualify as an MDE (American Psychiatric Association, 2013).

Depression Rates

The Psychological Health Center of Excellence (PHCoE) reported the rates of depressive disorders among U.S. ADSMs from 2005 to 2017 enrolled

---

[1]For a full discussion of military sexual trauma and resources, see Chapter 8 (this volume).

in TRICARE for a given year (PHCoE, 2019). Period prevalence included ADSMs who sought mental health care and were coded with a depressive disorder in the year of interest, whereas incidence indicated 6 months without delivered care for the same condition before the new encounter. Across all services, the rates of depressive disorders rose from 2005 to 2017 (point prevalence, 2.2% vs. 3.3%, and incidence, 1.6% vs. 2.1%). The Armed Forces Health Surveillance Branch (AFHSB) published findings in a *Medical Surveillance Monthly Report* on U.S. ADSMs between 2007 and 2016 from medical encounters reimbursed through the Military Health System (MHS; Stahlman & Oetting, 2018). Over the entire period, depressive disorders were the second most diagnosed of all incident mental health disorder diagnoses at 16.8%, with an incidence rate of 242.5 cases per 10,000 person-years. Between 2007 and 2016, rates of depressive disorders were highest among ADSMs aged 20 to 24 years old, females, and Army soldiers. The top three military occupations with the highest rates of depression across the entire period were (1) motor transport, (2) health care, and (3) combat-related (i.e., infantry, artillery, or combat engineering).

While incorporating the prevalence and incidence of depressive disorders based on health care evaluations might ensure valid estimates, an important limitation of the PHCoE and AFHSB summaries depended on patients who utilized medical care and, therefore, may underestimate the overall burden of depression on ADSMs. A study of 41,351 U.S. ADSMs examined the self-reported risk of depression at approximately 30 days and between 90 to 180 days returning from deployment to Iraq or Afghanistan (Mustillo et al., 2015). Furthermore, this study analyzed the frequency of depressive disorders listed in any TRICARE medical encounter within 6 months postdeployment. The service branch with the most positive screens for possible depression was the U.S. Marine Corps at 27.4% within 30 days and 23.1% between 90 to 180 days, whereas the Army had 12.2% and 9.9% screen positive at the previous time points, respectively. Conversely, 6.6% of Marine Corps and 5.8% of Army service members had a depressive disorder listed in a medical encounter within 6 months of returning from deployment. A report released by the Deployment Health Clinical Center (now PHCoE) among U.S. ADSMs from 2005 to 2016 showed an increasing trend of outpatient and inpatient health care encounters for depressive disorders in the MHS across the entire time span (Deployment Health Clinical Center, 2017). Nevertheless, further interventions may be warranted to reduce the disparity between ADSMs with probable depression and the utilization of services (Thériault et al., 2020).

An investigation of 1,885 U.S. veterans from the 2005 to 2016 National Health and Nutrition Survey found 9.6% of the sample had depression over the entire period, with the highest peak at 12.3% from the 2011 to 2012 cycle, and 7.2% at the most recent 2015 to 2016 cycle (Liu, Collins, Wang,

Xie, & Bie, 2019). In addition, female veterans have had higher rates of depression than men since 2009, and fewer than 12 years of education was associated with a greater prevalence of depression throughout most years of interest, including the most recent cycle from 2015 to 2016. Furthermore, a study of 2,732 U.S. veterans from the National Health and Resilience in Veterans Survey in 2011 found 10.2% had probable MDD based on an anonymous Web-based survey (Nichter, Norman, Haller, & Pietrzak, 2019). Taken together, ongoing evaluations for depression remain vital among U.S. service members and veterans. Understanding the contributing and protective factors of depression in the military is a pivotal component of informed case conceptualization.

Etiology

U.S. ADSMs contend with critical life events that increase their likelihood of depression in adulthood, such as deployment-related trauma (Meadows et al., 2017). An investigation of 17,252 U.S. service members deployed to Iraq or Afghanistan found military personnel with combat experience were two times more likely to have new-onset MDD (Porter et al., 2018). In particular, if the service member had witnessed a person's death; witnessed instances of physical abuse; felt as if he or she was in great danger of being killed; had been wounded or injured, or knew someone seriously injured or killed. Also, a study of 551 U.S. ADSMs found the limited exposure combat subgroup, defined strictly as being sent outside the wire, was more likely to be diagnosed with a depressive disorder when screened in a primary-care setting, whereas service members assigned to the medical exposure combat subgroup, characterized as caring for the injured or handling dead bodies, did not show a significant decrease in depression at 12-month follow-up (Kelber et al., 2019). The limited exposure subgroup consisted mainly of functional repair occupations, whereas health care-related specialties were largely made up of service members in the medical exposure subgroup. Moving forward, assessing for the type of combat exposure and military occupational specialty may inform treatment outcomes.

A history of traumatic experiences during childhood such as physical abuse was associated with depression severity among 1,488 U.S. veterans of Iraq or Afghanistan, even after controlling for combat exposure (Youssef et al., 2013). A study of U.S. Veterans Health Administration patients found women with a history of childhood abuse (sexual, physical, or both) were nearly three times more likely to have recurrent MDD, whereas trauma postmilitary was associated with recurrent MDD in men (Curry et al., 2019). Collecting data on adverse experiences when entering basic training may aid in recognizing those who might benefit from early interventions before exposure to military-related trauma (Duncan et al., 2020).

Psychological Factors

The ability to enhance and suppress emotions, known as expressive flexibility, might promote adaptive coping and attenuate depression. U.S. combat veterans with MDD were observed to have lower emotional enhancement but similar levels of emotional suppression compared to combat veterans without MDD (Rodin et al., 2017). Suppression ability might be a result of military training and adaptive to withstand stressful environments; however, impaired emotional expression may serve as a driver of MDD and thus a potential target for treatment. Effective treatments addressing emotional expression are discussed below (e.g., Walser, Sears, Chartier, & Karlin, 2012; Wenzel, Brown, & Karlin, 2011; see the "VA/DoD Depression Treatment Recommendations" section). A 2-year prospective study of 2,157 U.S. military veterans found 1.3% classified as resilient (high trauma/low psychological distress) and 50.4% categorized as distressed (high trauma/ high psychological distress) screened positive for MDD at baseline (Isaacs et al., 2017). In comparison to the distressed group, there were greater positive perceptions of the military's effect on one's life, extraversion, emotional stability, and altruism associated with resilient membership at baseline. Greater dispositional gratitude and a greater sense of purpose in life at baseline were independent predictors of resilient membership at 2-year follow-up compared to the distressed group. An investigation of 2,171 U.S. ADSMs found individuals with low resilience, characterized as having poor cognitive, emotional, and behavioral responses to stressful life events, were nearly three times more likely to have MDD based on self-report (Vyas et al., 2016). Increasing resilience at a follow-up assessment demonstrated a reduced likelihood of up to 54% for developing MDD alone and up to 93% for developing comorbid PTSD and MDD. A 2-year prospective study followed 70,664 Army soldiers and found a dose–response relationship with resilience, whereby strengths at baseline such as positive affect, lack of catastrophic thinking, and lack of loneliness reduced the odds of developing depression by 19–52% (Shrestha et al., 2018). U.S. military training programs may identify service members at risk for depression and intervene by enriching psychological resilience (Crane et al., 2019).

Unit Cohesion

Increased social bonding or greater unit cohesion, such as believing one can rely on other unit members or first-line leaders for support, weakened the link between combat experiences and depression in a sample of 5,283 Army and activated National Guard or Reserve soldiers (Reed-Fitzke & Lucier-Greer, 2020). A prospective study of 1,307 Marines found individuals with higher perceptions of cohesion (compared to members of the same unit) at predeployment lowered the risk of MDD at postdeployment

(Breslau, Setodji, & Vaughan, 2016). A longitudinal investigation of 4,645 Army soldiers measured unit cohesion at the individual level before deployment and 1 month, 3 months, and 9 months after returning from Afghanistan (Anderson et al., 2019). Greater perceived unit cohesion both before deployment and 1 month after deployment lowered the odds of an MDE at 3- or 9-months postdeployment, regardless of the level of deployment stress exposure. Overall, the findings recommend evaluating cohesion at an individual's perspective over one's assessment of the unit as a whole. Furthermore, clinicians may benefit from exploring social well-being and mental health among enlisted personnel transitioning to civilian life (Vogt et al., 2020).

Taken together, depression in military personnel can onset or recede due to a myriad of factors, including trauma exposure, psychological resilience, and perceived cohesion within military units. Also, ample evidence suggests biological factors such as genetic or neurological components are linked to depression (for an in-depth discussion of biological considerations, see Feliciano, Renn, & Segal, 2018). The findings support the diathesis–stress model, in which a higher vulnerability (diathesis) requires less stress due to life events to cause MDD, whereas a lower predisposition demands higher environmental stressors to induce MDD (Bartone & Homish, 2020; Colodro-Conde et al., 2018).

VA/DoD Depression Treatment Recommendations

The administration of the Patient Health Questionnaire-2 (PHQ-2; Kroenke, Spitzer, & Williams, 2003) is encouraged as a screening instrument for all patients not currently receiving treatment for depression. The PHQ-2 is a two-item depression screener that assesses for depressed mood and anhedonia over the past 2 weeks, and a total score greater than 3 (out of a possible 6) likely indicates MDD (Kroenke et al., 2003). If a patient is suspected to have depression, it is recommended that he or she complete a diagnostic evaluation using the DSM-5 criteria to establish a working diagnosis, as well as determine the functional status, medical history, past treatment history, and relevant family history. Furthermore, it is suggested that the Patient Health Questionnaire-9 (PHQ-9, Kroenke, Spitzer, & Williams, 2001) be administered to measure the initial severity of depression and to monitor progress during treatment. The PHQ-9 self-report form assesses for nine depressive symptoms over the past 2 weeks and has been validated among individuals with and without depressive disorders (Löwe, Kroenke, Herzog, & Gräfe, 2004). Ongoing monitoring of symptom intensity across treatment can help inform evaluations of treatment response and quantify remission of depression (i.e., PHQ-9 total score of 4 or less, maintained for at least 1 month) to help inform collaborative clinical decision making. See Figure 4.1 for the PHQ-2 and PHQ-9 self-report items.

Over the last 2 weeks, how often have you been bothered by any of the following problems?	Not at all	Several days	More than half the days	Nearly every day
1. Little interest or pleasure in doing things	0	1	2	3
2. Feeling down, depressed, or hopeless	0	1	2	3
3. Trouble falling or staying asleep, or sleeping too much	0	1	2	3
4. Feeling tired or having little energy	0	1	2	3
5. Poor appetite or overeating	0	1	2	3
6. Feeling bad about yourself, or that you are a failure or have let yourself or your family down	0	1	2	3
7. Trouble concentrating on things, such as reading the newspaper or watching television	0	1	2	3
8. Moving or speaking so slowly that other people could have noticed? Or the opposite, being so fidgety or restless that you have been moving around a lot more than usual	0	1	2	3
9. Thoughts that you would be better off dead or of hurting yourself in some way	0	1	2	3

If you checked off any problems, how difficult have these problems made it for you to do your work, take care of things at home, or get along with other people?

Not difficult at all	Somewhat difficult	Very difficult	Extremely difficult
☐	☐	☐	☐

FIGURE 4.1. Patient Health Questionnaire–9 (PHQ-9). The PHQ-9 (Kroenke et al., 2001) was developed by Drs. Robert L. Spitzer, Janet B. W. Williams, Kurt Kroenke, and colleagues, with an educational grant from Pfizer Inc. No permission required to reproduce, translate, display, or distribute. The Patient Health Questionnaire–2 (PHQ-2) includes the first two items of the PHQ-9 and the total score ranges from 0 to 6. The PHQ-9 total score includes all nine items and ranges from 0 to 27.

Treatment Settings

Strong evidence exists for incorporating the collaborative care model for the treatment of MDD in primary-care settings due to significantly reduced depressive symptoms, greater treatment adherence, and favorable recovery rates at 6- and 12-month follow-ups (Coventry et al., 2014; Thota et al., 2012). A systematic review of collaborative care for depression defined this model as a minimum of two health professionals working together, an assigned case manager tasked with coordinating or delivering services, a structured management plan offering pharmacological and psychotherapy interventions, monitored follow-ups, and enhanced interprofessional communication (Wood, Ohlsen, & Ricketts, 2017). Key identified barriers to establishing this multiprofessional approach were organizational disagreement on integration and poor interprofessional communication. A higher likelihood of successful implementation followed greater acceptability of the model's strength and quality due to education and supervision, as well as clearly defined roles for case managers to reduce the perception of added workload and personal stress. Further reports from patient views may enhance this model.

Delivering frontline treatments for MDD via telemental health (TMH; e.g., video conferencing) offers patients improved access to quality clinical care (Linde et al., 2015; Osenbach, O'Brien, Mishkind, & Smolenski, 2013). TMH provides services to underserved populations such as rural or remote areas, eliminates barriers due to travel or limited mobility, and expands care to patients who avoid military- or veteran-affiliated clinics (e.g., stigma, reminders of service-related trauma). However, an investigation of Army soldiers and U.S. military veterans found similar effectiveness for reducing hopelessness between TMH and in-person visits for mild to moderate symptom severities, whereas greater improvement for severe symptom profiles favored in-person psychotherapy (Smolenski, Pruitt, Vuletic, Luxton, & Gahm, 2017). This finding may account for the inherent social interaction and behavioral activation associated with attending in-person visits. From this perspective, further research on which patient profiles benefit from video compared to traditional office time appears warranted; nevertheless, TMH may extend sufficient care for those unable to attend in-person appointments.

Evidence-Based Treatments

Evidence-based psychotherapy for uncomplicated mild to moderate MDD (e.g., PHQ-9 total score of 10–19) includes acceptance and commitment therapy for depression (ACT-D; Walser et al., 2012), behavioral therapy/behavioral activation (BT/BA; Lejuez, Hopko, Acierno, Daughters, & Pagoto, 2011), cognitive-behavioral therapy for depression (CBT-D; Wenzel et al., 2011), interpersonal psychotherapy for depression (IPT; Clougherty et al., 2014), mindfulness-based cognitive therapy for depression (MBCT; Segal, Williams, & Teasdale, 2013), and problem-solving therapy (PST; Nezu, Nezu, & D'Zurilla, 2012). BT/BA is a time-effective behavioral intervention that can vary between 5 to 10 sessions (depending on the number of additional sessions needed for implementation and termination planning) and targets adaptive reinforcement behaviors using a successive approximation approach. Like BT/BA, CBT-D enhances behaviors conducive to improving mood; however, this intervention also identifies and modifies problematic beliefs associated with depression. ACT-D is a 12-session, third-wave behavioral intervention that focuses on helping patients accept internal experiences and commit to actions that embody their personal values. IPT is based on attachment theory and treats MDD using a 16-session, manualized intervention to address the following primary areas related to interpersonal functioning: role transitions, role disputes, interpersonal loss, and interpersonal skills. Like CBT-D, MBCT focuses on recognizing maladaptive beliefs (and other internal experiences); however, this treatment encourages patients to detach and observe thoughts, rather than attempt to eliminate them. PST is a time-limited, cognitive-behavioral approach that prioritizes collaborating with patients to promote self-efficacy and learn coping skills with specific problem areas contributing to depression. When deciding on treatment modality, it is vital to align intervention mechanisms of change to patient-specific drivers of MDD and ascertain patient preferences to increase collaboration.

For uncomplicated mild to moderate MDD, evidence-based pharmacotherapy includes two classes of antidepressant medications—namely, an SSRI (except fluvoxamine) and serotonin and norepinephrine reuptake inhibitors (SNRIs) (Khan, Faucett, Lichtenberg, Kirsch, & Brown, 2012). Bupropion and mirtazapine are first-line treatments for MDD and may provide an option for patients unwilling to take antidepressants due to unwanted sexual side effects such as decreased libido. It is recommended that one use an alternative monotherapy or augment with a second medication or psychotherapy if a patient shows partial or no response to the initial medication (maximized) after 4 to 6 weeks of delivery (Trivedi et al., 2006). Furthermore, the offer of computer-based CBT (Richards & Richardson, 2012) or PST (Bedford, Dietch, Taylor, Boals, & Zayfert, 2018) is encouraged for mild to moderate MDD as an adjunctive intervention or if standard psychotherapy is not available.

When a patient presents with complex MDD (e.g., a PHQ-9 total score of 20 or greater, recurrent episodes, or need for hospitalization), the use of a combination of evidence-based psychotherapy and pharmacotherapy is suggested (Cuijpers et al., 2014). Furthermore, electroconvulsive therapy (ECT) with or without psychotherapy in patients with severe MDD is recommended for specific conditions such as catatonia, psychotic depression, severe suicidality, and a history of poor response to multiple antidepressants (Anderson, McAllister-Williams, Downey, Elliott, & Loo, 2020; The UK ECT Review Group, 2003).

Following remission of MDD, psychotherapy and medication options exist for planning continuation and maintenance treatments. When a patient responds to antidepressant medication, continued antidepressant use for at least 6 months is recommended to reduce the rate of relapse (e.g., recurrent MDE). If a patient reports an unstable remission status, it is recommended that one offer maintenance pharmacotherapy for 12 months and possibly indefinitely; or if psychotherapy is preferred, it is advised that one provide CBT-D, IPT, or MBCT for approximately 3 to 6 months after remission is achieved to prevent relapse.

Case 4.2. The Depressed Medic

The Sergeant (SGT), an Army Infantry Branch medic, presented to treatment stating she was extremely unhappy with her occupation and that she had lost her sense of purpose in life. During her adolescence, she reported having depressive episodes that remitted without treatment. Over the past year, she had noticed a drastic change in her mood following combat exposure and low perceived support from her leaders. She reported that she did not believe others trusted her to do her job. Within the past 2 weeks, she had experienced the following symptoms: depressed mood, minimal desire to initiate enjoyable activities, feelings of worthlessness, insomnia, difficulties concentrating, and hopelessness about the future. Although she occasionally thought she was better off dead, she believed ending her life was not an option and denied having any such plan. Her total score on the PHQ-9 was 16, which fell within the range of moderately severe depression. She indicated that her symptoms of depression significantly impaired her work performance and social relationships. With all of this information taken together, she met the diagnostic criteria for MDD, recurrent type, moderate severity. After consideration of her symptoms and collaboration on her treatment preferences, ACT-D was conducted to disentangle her from getting "caught up" in thoughts that she was a failure, to increase her ability to contact the present moment, and to rebuild her sense of purpose. Although she was still mildly symptomatic with intermittent sadness following 12 weeks of ACT-D, she voiced significant improvement in her work and social relationships by attending to the present moment, tolerating unpleasant thoughts and emotions, and refocusing her decisions and actions to live a meaningful life.

ANXIETY DISORDERS

Anxiety disorders are a group of diagnoses that involve excessive fear and anxiety. Some anxiety disorders involve excessive anxiety to a *perceived imminent threat,* with a corresponding fight or flight response and escape or avoidant behaviors to cope. Other anxiety disorders involve excessive *anticipation of threats in the future,* with physiological and cognitive preparations to cope. In this section, we review GAD, including diagnostic features, risk factors for GAD among military personnel, and effective treatments.

Diagnostic Criteria for GAD

GAD involves excessive anxiety and worry that is difficult to control and relates to multiple areas of life, such as occupational or academic performance (American Psychiatric Association, 2013). The excessive apprehension occurs for at least 6 months and is present more days than not, causing significant distress or impaired functioning. At least three of six symptoms must be present and related to the worry and anxiety: restlessness or feeling keyed up, easily fatigued, problems with concentration, irritability, muscle tension, and sleep disturbance. The anxiety and associated symptoms must not be related to the use of a substance or other medical/mental health condition.

Prevalence of Anxiety and GAD

In the United States, the lifetime prevalence of GAD is 9% in adults, with a 1-year prevalence of 0.9% (DSM-5). Women are at twice the risk of GAD, relative to men (American Psychiatric Association, 2013). Compared to the general U.S. population, rates of anxiety appear to be higher among military personnel. A military surveillance report of service members who served from 2007 to 2016 characterized the crude incidence rates of mental health disorders diagnosed during the medical encounters of the force (Stahlman & Oetting, 2018). These data are limited by the number of military personnel seeking treatment and the unknown number of those with mental health conditions not seeking care. Regardless, the overall crude incidence rate of anxiety disorders for the 10 years from 2007 to 2016 among active component military personnel was 212.0 per 10,000 person-years. Consistent with the general U.S. population, rates of anxiety disorders were higher among women. Army soldiers had higher rates of anxiety disorders relative to the U.S. Navy, U.S. Air Force, and Marine Corps service members. Of the more than 853,000 military personnel diagnosed with a mental health condition, 14.9% were anxiety disorders, as defined by ICD-9 and ICD-10. Unfortunately, the study did not separate rates by specific diagnoses.

Data from the MHS Data Repository found that the 2017 prevalence of anxiety disorders (i.e., new-onset and continuing cases) among ADSMs was 3.5% (PHCoE, 2019). The prevalence was highest in the Army (4.4%) and lowest among the Marine Corps (2.3%). Across the years, the 1-year prevalence rate for all services from 2005 to 2017 ranged from 1.0% to 3.7%. A similar rate (2.0%) was reported for the prevalence of other anxiety syndrome in a large, longitudinal study of health outcomes in the military (Riddle et al., 2007).

Interestingly, rates are much higher among health care-seeking veterans who are no longer serving in uniform. A 12% GAD prevalence rate was found among primary-care patients in the VA (Milanak, Gros, Magruder,

Brawman-Mintzer, & Frueh, 2013). In a sample of over 8,300 Canadian military personnel, the prevalence of GAD was 1.7% for the past year and 4.4% over a lifetime (Erickson et al., 2015).

Etiology

Several factors and theories have been promulgated to help explain the etiology of GAD. Like all mental illnesses, anxiety is likely the result of a combination of genes, environment, and stress. First, heritability studies highlight the role of genetic risk. Research suggests that GAD likely shares genetic origins with other anxiety disorders and depression (Purves et al., 2019), and that the heritability of GAD sits at approximately 30% (Gottschalk & Domschke, 2017).

As genetics do not entirely account for GAD onset, research on cognitive-behavioral theories helps describe additional factors contributing to the development of GAD. A leading model, Borkovec's cognitive avoidance theory of worry (Borkovec, 1994; Borkovec, Alcaine, & Behar, 2004) builds on Foa and Kozak's (1986) emotional processing theory and posits that worry represents a cognitive avoidance approach to perceived future threats by employing verbal linguistic, thought-based activity, which prevents distress and thus inhibits emotional processing. Specifically, worry facilitates the opportunity to identify strategies to prevent feared events from happening, but also avoids the physical and emotional effects of approaching the feared stimuli and associated distress. Furthermore, the verbal linguistic nature of worry prevents distressing mental imagery and emotions. According to the cognitive avoidance theory of worry, worry is thus negatively reinforced (by reducing or avoiding distress) and thus is more likely to occur with future stressors.

A second approach, the intolerance of uncertainty theory, posits that individuals with GAD are distressed by uncertainty, and such situations set off a chain of worry and anxiety (Dugas, Gagnon, Ladouceur, & Freeston, 1998; Koerner & Dugas, 2006). Worry is used to help cope with the stressful situation or to prevent the situation from happening. Anxiety about the uncertainty triggers cognitive avoidance and leads to a negative problem orientation. Those who experience a negative problem orientation do not believe they solve problems effectively, see problems as threats, have limited frustration tolerance when addressing problems, and are pessimistic about the probable outcomes of problems. This negative problem orientation and cognitive avoidance result in stress and increased worry and anxiety, contributing to the maladaptive cycle.

Risk and Protective Factors among Military Personnel

In addition to the factors highlighted by theories of anxiety, military-specific factors can influence the risk for GAD as well. For example, military units are made up of teams of men and women who typically train and deploy together. The cohesion and leadership of such teams can have an impact on the functioning of individuals. A longitudinal study of soldiers before, during, and after deployment found that soldiers who reported stronger unit cohesion 1 to 2 months before deployment to Afghanistan had a lower risk of GAD postdeployment (Anderson et al., 2019).

Childhood adversity increases the risk of mental health problems in adulthood, which is often referred to as the stress sensitization hypothesis (Hammen, Henry, & Daley, 2000). Adults with several childhood adversities are at greater risk of depression, anxiety, and PTSD when they encounter major life stressors (McLaughlin, Conron, Koenen, & Gilman, 2010). Those who enter the military are no different. Consistent with the stress sensitization hypothesis, new Army recruits were at greater risk of GAD following recent stressful events if they were exposed to childhood maltreatment (Bandoli et al., 2017).

Two other factors contributing to the risk of GAD in military personnel are TBI and marital distress. TBI that occurred during deployment has been found to increase the risk of GAD, even after controlling for predeployment mental health status, the severity of deployment stress, and prior TBI history (Stein et al., 2015). Given the role of social support in buffering the effects of stress, it is not surprising that research on military personnel found that marital distress was positively associated with GAD, panic disorder, and substance use disorder in the previous 30 days (Whisman, Salinger, Labrecque, Gilmour, & Snyder, 2020).

Differential Diagnosis in Military Personnel: Agoraphobia and Specific Phobia

A detailed review of all anxiety disorders is beyond the scope of a single chapter. However, given the prevalence of PTSD among military personnel, certain predictable assessment challenges merit discussion regarding the attribution of symptoms to trauma versus an anxiety disorder. Agoraphobia involves marked anxiety about at least two of five situations: public transportation, open spaces, enclosed places, crowds, or being outside the home alone (American Psychiatric Association, 2013). DSM-5 diagnostic criteria require that the anxiety is associated with cognitions regarding the difficulty of escape or apprehension about accessing help should panic or embarrassing symptoms occur. For this chapter's purposes, the key factor related to the discussion of agoraphobia in military populations is the consideration of whether manifestations of avoidance should be counted as a symptom for PTSD or agoraphobia. Consider the case of a soldier, recently returned from combat deployment, who rarely leaves his home and avoids public shopping centers due to his anxiety. Is this symptom attributed to the avoidance criteria of PTSD or rather agoraphobia?

Schillaci and colleagues (2009) discussed the problem and the criterion they developed for their assessments, prior to the establishment of the DSM-5. In their study of 115 combat veterans with PTSD and depression, the authors found it necessary to distinguish symptoms of agoraphobia from trauma-related avoidance and hypervigilance. They determined that avoidance of situations from which escape could be difficult was considered a PTSD symptom when it clearly related to the trauma theme and was otherwise considered a symptom of agoraphobia. Using this criterion, the authors found that 12% of their sample of veterans had PTSD with comorbid panic disorder with agoraphobia. The establishment of DSM-5 has clarified this dilemma. According to DSM-5, agoraphobia is considered if the fear, anxiety, or avoidance is *not* restricted to trauma reminders.

A similar dilemma emerges regarding certain phobias after trauma. The diagnosis of specific phobia involves significant fear or anxiety about a specific object or situation, which almost always provokes the distressing emotional response and is, therefore, avoided (American Psychiatric Association, 2013). It is not uncommon for sexual assault survivors with PTSD to avoid sex (Foa & Rothbaum, 2001). If we consider a sailor who has been sexually assaulted, and now avoids sex, is this presentation a reminder of assault that is avoided as a symptom of PTSD, or has he or she developed a symptom of specific phobia? According to DSM-5, if the specific phobia developed following trauma, the diagnosis of specific phobia is only made if full criteria for PTSD are not met.

Additional Assessment Considerations among Military Personnel

Given the central role of fear in anxiety disorders, it is worth noting that service members may not always perceive, or at least report, the emotion of fear. Military training prepares service members to obey lawful orders, regardless of personal risk. Fear is sometimes unhelpful to the goal of supporting the mission in the face of danger. Accordingly, asking about constructs such as "stress," "worry," or "anxiety" may be more productive during assessment for anxiety among some military personnel, even if these terms are not perfect synonyms.

Evidence-Based Treatments for GAD

The VA/DoD library of Clinical Practice Guidelines does not include a treatment guideline for GAD or anxiety. However, the Anxiety and Depression Association of America's GAD Clinical Practice Review Task Force produced a practice guideline that provides an evidence-based review (Powers, Becker, Gorman, Kissen, & Smits, 2015), and several practice guidelines are also available in the scientific literature (Andrews et al., 2018; Katzman et al., 2014). Generally, recommended treatments include CBT and Food and Drug Administration–approved SSRIs and SNRIs, which are discussed below.

Several CBT psychotherapy treatment protocols for GAD have shown efficacy, and these psychotherapy protocols typically include multiple components designed to address factors theoretically linked to anxiety. Common features include psychoeducation about anxiety, relaxation exercises or stress management, progressive exposure to anxiety-provoking situations or circumstances, inhibition of safety behaviors used to manage anxiety, and cognitive restructuring, or other skills to address overestimations of threat or catastrophizing. Problem-solving skills are also common. Several meta-analytic reviews of the scientific literature have concluded that CBT for GAD is efficacious (e.g., Hofmann & Smits, 2008; Mitte, 2005). A recent meta-analysis examined CBT relative to wait lists, treatment as usual, or psychological placebo control and found that CBT for GAD outperformed comparators with a medium to large effect size (Carl et al., 2020).

Computerized CBT for GAD has also been shown to be effective. These programs typically provide Internet-based delivery of CBT treatment components to help ensure access to treatment, particularly to support those living in rural areas. A meta-analysis of Internet-based CBT for anxiety found that the five reviewed studies addressing GAD demonstrated a large effect, relative to control conditions (Olthuis, Watt, Bailey, Hayden, & Stewart, 2016).

Finally, a recent review of recommended treatments for GAD highlighted SSRIs and SNRIs as first-line pharmacotherapy (Craske & Bystritsky, 2020). Recommended SSRIs in this treatment guide include citalopram, escitalopram, sertraline, paroxetine, fluoxetine, and fluvoxamine. Recommended SNRIs include duloxetine and venlafaxine (extended-release). As head-to-head comparisons of medications for GAD are lacking, most prescribers work with their patients to select medications based on side effect profiles, considering other medications the patient is already taking, or based on patient preferences or past treatment experiences (Craske & Bystritsky, 2020). Military personnel may want to work with their prescriber to consider impacts of medication side effects on job-specific functioning requirements. Better outcomes have been found when medication is combined with CBT for children (Walkup et al., 2008) and older adults (Wetherell et al., 2013). To conclude this section, let us examine one more case.

Case 4.3. The Soldier Who Worried about Everything

The specialist (SPC) spends considerable time and energy worrying about things that could go wrong with his job performance. He consistently anticipates bad outcomes to support his preparatory planning and to ensure he does not fail. His physician first spoke with him about his anxiety after routine screening. His referral to a behavioral health provider resulted in an intake interview, during which symptoms for GAD were evaluated and the clinician ruled out other possible explanations for the symptoms. When discussing treatment options for GAD, the SPC declined a referral to a prescriber, explaining that changes in medication can affect readiness to deploy and he was concerned about the side effects of some of the medications discussed. He initiated CBT for GAD and was surprised that it did not resemble the psychotherapy he had seen on TV. Instead, his therapist had a specific plan for each session, teaching him about his anxiety, his thinking, and skills he could use to manage his anxiety. Although he was apprehensive about anxiety-provoking assignments, like intentionally entering into anxiety-provoking situations, he rapidly learned that his feared catastrophes did not come to pass, and he had a sense of control from choosing to voluntarily engage. As he completed more of these exercises, he started to feel better about himself for doing so, and his mood improved. He attended therapy for 13 sessions and developed a special appreciation for the changes in how he thought about situations and the relaxation exercises he learned. Although he felt as if he still worried more than most soldiers at the conclusion of treatment, he was much less anxious and had the tools to manage his anxiety.

CONCLUSION

Service members and their families make significant sacrifices before, during, and after military deployments. Behavioral health disorders are part of the price paid by some, with PTSD, depression, and anxiety among the most common. Significant work has been undertaken in DoD to ensure that help is available to those who need it, whether through TMH or face-to-face care. Furthermore, reviewed research suggests that effective treatments are available for many deployment-related problems. This is encouraging. However, significant questions remain. There is limited clinical research on the comparative efficacy of many evidence-based psychological treatments generally, and certainly for the subgroup of active-duty military personnel. Preemptively selecting the evidence-based treatment that would be most effective for a given service member is not currently possible, and continued research into precision medicine is warranted. Many questions also remain about the relationship between military deployments and future mental health. In particular, limited information is known about the long-term mental health implications of deployments to Iraq and Afghanistan. Longitudinal studies of representative samples are needed to address these and related questions.

REFERENCES

Aldea, M. A., Michael, K., Alexander, K., & Kison, S. (2019). Obsessive–compulsive tendencies in a sample of veterans with posttraumatic stress disorder. *Journal of Cognitive Psychotherapy, 33*(1), 33–45.

American Psychiatric Association. (1994). *Diagnostic and statistical manual of mental disorders* (4th ed.). Washington, DC: Author.

American Psychiatric Association. (2013). *Diagnostic and statistical manual of mental disorders* (5th ed.). Arlington, VA: Author.

Anderson, I. M., McAllister-Williams, R. H., Downey, D., Elliott, R., & Loo, C. (2020). Cognitive function after electroconvulsive therapy for depression: Relationship to clinical response. *Psychological Medicine,* 1–10.

Anderson, L., Campbell-Sills, L., Ursano, R. J., Kessler, R. C., Sun, X., Heeringa, S. G., et al. (2019). Prospective associations of perceived unit cohesion with postdeployment mental health outcomes. *Depression and Anxiety, 36*(6), 511–521.

Andrews, G., Bell, C., Boyce, P., Gale, C., Lampe, L., Marwat, O., et al. (2018). Royal Australian and New Zealand College of Psychiatrists clinical practice guidelines for the treatment of panic disorder, social anxiety disorder and generalised anxiety disorder. *Australian & New Zealand Journal of Psychiatry, 52*(12), 1109–1172.

Armenta, R. F., Rush, T., LeardMann, C. A., Millegan, J., Cooper, A., Hoge, C. W., et al. (2018). Factors associated with persistent posttraumatic stress disorder among U.S. military service members and veterans. *Bio Med Central Psychiatry, 18*(48), 1–11.

Back, S. E., Killeen, T., Badour, C. L., Flanagan, J. C., Allan, N. P., Ana, E. S., et al. (2019). Concurrent treatment of substance use disorders and PTSD using prolonged exposure: A randomized clinical trial in military veterans. *Addictive Behaviors, 90,* 369–377.

Badour, C. L., Bown, S., Adams, T. G., Bunaciu, L., & Feldner, M. T. (2012). Specificity of fear and disgust experienced during traumatic interpersonal victimization in predicting posttraumatic stress and contamination-based obsessive–compulsive symptoms. *Journal of Anxiety Disorders, 26*(5), 590–598.

Bandoli, G., Campbell-Sills, L., Kessler, R. C., Heeringa, S. G., Nock, M. K., Rosellini, A. J., et al. (2017). Childhood adversity, adult stress, and the risk of major depression or generalized anxiety disorder in U.S. soldiers: A test of the stress sensitization hypothesis. *Psychological Medicine, 47*(13), 2379–2392.

Bartone, P. T., & Homish, G. G. (2020). Influence of hardiness, avoidance coping, and combat exposure on depression in returning war veterans: A moderated-mediation study. *Journal of Affective Disorders, 265,* 511–518.

Bedford, L. A., Dietch, J. R., Taylor, D. J., Boals, A., & Zayfert, C. (2018). Computer-guided problem-solving treatment for depression, PTSD, and insomnia symptoms in student veterans: A pilot randomized controlled trial. *Behavior Therapy, 49*(5), 756–767.

Borkovec, T. D. (1994). The nature, functions, and origins of worry. In G. C. L. Davey & F. Tallis (Eds.), *Worrying: Perspectives on theory, assessment and treatment* (pp. 5–33). Hoboken, NJ: John Wiley & Sons.

Borkovec, T. D., Alcaine, O. M., & Behar, E. (2004). Avoidance theory of worry and generalized anxiety disorder. In R. G. Heimberg, C. L. Turk, & D. S. Mennin (Eds.), *Generalized anxiety disorder: Advances in research and practice* (pp. 77–108). New York: Guilford Press.

Bradley, R., Greene, J., Russ, E., Dutra, L., & Westen, D. (2005). A multidimensional meta-analysis of psychotherapy for PTSD. *American Journal of Psychiatry, 162*(2), 214–227.

Breslau, J., Setodji, C. M., & Vaughan, C. A. (2016). Is cohesion within military units associated with post-deployment behavioral and mental health outcomes? *Journal of Affective Disorders, 198*, 102–107.

Breslau, N., Davis, G. C., Andreski, P., & Peterson, E. (1991). Traumatic events and posttraumatic stress disorder in an urban population of young adults. *Archives of General Psychiatry, 48*(3), 216–222.

Brewin, C. R., Andrews, B., & Valentine, J. D. (2000). Meta-analysis of risk factors for posttraumatic stress disorder in trauma-exposed adults. *Journal of Consulting and Clinical Psychology, 68*(5), 748–766.

Brown, T. A., Campbell, L. A., Lehman, C. L., Grisham, J. R., & Mancill, R. B. (2001). Current and lifetime comorbidity of the DSM-IV anxiety and mood disorders in a large clinical sample. *Journal of Abnormal Psychology, 110*(4), 585–599.

Bryant, R. A. (2019). Post-traumatic stress disorder: A state-of-the-art review of evidence and challenges. *World Psychiatry, 18*(3), 259–269.

Bryant, R. A., O'Donnell, M. L., Creamer, M., McFarlane, A. C., & Silove, D. (2013). A multisite analysis of the fluctuating course of posttraumatic stress disorder. *Journal of the American Medical Association Psychiatry, 70*(8), 839–846.

Carl, E., Witcraft, S. M., Kauffman, B. Y., Gillespie, E. M., Becker, E. S., Cuijpers, P., et al. (2020). Psychological and pharmacological treatments for generalized anxiety disorder (GAD): A meta-analysis of randomized controlled trials. *Cognitive Behaviour Therapy, 49*(1), 1–21.

Cloitre, M., Garvert, D. W., Brewin, C. R., Bryant, R. A., & Maercker, A. (2013). Evidence for proposed ICD-11 PTSD and complex PTSD: A latent profile analysis. *European Journal of Psychotraumatology, 4*(20706), 1–12.

Clougherty, K. F., Kinrichsen, G. A., Steele, J. L., Miller, S. A., Raffa, S. D., Stewart, M. O., et al. (2014). *Therapist guide to interpersonal psychotherapy for depression in veterans*. Washington, DC: U.S. Department of Veterans Affairs.

Colodro-Conde, L., Couvy-Duchesne, B., Zhu, G., Coventry, W. L., Byrne, E. M., Gordon, S., et al. (2018). A direct test of the diathesis–stress model for depression. *Molecular Psychiatry, 23*(7), 1590–1596.

Corrigan, J.-P., Fitzpatrick, M., Hanna, D., & Dyer, K. F. W. (2020). Evaluating the effectiveness of phase-oriented treatment models for PTSD—A meta-analysis. *Traumatology*, 1–8.

Coventry, P. A., Hudson, J. L., Kontopantelis, E., Archer, J., Richards, D. A., Gilbody, S., et al. (2014). Characteristics of effective collaborative care for treatment of depression: A systematic review and meta-regression of 74 randomised controlled trials. *PLoS One, 9*(9), e108114.

Coyle, L., Hanna, D., Dyer, K. F. W., Read, J., Curran, D., & Shannon, C. (2019).

Does trauma-related training have a relationship with, or impact on, mental health professionals' frequency of asking about, or detection of, trauma history? A systematic literature review. *Psychological Trauma: Theory, Research, Practice, and Policy, 11*(7), 802–809.

Crane, M. F., Boga, D., Karin, E., Gucciardi, D. F., Rapport, F., Callen, J., et al. (2019). Strengthening resilience in military officer cadets: A group-randomized controlled trial of coping and emotion regulatory self-reflection training. *Journal of Consulting and Clinical Psychology, 87*(2), 125–140.

Craske, M., & Bystritsky, A. (2020). *Approach to treating generalized anxiety disorder in adults* (M. B. Stein & M. Friedman, Eds.). UpToDate. Retrieved from *www.uptodate.com/contents/approach-to-treating-generalized-anxiety-disorder-in-adults*.

Creamer, M., Burgess, P., & Mcfarlane, A. C. (2001). Post-traumatic stress disorder: Findings from the Australian National Survey of Mental Health and Well-being. *Psychological Medicine, 31*(7), 1237–1247.

Cuijpers, P., Sijbrandij, M., Koole, S. L., Andersson, G., Beekman, A. T., & Reynolds, C. F. (2014). Adding psychotherapy to antidepressant medication in depression and anxiety disorders: A meta-analysis. *Focus, 12*(3), 347–358.

Curry, J. F., Shepherd-Banigan, M., Van Voorhees, E., Wagner, H. R., Kelley, M. L., Strauss, J., et al. (2019). Sex differences in predictors of recurrent major depression among current-era military veterans. *Psychological Services, 1*–10.

Department of the Army. (2016). *A leader's guide to soldier health and fitness* (Army techniques publication no. 6–22.5). Arlington, VA: Author.

Department of Veterans Affairs/Department of Defense. (2016). *VA/DoD clinical practice guideline for management of major depressive disorder* (Version 3.0). Washington, DC: Author.

Department of Veterans Affairs/Department of Defense. (2017). *VA/DoD clinical practice guideline for the management of posttraumatic stress disorder and acute stress disorder* (Version 3.0). Washington, DC: Author.

Deployment Health Clinical Center. (2017). *Mental health care utilization by active duty service members in the Military Health System, fiscal years 2005–2016.* Alexandria, VA: Defense Center of Excellence for Psychological Health and Traumatic Brain Injury Center. Retrieved from *https://pdhealth.mil/research-analytics/psychological-health-numbers/mental-health-care-utilization*.

Dohrenwend, B. P., Turner, J. B., Turse, N. A., Adams, B. G., Koenen, K. C., & Marshall, R. (2006). The psychological risks of Vietnam for U.S. veterans: A revisit with new data and methods. *Science, 313*(5789), 979–982.

Donoho, C. J., Bonanno, G. A., Porter, B., Kearney, L., & Powell, T. M. (2017). A decade of war: Prospective trajectories of posttraumatic stress disorder symptoms among deployed U.S. military personnel and the influence of combat exposure. *American Journal of Epidemiology, 186*(12), 1310–1318.

Dugas, M. J., Gagnon, F., Ladouceur, R., & Freeston, M. H. (1998). Generalized anxiety disorder: A preliminary test of a conceptual model. *Behaviour Research and Therapy, 36*(2), 215–226.

Duncan, J. M., Reed-Fitzke, K., Ferraro, A. J., Wojciak, A. S., Smith, K. M., & Sánchez, J. (2020). Identifying risk and resilience factors associated with the likelihood of seeking mental health care among U.S. Army soldiers-in-training. *Military Medicine, 185*(7–8), e1247–e1254.

Dutra, S. J., & Wolf, E. J. (2017). Perspectives on the conceptualization of the dissociative subtype of PTSD and implications for treatment. *Current Opinion in Psychology, 14*, 35–39.

Ehlers, A., Clark, D. M., Hackmann, A., McManus, F., Fennell, M., Herbert, C., et al. (2003). A randomized controlled trial of cognitive therapy, a self-help booklet, and repeated assessments as early interventions for posttraumatic stress disorder. *Archives of General Psychiatry, 60*(10), 1024–1032.

Elwood, L. S., Hahn, K. S., Olatunji, B. O., & Williams, N. L. (2009). Cognitive vulnerabilities to the development of PTSD: A review of four vulnerabilities and the proposal of an integrative vulnerability model. *Clinical Psychology Review, 29*(1), 87–100.

Erickson, J., Kinley, D. J., Afifi, T. O., Zamorski, M. A., Pietrzak, R. H., Stein, M. B., et al. (2015). Epidemiology of generalized anxiety disorder in Canadian military personnel. *Journal of Military, Veteran and Family Health, 1*(1), 26–36.

Feliciano, L., Renn, B. A., & Segal, D. L. (2018). Depressive disorders. In D. C. Beidel & B. C. Frueh (Eds.), *Adult psychopathology and diagnosis* (8th ed., pp. 247–298). Hoboken, NJ: John Wiley & Sons.

Ferdinand, L. G., Kelly, U. A., Skelton, K., Stephens, K. J., & Bradley, B. (2011). An evolving integrative treatment program for military sexual trauma (MST) and one veteran's experience. *Issues in Mental Health Nursing, 32*(9), 552–559.

Foa, E. B., Hembree, E., Rothbaum, B. O., & Rauch, S. A. M. (2019). *Prolonged exposure therapy for PTSD: Emotional processing of traumatic experiences therapist guide* (2nd ed.). New York: Oxford University Press.

Foa, E. B., & Kozak, M. J. (1986). Emotional processing of fear: Exposure to corrective information. *Psychological Bulletin, 99*(1), 20–35.

Foa, E. B., & Rothbaum, B. O. (2001). *Treating the trauma of rape: Cognitive-behavioral therapy for PTSD*. New York: Guilford Press.

Foa, E. B., Yadin, E., & Lichner, T. K. (2012). *Exposure and response (ritual) prevention for obsessive compulsive disorder: Therapist guide* (2nd ed.). New York: Oxford University Press.

Folke, S., Nielsen, A. B. S., Andersen, S. B., Karatzias, T., & Karstoft, K.-I. (2019). ICD-11 PTSD and complex PTSD in treatment-seeking Danish veterans: A latent profile analysis. *European Journal of Psychotraumatology, 10*(1686806), 1–10.

Forbes, D., Lockwood, E., Phelps, A., Wade, D., Creamer, M., Bryant, R. A., et al. (2014). Trauma at the hands of another: Distinguishing PTSD patterns following intimate and nonintimate interpersonal and noninterpersonal trauma in a nationally representative sample. *The Journal of Clinical Psychiatry, 75*(2), 147–153.

Ford, J. D., Courtois, C. A., Steele, K., Hart, O. van der, & Nijenhuis, E. R. S. (2005). Treatment of complex posttraumatic self-dysregulation. *Journal of Traumatic Stress, 18*(5), 437–447.

Fulton, J. J., Calhoun, P. S., Wagner, H. R., Schry, A. R., Hair, L. P., Feeling, N., et al. (2015). The prevalence of posttraumatic stress disorder in Operation Enduring Freedom/Operation Iraqi Freedom (OEF/OIF) veterans: A meta-analysis. *Journal of Anxiety Disorders, 31*, 98–107.

Gershuny, B. S., Baer, L., Jenike, M. A., Minichiello, W. E., & Wilhelm, S. (2002).

Comorbid posttraumatic stress disorder: Impact on treatment outcome for obsessive–compulsive disorder. *American Journal of Psychiatry, 159*(5), 852–854.

Gershuny, B. S., Baer, L., Parker, H., Gentes, E. L., Infield, A. L., & Jenike, M. A. (2008). Trauma and posttraumatic stress disorder in treatment-resistant obsessive–compulsive disorder. *Depression and Anxiety, 25*(1), 69–71.

Gersons, B. P. R., Carlier, I. V. E., Lamberts, R. D., & van der Kolk, B. A. (2000). Randomized clinical trial of brief eclectic psychotherapy for police officers with posttraumatic stress disorder. *Journal of Traumatic Stress, 13*(2), 333–347.

Gottschalk, M. G., & Domschke, K. (2017). Genetics of generalized anxiety disorder and related traits. *Dialogues in Clinical Neuroscience, 19*(2), 159–168.

Hammen, C., Henry, R., & Daley, S. E. (2000). Depression and sensitization to stressors among young women as a function of childhood adversity. *Journal of Consulting and Clinical Psychology, 68*(5), 782–787.

Held, P., Klassen, B. J., Boley, R. A., Wiltsey Stirman, S., Smith, D. L., Brennan, M. B., et al. (2020). Feasibility of a 3-week intensive treatment program for service members and veterans with PTSD. *Psychological Trauma: Theory, Research, Practice, and Policy, 12*(4), 422–430.

Hofmann, S. G., & Smits, J. A. J. (2008). Cognitive-behavioral therapy for adult anxiety disorders: A meta-analysis of randomized placebo-controlled trials. *The Journal of Clinical Psychiatry, 69*(4), 621–632.

Isaacs, K., Mota, N. P., Tsai, J., Harpaz-Rotem, I., Cook, J. M., Kirwin, P. D., et al. (2017). Psychological resilience in U.S. military veterans: A 2-year, nationally representative prospective cohort study. *Journal of Psychiatric Research, 84,* 301–309.

Iverson K. M., Mercado R., Carpenter S. L., & Street A. E. (2013). Intimate partner violence among women veterans: Previous interpersonal violence as a risk factor. *Journal of Traumatic Stress, 26*(6), 767–771.

Jaffe, A. E., Steel, A. L., DiLillo, D., Hoffman, L., Gratz, K. L., & Messman-Moore, T. L. (2017). Victim alcohol intoxication during a sexual assault: Relations with subsequent PTSD symptoms. *Violence and Victims, 32*(4), 642–657.

Joellenbeck, L. M., Russell, P. K., & Guze, S. B. (Eds.). (1999). *Strategies to protect the health of deployed U.S. forces: Medical surveillance, record keeping, and risk reduction.* Washington, DC: Institute of Medicine (U.S.) Medical Follow-Up Agency/National Academies Press. Retrieved from *www.ncbi.nlm.nih. gov/books/NBK225094.*

Karstoft, K.-I., Armour, C., Elklit, A., & Solomon, Z. (2013). Long-term trajectories of posttraumatic stress disorder in veterans: The role of social resources. *The Journal of Clinical Psychiatry, 74*(12), e1163–e1168.

Katzman, M. A., Bleau, P., Blier, P., Chokka, P., Kjernisted, K., & Van Ameringen, M. (2014). Canadian clinical practice guidelines for the management of anxiety, posttraumatic stress and obsessive–compulsive disorders. *BioMed Central Psychiatry, 14*(S1), 1–83.

Keane, T. M., Marshall, A. D., & Taft, C. T. (2006). Posttraumatic stress disorder: Etiology, epidemiology, and treatment outcome. *Annual Review of Clinical Psychology, 2*(1), 161–197.

Kelber, M. S., Smolenski, D. J., Workman, D. E., Morgan, M. A., Garvey Wilson, A. L., Campbell, M. S., et al. (2019). Typologies of combat exposure and their effects on posttraumatic stress disorder and depression symptoms. *Journal of Traumatic Stress, 32*(6), 946–956.

Kessler, R. C., Sonnega, A., Bromet, E., Hughes, M., & Nelson, C. B. (1995). Posttraumatic stress disorder in the National Comorbidity Survey. *Archives of General Psychiatry, 52*(12), 1048–1060.

Khan, A., Faucett, J., Lichtenberg, P., Kirsch, I., & Brown, W. A. (2012). A systematic review of comparative efficacy of treatments and controls for depression. *PLoS One, 7*(7), e41778.

Knefel, M., Lueger-Schuster, B., Bisson, J., Karatzias, T., Kazlauskas, E., & Roberts, N. P. (2020). A cross-cultural comparison of ICD-11 complex posttraumatic stress disorder symptom networks in Austria, the United Kingdom, and Lithuania. *Journal of Traumatic Stress, 33*(1), 41–51.

Koerner, N., & Dugas, M. J. (2006). A cognitive model of generalized anxiety disorder: The role of intolerance uncertainty. In G. C. L. Davey & A. Wells (Eds.), *Worry and its psychological disorders: Theory, assessment and treatment* (1st ed., pp. 201–216). Hoboken, NJ: John Wiley & Sons.

Kroenke, K., Spitzer, R. L., & Williams, J. B. W. (2001). The PHQ-9: Validity of a brief depression severity measure. *Journal of General Internal Medicine, 16*(9), 606–613.

Kroenke, K., Spitzer, R. L., & Williams, J. B. W. (2003). The Patient Health Questionnaire-2: Validity of a two-Item depression screener. *Medical Care, 41*(11), 1284–1292.

LeardMann, C. A., Pietrucha, A., Magruder, K. M., Smith, B., Murdoch, M., Jacobson, I. G., et al. (2013). Combat deployment is associated with sexual harassment or sexual assault in a large, female military cohort. *Women's Health Issues, 23*(4), e215–e223.

Leeies, M., Pagura, J., Sareen, J., & Bolton, J. M. (2010). The use of alcohol and drugs to self-medicate symptoms of posttraumatic stress disorder. *Depression and Anxiety, 27*(8), 731–736.

Lehavot, K., Katon, J. G., Chen, J. A., Fortney, J. C., & Simpson, T. L. (2018). Post-traumatic stress disorder by gender and veteran status. *American Journal of Preventive Medicine, 54*(1), e1–e9.

Lejuez, C. W., Hopko, D. R., Acierno, R., Daughters, S. B., & Pagoto, S. L. (2011). Ten year revision of the brief behavioral activation treatment for depression: Revised treatment manual. *Behavior Modification, 35*(2), 111–161.

Letica-Crepulja, M., Stevanović, A., Protuđer, M., Juretić, T. G., Rebić, J., & Frančišković, T. (2020). Complex PTSD among treatment-seeking veterans with PTSD. *European Journal of Psychotraumatology, 11*(1716593), 1–10.

Linde, K., Sigterman, K., Kriston, L., Rücker, G., Jamil, S., Meissner, K., et al. (2015). Effectiveness of psychological treatments for depressive disorders in primary care: Systematic review and meta-analysis. *The Annals of Family Medicine, 13*(1), 56–68.

Littleton, H., Grills-Taquechel, A., & Axsom, D. (2009). Impaired and incapacitated rape victims: Assault characteristics and post-assault experiences. *Violence and Victims, 24*(4), 439–457.

Liu, Y., Collins, C., Wang, K., Xie, X., & Bie, R. (2019). The prevalence and trend of depression among veterans in the United States. *Journal of Affective Disorders, 245*, 724–727.

Löwe, B., Kroenke, K., Herzog, W., & Gräfe, K. (2004). Measuring depression outcome with a brief self-report instrument: Sensitivity to change of the Patient Health Questionnaire (PHQ-9). *Journal of Affective Disorders, 81*(1), 61–66.

Markowitz, J. C., Petkova, E., Neria, Y., Van Meter, P. E., Zhao, Y., Hembree, E., et al. (2015). Is exposure necessary? A randomized clinical trial of interpersonal psychotherapy for PTSD. *American Journal of Psychiatry, 172*(5), 430–440.

Marshall, R. D., Olfson, M., Hellman, F., Blanco, C., Guardino, M., & Struening, E. L. (2001). Comorbidity, impairment, and suicidality in subthreshold PTSD. *American Journal of Psychiatry, 158*(9), 1467–1473.

McLaughlin, K. A., Conron, K. J., Koenen, K. C., & Gilman, S. E. (2010). Childhood adversity, adult stressful life events, and risk of past-year psychiatric disorder: A test of the stress sensitization hypothesis in a population-based sample of adults. *Psychological Medicine, 40*(10), 1647–1658.

McLaughlin, K. A, & Lambert, H. K. (2017). Child trauma exposure and psychopathology: Mechanisms of risk and resilience. *Current Opinion in Psychology, 14*, 29–34.

Meadows, S. O., Tanielian, T., Karney, B., Schell, T., Griffin, B. A., Jaycox, L. H., et al. (2017). The deployment life study: Longitudinal analysis of military families across the deployment cycle. *RAND Health Quarterly, 6*(2), 1–28.

Meichenbaum, D. H., & Deffenbacher, J. L. (1988). Stress inoculation training. *The Counseling Psychologist, 16*(1), 69–90.

Milanak, M. E., Gros, D. F., Magruder, K. M., Brawman-Mintzer, O., & Frueh, B. C. (2013). Prevalence and features of generalized anxiety disorder in Department of Veteran Affairs primary care settings. *Psychiatry Research, 209*(2), 173–179.

Mitte, K. (2005). Meta-analysis of cognitive-behavioral treatments for generalized anxiety disorder: A comparison with pharmacotherapy. *Psychological Bulletin, 131*(5), 785–795.

Mustillo, S. A., Kysar-Moon, A., Douglas, S. R., Hargraves, R., Wadsworth, S. M., Fraine, M., et al. (2015). Overview of depression, post-traumatic stress disorder, and alcohol misuse among active duty service members returning from Iraq and Afghanistan, self-report and diagnosis. *Military Medicine, 180*(4), 419–427.

Najavits, L. M. (2015). The problem of dropout from "gold standard" PTSD therapies. *F1000Prime Reports, 7*(43), 1–8.

Neuner, F., Elbert, T., & Schauer, M. (2020). Narrative exposure therapy for PTSD. In L. F. Bufka, C. V. Wright, & R. W. Halfond (Eds.), *Casebook to the APA clinical practice guideline for the treatment of PTSD* (pp. 187–205). Washington, DC: American Psychological Association.

Nezu, A. M., Nezu, C. M., & D'Zurilla, T. (2012). *Problem-solving therapy: A treatment manual.* New York: Springer.

Nichter, B., Norman, S., Haller, M., & Pietrzak, R. H. (2019). Psychological burden of PTSD, depression, and their comorbidity in the US veteran population: Suicidality, functioning, and service utilization. *Journal of Affective Disorders, 256*, 633–640.

Olthuis, J. V., Watt, M. C., Bailey, K., Hayden, J. A., & Stewart, S. H. (2016). Therapist-supported Internet cognitive behavioural therapy for anxiety disorders in adults. *Cochrane Database of Systematic Reviews, 3*, 1–195.

Osenbach, J. E., O'Brien, K. M., Mishkind, M., & Smolenski, D. J. (2013). Synchronous telehealth technologies in psychotherapy for depression: A meta-analysis. *Depression and Anxiety, 30*(11), 1058–1067.

Panagioti, M., Gooding, P. A., & Tarrier, N. (2012). A meta-analysis of the association between posttraumatic stress disorder and suicidality: The role of comorbid depression. *Comprehensive Psychiatry, 53*(7), 915–930.

Porter, B., Hoge, C. W., Tobin, L. E., Donoho, C. J., Castro, C. A., Luxton, D. D., et al. (2018). Measuring aggregated and specific combat exposures: Associations between combat exposure measures and posttraumatic stress disorder, depression, and alcohol-related problems. *Journal of Traumatic Stress, 31*(2), 296–306.

Possemato, K., McKenzie, S., McDevitt-Murphy, M. E., Williams, J. L., & Ouimette, P. (2014). The relationship between postdeployment factors and PTSD severity in recent combat veterans. *Military Psychology, 26*(1), 15–22.

Powers, M., Becker, E., Gorman, J., Kissen, D., & Smits, J. (2015). *Clinical practice review for GAD.* Anxiety and Depression Association of America. Retrieved from *https://adaa.org/resources-professionals/practice-guidelines-gad*.

Psychological Health Center of Excellence. (2019). *Psychological health by the numbers: Mental health disorder prevalence and incidence among active duty service members, 2005–2017.* Falls Church, VA: Defense Health Agency. Retrieved from *www.pdhealth.mil/research-analytics/psychological-health-numbers/mental-health-disorder-prevalence-and-incidence*.

Purves, K. L., Coleman, J. R. I., Meier, S. M., Rayner, C., Davis, K. A. S., Cheesman, R., et al. (2019). A major role for common genetic variation in anxiety disorders. *Molecular Psychiatry,* 1–12.

Reed-Fitzke, K., & Lucier-Greer, M. (2020). The buffering effect of relationships on combat exposure, military performance, and mental health of U.S. military soldiers: A vantage point for CFTs. *Journal of Marital and Family Therapy, 46*(2), 321–336.

Resick, P. A., Monson, C. M., & Chard, K. M. (2016). *Cognitive processing therapy for PTSD: A comprehensive manual.* New York: Guilford Press.

Resick, P. A., Wachen, J. S., Mintz, J., Young-McCaughan, S., Roache, J. D., Borah, A. M., et al. (2015). A randomized clinical trial of group cognitive processing therapy compared with group present-centered therapy for PTSD among active duty military personnel. *Journal of Consulting and Clinical Psychology, 83*(6), 1058–1068.

Richards, D., & Richardson, T. (2012). Computer-based psychological treatments for depression: A systematic review and meta-analysis. *Clinical Psychology Review, 32*(4), 329–342.

Riddle, J. R., Smith, T. C., Smith, B., Corbeil, T. E., Engel, C. C., Wells, T. S., et al. (2007). Millennium Cohort: The 2001–2003 baseline prevalence of mental disorders in the U.S. military. *Journal of Clinical Epidemiology, 60*(2), 192–201.

Rodin, R., Bonanno, G. A., Rahman, N., Kouri, N. A., Bryant, R. A., Marmar,

C. R., et al. (2017). Expressive flexibility in combat veterans with posttraumatic stress disorder and depression. *Journal of Affective Disorders, 207,* 236–241.

Rosen, V., & Ayers, G. (2020). An update on the complexity and importance of accurately diagnosing post-traumatic stress disorder and comorbid traumatic brain injury. *Neuroscience Insights, 15,* 1–8.

Sareen, J. (2014). Posttraumatic stress disorder in adults: Impact, comorbidity, risk factors, and treatment. *The Canadian Journal of Psychiatry, 59*(9), 460–467.

Schiavone, F. L., Frewen, P., McKinnon, M., & Lanius, R. (2018). The dissociative subtype of PTSD: An update of the literature. *PTSD Research Quarterly, 29*(3), 1–13.

Schillaci, J., Yanasak, E., Adams, J. H., Dunn, N. J., Rehm, L. P., & Hamilton, J. D. (2009). Guidelines for differential diagnoses in a population with posttraumatic stress disorder. *Professional Psychology: Research and Practice, 40*(1), 39–45.

Segal, Z. V., Williams, J. M. G., & Teasdale, J. D. (2013). *Mindfulness-based cognitive therapy for depression* (2nd ed.). New York: Guilford Press.

Shapiro, F. (1989). Eye movement desensitization: A new treatment for post-traumatic stress disorder. *Journal of Behavior Therapy and Experimental Psychiatry, 20*(3), 211–217.

Shrestha, A., Cornum, B. R., Vie, L. L., Scheier, L. M., Lester, M. P. B., & Seligman, M. E. (2018). Protective effects of psychological strengths against psychiatric disorders among soldiers. *Military Medicine, 183*(Suppl. 1), 386–395.

Sloan, D. M., & Marx, B. P. (2019). *Written exposure therapy for PTSD: A brief treatment approach for mental health professionals.* Washington, DC: American Psychological Press.

Sloan, D. M., Marx, B. P., Lee, D. J., & Resick, P. A. (2018). A brief exposure-based treatment vs. cognitive processing therapy for posttraumatic stress disorder: A randomized noninferiority clinical trial. *Journal of the American Medical Association Psychiatry, 75*(3), 233–239.

Smolenski, D. J., Pruitt, L. D., Vuletic, S., Luxton, D. D., & Gahm, G. (2017). Unobserved heterogeneity in response to treatment for depression through videoconference. *Psychiatric Rehabilitation Journal, 40*(3), 303–308.

Stahlman, S., & Oetting, A. A. (2018). Mental health disorders and mental health problems, active component, U.S. Armed Forces, 2007–2016. *Medical Surveillance Monthly Report, 25*(3), 2–11.

Stein, M. B., Kessler, R. C., Heeringa, S. G., Jain, S., Campbell-Sills, L., Colpe, L. J., et al. (2015). Prospective longitudinal evaluation of the effect of deployment-acquired traumatic brain injury on posttraumatic stress and related disorders: Results from the Army study to assess risk and resilience in servicemembers (Army STARRS). *American Journal of Psychiatry, 172*(11), 1101–1111.

Surís, A., Lind, L., Kashner, T. M., Borman, P. D., & Petty, F. (2004). Sexual assault in women veterans: An examination of PTSD risk, health care utilization, and cost of care. *Psychosomatic Medicine, 66*(5), 749–756.

The UK ECT Review Group. (2003). Efficacy and safety of electroconvulsive therapy in depressive disorders: A systematic review and meta-analysis. *The Lancet, 361*(9360), 799–808.

Thériault, F. L., Gardner, W., Momoli, F., Garber, B. G., Kingsbury, M., Clayborne, Z., et al. (2020). Mental health service use in depressed military personnel: A systematic review. *Military Medicine, 185*(7–8), e1255–e1262.

Thota, A. B., Sipe, T. A., Byard, G. J., Zometa, C. S., Hahn, R. A., McKnight-Eily, L. R., et al. (2012). Collaborative care to improve the management of depressive disorders: A community guide systematic review and meta-analysis. *American Journal of Preventive Medicine, 42*(5), 525–538.

Tolin, D. F., & Foa, E. B. (2006). Sex differences in trauma and posttraumatic stress disorder: A quantitative review of 25 years of research. *Psychological Bulletin, 132*(6), 959–992.

Trivedi, M. H., Rush, A. J., Wisniewski, S. R., Nierenberg, A. A., Warden, D., Ritz, L., et al. (2006). Evaluation of outcomes with citalopram for depression using measurement-based care in STARD: Implications for clinical practice. *American Journal of Psychiatry, 163*(1), 28–40.

Villalta, L., Khadr, S., Chua, K.-C., Kramer, T., Clarke, V., Viner, R. M., et al. (2020). Complex post-traumatic stress symptoms in female adolescents: The role of emotion dysregulation in impairment and trauma exposure after an acute sexual assault. *European Journal of Psychotraumatology, 11*(1710400), 1–11.

Vogt, D. S., Tyrell, F. A., Bramande, E. A., Nillni, Y. I., Taverna, E. C., Finley, E. P., et al. (2020). U.S. military veterans' health and well-being in the first year after service. *American Journal of Preventive Medicine, 58*(3), 352–360.

Vyas, K. J., Fesperman, S. F., Nebeker, B. J., Gerard, S. K., Boyd, N. D., Delaney, E. M. (2016). Preventing PTSD and depression and reducing health care costs in the military: A call for building resilience among service members. *Military Medicine, 181*(10), 1240–1247.

Walkup, J. T., Albano, A. M., Piacentini, J., Birmaher, B., Compton, S. N., Sherrill, J. T., et al. (2008). Cognitive behavioral therapy, sertraline, or a combination in childhood anxiety. *New England Journal of Medicine, 359*(26), 2753–2766.

Walser, R. D., Sears, K., Chartier, M., & Karlin, B. E. (2012). *Acceptance and commitment therapy for depression in veterans: Therapist manual.* Washington, DC: Department of Veterans Affairs.

Walter, K. H., Levine, J. A., Highfill-McRoy, R. M., Navarro, M., & Thomsen, C. J. (2018). Prevalence of posttraumatic stress disorder and psychological comorbidities among U.S. active duty service members, 2006–2013. *Journal of Traumatic Stress, 31*(6), 837–844.

Wenzel, A., Brown, G. K., & Karlin, B. E. (2011). *Cognitive behavioral therapy for depression in veterans and military service members: Therapist manual.* Washington, DC: Department of Veterans Affairs.

Wetherell, J. L., Petkus, A. J., White, K. S., Nguyen, H., Kornblith, S., Andreescu, C., et al. (2013). Antidepressant medication augmented with cognitive-behavioral therapy for generalized anxiety disorder in older adults. *American Journal of Psychiatry, 170*(7), 782–789.

Whisman, M. A., Salinger, J. M., Labrecque, L. T., Gilmour, A. L., & Snyder, D. K. (2020). Couples in arms: Marital distress, psychopathology, and suicidal ideation in active-duty Army personnel. *Journal of Abnormal Psychology, 129*(3), 248–255.

Wood, E., Ohlsen, S., & Ricketts, T. (2017). What are the barriers and facilitators to implementing collaborative care for depression? A systematic review. *Journal of Affective Disorders, 214,* 26–43.

World Health Organization. (2018). *International classification of diseases for mortality and morbidity statistics* (11th revision, ICD-11). Zurich, Switzerland: Author.

Xue, C., Ge, Y., Tang, B., Liu, Y., Kang, P., Wang, M., et al. (2015). A meta-analysis of risk factors for combat-related PTSD among military personnel and veterans. *PLoS One, 10*(3), e0120270.

Youssef, N. A., Green, K. T., Dedert, E. A., Hertzberg, J. S., Calhoun, P. S., Dennis, M. F., et al. (2013). Exploration of the influence of childhood trauma, combat exposure, and the resilience construct on depression and suicidal ideation among US Iraq/Afghanistan era military personnel and veterans. *Archives of Suicide Research, 17*(2), 106–122.

Zalta, A. K., Held, P., Smith, D. L., Klassen, B. J., Lofgreen, A. M., Normand, P. S., et al. (2018). Evaluating patterns and predictors of symptom change during a three-week intensive outpatient treatment for veterans with PTSD. *Bio Med Central Psychiatry, 18*(242), 1–15.

Zinzow, H. M., Grubaugh, A. L., Monnier, J., Suffoletta-Maierle, S., & Frueh, B. C. (2007). Trauma among female veterans: A critical review. *Trauma, Violence, & Abuse, 8*(4), 384–400.

CHAPTER 5

Behavioral Health Services within Primary-Care Clinics

Kevin Michael Wilfong, Jeffrey L. Goodie,
Donald D. McGeary, and Alan L. Peterson

Primary-care clinics operate as the de facto setting for mental health treatment, providing some form of health care services to more than half of individuals with mental health conditions (Centers for Disease Control and Prevention [CDC], 2014; Kessler & Stafford, 2008). Efforts to improve services delivered by primary care, guided by ideals such as the Military Health System (MHS) quadruple aim (i.e., readiness, population health, experience of care, and per capita cost), have paved a landscape for integrating behavioral health services as an essential component of routine care. Currently, psychologists and social workers have been integrated into most primary-care clinics in the military that have at least 3,000 enrollees. This chapter will provide a brief history of integrated behavioral health in the military as well as models of integration, ethical considerations for care, recommended training, and common interventions in the primary-care behavioral health (PCBH) model of service delivery.

BRIEF HISTORY OF INTEGRATED BEHAVIORAL HEALTH IN PRIMARY CARE IN THE MILITARY

Behavioral health services of various kinds within primary-care and family medicine clinics have been provided for many decades (Engel, Kroenke, & Katon, 1994; Williams, Bishop, Hennen, & Johnson, 1974). The first formal initiation of a servicewide clinical and training program to integrate military behavioral health providers into military primary-care clinics began in 2000 at the three U.S. Air Force psychology internship sites (Hunter & Goodie, 2012; Hunter & Peterson, 2001). At that time, the Air Force had initiated a major redesign of its primary-care clinics called the Primary Care Optimization Project. The aspect of this program specifically related to behavioral health providers was called the Behavioral Health Optimization Project (BHOP); the goal of this project was to offer services in primary care that satisfied patients and providers, improved access to care, promoted team-based care, addressed a broad range of presenting problems, and enhanced early identification and treatment of behavioral health conditions (Hunter, Goodie, Dobmeyer, & Dorrance, 2014). Although a variety of behavioral health providers have been trained and have worked in military primary-care clinics (e.g., psychologists, social workers, psychiatrists, psychiatric nurse practitioners), the initial Air Force training program focused specifically on clinical and counseling psychologists.

In 2000, Kirk Strosahl, a pioneer in the integration of psychologists into primary-care settings, was contracted by the Air Force to help initiate this new BHOP program (Peterson, 2018). Dr. Strosahl was charged with the establishment of a training program as well as developing clinical competencies required for psychologists to work in primary-care settings. His involvement also included the establishment of a specific model for the integration of psychologists into military primary care; one emphasis of this model was the adaptation for primary care of empirically supported treatments that had been established in specialty care settings. The model was called the primary-care mental health model (now referred to as the primary-care behavioral health [PCBH] model; Reiter, Dobmeyer, & Hunter, 2018; Strosahl & Sobel, 1996).

In total, Dr. Strosahl provided extensive training to six psychologists and a clinical social worker at the Air Force's three psychology internship sites. These individuals were designated as "expert trainers" for the purpose of training other psychology and social worker interns in integrated primary-care techniques. Across the three Air Force psychology internship sites, about 24 clinical psychology interns per year were trained to work as behavioral health consultants (BHCs). Upon graduation from the internship programs, these new psychologists were assigned to 1 of about 75 Air Force medical treatment facilities located around the world to disseminate the PCBH model at their individual military treatment facilities. This extensive training pipeline for psychology interns and licensed psychologists and social workers was key to the rapid dissemination and implementation of the PCBH model throughout the Air Force (Peterson, 2018).

In 2008, the Department of Defense (DoD) established the Mental Health Integration Working Group (MHIWG), which included representation from the Air Force, U.S. Navy, and U.S. Army and multiple specialties (i.e., family medicine, psychology, social work, and psychiatry), and was led by Dr. Christopher Hunter, who was one of the original Air Force expert trainers (Hunter et al., 2014). Building on the recommendations made by the MHIWG and after funding was secured, the DoD formulated Department of Defense Instruction 6490.15, which shaped the implementation of the PCBH model of delivery throughout the MHS (Hunter et al. 2014). As of 2020, there were 312 behavioral health consultant positions across the MHS.

MODELS OF INTEGRATED PRIMARY CARE

Behavioral health services can be delivered in primary care using a continuum of integration. To better understand the ethical issues, training curriculum, and evidence-based interventions outlined below, it is important to distinguish between medical-provided behavioral health care, specialty behavioral health colocated within primary care, and having behavioral health providers integrated into the primary-care system.

Medical-Provided Behavioral Health Care

Medical-provided behavioral health care refers to a delivery model in which medical providers (i.e., physicians, nurses) with limited required training in behavioral health interventions provide these interventions without direct consultation or collaboration with a behavioral health provider. Medical providers may employ behavioral health screening tools or implement programs such as the screening, brief intervention, referral and treatment (SBIRT) model (Collins, Hewson, Munger, & Wade, 2010). Although this model provides some evidence for effectively reducing behaviors such as risky drinking behavior (Moyer, 2013), treatment in primary care is most often reliant on psychoeducation and pharmacotherapy. Furthermore, individuals presenting to primary care without designated behavioral health assets are often not being identified or are undertreated for their mental health concerns (Mitchell, Rao, & Vaze, 2010).

Colocated Specialty Behavioral Health

To enhance the quality of assessment and intervention of behavioral health care, some systems colocate independent behavioral health clinics near or within primary care. Operationally, these behavioral health clinics resemble specialty behavioral health with 50-minute appointments, enhanced privacy on medical records, and a care plan executed independently from medical care. Colocation of behavioral health services and primary care includes several apparent benefits. These include more likely collaboration between medical and behavioral health teams, the potential for reduced stigma that is often associated with siloed specialty care, and perceptions by the medical team of improved access to behavioral health treatment through familiar providers (Collins et al., 2010; Strosahl, 2005). However, colocated care still does not fully address the MHS quadruple aim (Defense Health Agency, 2020). That is, colocation may improve the *experience of care,* but optimizing *readiness, improving population health,* and *managing total health care cost* require a stepped-care approach that can ensure the total military force is medically ready by making behavioral health a scalable resource that is routinely available.

Integrated Primary Care

Opposite the continuum from medical-provided behavioral health care is the complete integration of behavioral health providers as part of the primary-care team. Currently, there is more than one model showing valuable outcomes for improving mental health. One such method of delivery is the collaborative care model (CoCM). This model integrates a behavioral health care manager who is trained in managing common behavioral health disorders, as part of the primary-care team to actively coordinate patient care between medical and behavioral health providers. Given this model's historical emphasis on augmenting the primary-care team to address common behavioral health concerns, implementation of the CoCM largely focuses on patients with depression and anxiety. The positive outcomes across 79 randomized controlled trials have highlighted the model's impact for effective intervention of anxiety and depression (Archer et al., 2012). Another delivery model used in military health systems looks to further the effectiveness of the primary-care team by addressing both the behavioral health and health behavior needs of the patient.

Primary-Care Behavioral Health

The integration model used in most military health systems is the PCBH model. This model of delivery was selected for its considerable changes to how behavioral health providers assess and intervene with patients. The changes allow an increased number of individuals in the population access to a behavioral health clinician. The PCBH model aims to provide brief, targeted, and evidence-based assessment and intervention in a primary-care setting (Hunter et al., 2017). In this model, licensed psychologists and social workers serve as BHCs for the primary-care team. The BHC helps the team and its patients target behavioral health concerns (e.g., depression, insomnia, posttraumatic stress disorder), as well as challenging health–behavior change (e.g., tobacco use, physical activity) and management of disease processes with significant biopsychosocial components (e.g., chronic pain, obesity, diabetes). The current operational definition of the BHC was developed by Reiter and colleagues (2018) in consultation with other subject matter experts using the acronym GATHER to outline essential competencies:

> The BHC assists in the care of patients of any age and with any health condition (Generalist); strives to intervene with all patients on the day they are referred (Accessible); shares clinic space and resources and assists the team in various ways (Team-based); engages with a large percentage of the clinic population (High volume); helps improve the team's biopsychosocial assessment and intervention skills and processes (Educator); and is a routine part of biopsychosocial care (Routine). (p. 112)

In the PCBH model, patients are typically seen by the BHC for one to four appointments lasting 15 to 30 minutes each. During an episode of care, notes are entered in the medical record, and the patient's primary-care provider (PCP) receives direct feedback about the plan for the patient. In this model of delivery, ownership of care is maintained by the PCP, and follow-up is based on a consultant approach, meaning "patients are followed by the BHC and PCP until functioning or symptoms begin improving; at that point, the PCP resumes sole oversight of care but re-engages the BHC at any time, as needed" (Reiter et al., 2018, p. 112). For most patients, data have shown that the greatest functional improvement occurs in the first four appointments (Bryan et al., 2014); if patients do not begin to show improvement after approximately four appointments in this setting, the BHC assists the team with a referral to the appropriate resources in specialty care (e.g., outpatient mental health clinic). For some patients, more than four appointments with the BHC may be appropriate to help the primary-care team and patient manage chronic concerns that do not warrant the regularity of specialty behavioral health. Overall, the PCBH approach is intended to augment the existing delivery of behavioral health services in primary care to improve the biopsychosocial management of health, not to replace services provided in any other setting (Reiter et al., 2018).

Ethical Issues

Working in a primary-care setting requires a different standard of care compared to working in specialty behavioral health clinics, which has important implications for ethical practice. The topic of behavioral health providers adapting ethical standards for primary-care settings has been addressed by multiple authors (Dobmeyer, 2013; Goodie, Kanzler, Hunter, Glotfelter, & Bodart, 2013; Kanzler, Goodie, Hunter, Glotfelter, & Bodart, 2013; Runyan, Robinson, & Gould, 2013; Runyan, Carter-Henry, & Ogbeide, 2018). Runyan and colleagues' (2018) adaptation of ethical principles provides an interprofessional collaborative primary-care model that aims to consider the ethical standards of the entire care team. Its fundamental principle is to "help/do no harm," with additional principles focused on patient-centered informed consent, transparent documentation, and transparency in consultation with patients and colleagues. The model helps to bridge the gap between multiple, sometimes competing, ethical considerations. The following will identify unique aspects of common ethical challenges including boundaries of clinical competence, multiple relationships, informed consent, documentation, and confidentiality. The reader is also directed to Chapter 17 (this volume) for further discussion of ethics in military settings.

Boundaries of Competence

In primary-care settings, BHCs are expected to practice as generalists, suggesting they are prepared to see anyone who walks through the door. Although it is not the responsibility of BHCs to provide an intervention for every condition, they must be able to identify and begin interventions for a wide range of conditions. For military psychology, this is not an unfamiliar expectation; unique to BHCs is the expectation that they also be well versed in managing health–behavior change and disease processes to augment medical care as part of the primary-care team. For those conditions that BHCs cannot treat, they facilitate appropriate referrals. As in all settings, BHCs are expected to practice and consult within their boundaries of competence.

Multiple Relationships

In military medical settings, it is common for medical providers to assist in the care of their peers (Kanzler et al., 2013). These attitudes toward caring for peers stand in sharp contrast to the encouragement from the American Psychological Association (APA, 2017) to avoid multiple relationships. In primary care, particularly in a wide range of military settings, behavioral health providers may be faced with challenging decisions regarding how to engage with primary-care peers. Following Runyan et al.'s model (2018) focusing on the principle of helping and not harming, it can be culturally and ethically appropriate to provide informal guidance and consultation to peers within the context of primary-care clinics. Nevertheless, it is important for providers to set boundaries with their peers if providing consultation or other care would interfere with the working relationships needed.

Informed Consent

In specialty behavioral health clinics, it is common and expected practice to spend time assuring that patients consent to treatment and understand the limits of that treatment through a verbal discussion and signed document outlining the limits of confidentiality. When receiving integrated behavioral health services in primary care, it is typical for the consent to care to be a verbal description of the services that will be provided (e.g., Hunter et al., 2017). This description includes information about the role of the BHC, the structure of the appointment, possible outcomes, how the encounter will be documented in the medical record, how the outcome will be communicated to the PCP, and limits of confidentiality. In the military setting, this includes a brief description of the applicability of the Uniformed Code of Military Justice. When using the PCBH model, the consent process is usually limited to about 2 minutes and is accompanied by a handout describing the BHC's role.

Documentation

In primary care, and more broadly across medical settings, information from appointments is recorded in the electronic health record. In contrast, the documentation of appointments in specialty behavioral health care settings is often protected behind additional security firewalls of the electronic health record that limit access to individuals who are authorized to read the behavioral health record. In primary-care settings, information from BHC encounters is included like other medical records. There are no additional privacy settings that obscure the content of those records. This practice requires BHCs to be mindful of what they include in the medical record.

Privacy and Confidentiality

As alluded to in the previous sections, expectations regarding privacy and confidentiality are different in primary-care settings compared to specialty behavioral health settings. Although patients should expect that their information will remain private and confidential within the context of the primary-care clinic, those seen by BHCs should expect that the broad descriptions of what was discussed during appointments and the plans for their care will be part of the medical record and will be discussed with their PCP.

Recommended Training Curriculum

Training in integrated primary care for psychologists may occur during doctoral, internship, or postdoctoral programs (Larkin, Bridges, Fields, & Vogel, 2016) or following formal training. The APA maintains a list of training programs and other resources for integrated primary care at *www.apa.org/ed/graduate/primary-care-psychology*. It is important to note that what is considered *integrated primary care* can vary widely between training programs.

As described earlier, across the military services, the Air Force has had one of the most robust, longest-running trainings in integrated primary care (Peterson, 2018). Although some psychology internship sites throughout the services offer PCBH training, the majority of BHCs are now civilian social workers and psychologists trained through the Defense Health Agency (DHA). The DHA has established one of the most comprehensive systems for training BHCs (Dobmeyer et al., 2016). The training uses a phased system that includes pretraining self-guided activities, Phase I "classroom training" consisting of didactics and simulated patient care, and Phase II training that requires site visits and observation of their practice in clinic (Dobmeyer et al., 2016). During Phase I and II, trainees are evaluated by an expert BHC who uses a standardized measure of core competencies to rate and provide feedback on their performance.

Outside of the DHA, other large health care systems have created their own trainings. The U.S. Department of Veterans Affairs (VA) also uses a phased model with requirements for learners to demonstrate standardized competencies during role-plays and with actual patients (Kearney et al., 2019). The training model used by the VA has been shown to improve fidelity to the integrated primary-care model through self-report, role-plays, and provider behavior (Kearney et al., 2019). The DHA and VA also both emphasize the importance of developing a train-the-trainer model to ensure that enough providers are proficient in the integrated primary-care competencies (Dobmeyer et al., 2016; Kearney et al., 2019).

Clinical Competencies

The Interorganizational Working Group on Competencies for Primary-Care Psychology Practice established a set of competencies for behavioral health providers working in these settings (McDaniel et al., 2014). The work group also lists essential components and sample behavioral anchors for clinical competencies in *science, systems, professionalism, relationships, application,* and *education.* Although full descriptions are too long to fully replicate for this chapter, Table 5.1 summarizes the clusters and associated competencies more completely described by McDaniel and colleagues (2014).

BHCS EVIDENCE-BASED INTERVENTIONS IN PRIMARY CARE

For many, the PCBH model of integrated primary care likely presents a substantial shift in the model, competencies, and ethical considerations associated with standards of care. Even providing behavioral health in a medical exam room can seem a far departure. Although the expectations and encounters of a BHC are unlike those of a provider in specialty behavioral health, evidence-based interventions remain an essential component

TABLE 5.1. Primary Care Competency Clusters

Cluster	Competency groups
Science	Science related to the biopsychosocial approach Research and evaluation
Systems	Leadership and administration Interdisciplinary systems Advocacy
Professionalism	Professional values and attitudes Individual, cultural, and disciplinary diversity Ethics in primary care Reflective practice/self-assessment/self-care
Relationships	Interprofessionalism Building and sustaining relationships in primary care
Application	Practice management Assessment Intervention Clinical consultation
Education	Teaching Supervision

of quality care. The following discussion will describe typical presenting problems as well as a brief review of the existing literature for evidence-based interventions by a BHC in a military primary-care clinic.

In addition, consultation examples are provided to illustrate usual care in the PCBH model. It is important to note that although patients typically are seen for one to four appointments, the modal number of appointments is one. This means the initial consultation with the BHC is vital for both assessment and intervention. One recommendation for structuring the initial consultation is the use of the 5 A's model of behavior change in primary care (Whitlock, Orleans, Pender, & Allan, 2002). Using this model, an initial 30-minute consultation could include 15 minutes to *assess* the problem, 3 minutes to *advise* the patient of possible interventions and *agree* on a plan, 10 minutes to *assist* with preparing the patient to carry out the intervention, and 2 minutes to *arrange* a follow-up plan between the patient, PCP, and BHC (Hunter et al., 2017). Although the time allotted for each component may vary from one consultation to the next, each of the interventions outlined below will employ this structure.

Insomnia

Sleeping complaints in primary care are pervasive, with as many as 69% of individuals who present to primary care reporting some form of insomnia (Isler, Peterson, & Isler, 2005). For 19% of individuals, these sleep complaints constitute chronic insomnia (Ram, Seirawan, Kumar, & Clark,

2010). The prevalence of sleep-related disorders in military populations can reach upwards of 9 out of 10 individuals, particularly postdeployment (Mysliwiec et al., 2013). In addition to the direct effects of insomnia, chronic sleep problems are associated with functional impairment, exacerbation of medical conditions, reduced quality of life, and development of other psychological conditions (Gagnon, Bélanger, Ivers, & Morin, 2013). Furthermore, service members with untreated sleep problems are at increased risk compared to their well-rested counterparts for developing additional behavioral disorders such as posttraumatic stress disorder, depression, and suicidality when exposed to austere conditions such as deployment, highlighting the importance of early detection and treatment in military populations (Gehrman et al., 2013).

Assessment of Sleep-Related Problems

Compared to specialty behavioral health, the brevity of assessment and intervention in primary care limits the time required for tools such as sleep diaries. Assessment of sleep in primary care is often reliant on focused functional assessment of sleep in combination with standardized self-report measures. The Insomnia Severity Index (ISI; Bastien, Vallières, & Morin, 2001) is one commonly used self-report measure targeting perceptions of sleep-related distress and severity of symptoms. Items are intended to capture sleep onset, maintenance, and satisfaction, as well as noticeability, interference, and experienced distress in daily life functioning (Bastien et al., 2001). The ISI is validated in a primary-care setting using a cutoff score of 14 for detecting clinical insomnia and provides a sensitivity of 82.4% and specificity of 82.1% (Gagnon et al., 2013). It is also important to screen for sleep disturbances that may be explained by medical conditions such as obstructive sleep apnea (OSA). The Berlin Questionnaire (Netzer, Stoohs, Netzer, Clark, & Strohl, 1999) and STOP-Bang Questionnaire (Chung et al., 2008) are two brief measures used in primary care that target common symptoms and risk factors associated with OSA, such as snoring, daytime sleepiness, observed cessation of breathing and body mass index. Beyond standardized screeners, a functional assessment of sleep is vital to better understand areas of focus for intervention. Functional assessment of sleep in primary care should include collecting a history of sleep problems, pertinent information about the current sleep environment, preparatory sleep behaviors, time spent in bed, functional impact of sleep, and at least a cursory review of related conditions (e.g., sleep apnea, narcolepsy, bruxism, substance misuse).

Primary-Care Intervention for Insomnia

Cognitive-behavioral therapy for insomnia (CBT-I) is a well-established, first-line intervention for insomnia, with outcomes outperforming the longitudinal effects of sleep medications once treatment is discontinued (Riemann & Perlis, 2009). When the core interventions from CBT-I are distilled and adapted for a primary-care setting, publications have repeatedly demonstrated successful results (Buysse et al., 2011; Falloon, Elley, Fernando, Lee, & Arroll, 2015; Fernando, Arroll, & Falloon, 2013). One pragmatic trial using these primary-care adaptations in the PCBH model revealed that 83% of participants attained greater than 85% sleep efficiency regardless of comorbidities (Goodie, Isler, Hunter, & Peterson, 2009).

CBT-I includes an array of strategies and tools for addressing different aspects of sleep. For primary-care settings, a brief behavioral treatment for insomnia protocol has been developed (Troxel, Germain, & Buysse, 2012) including interventions selected from the larger CBT-I repertoire to fit the nature of the sleep problem. Common strategies in primary care include alterations to sleep hygiene, stimulus control, sleep restriction, and relaxation techniques. These interventions are typically supplemented by a handout with examples of helpful strategies for relaxation, ways to improve sleep hygiene, a summary of healthy stimulus control, or a guide to effective sleep restriction. Patients may also be recommended resources such as an app by VA Mobile called CBT-i Coach (*https://mobile.va.gov/app/cbt-i-coach*) to aid with the selected intervention. Often, the functional assessment provides the necessary information to identify and prioritize which strategy will have the greatest impact leaving the initial consultation.

Let's review a sample case to demonstrate the BHC's' role and approach to a soldier who expressed concerns about daytime sleepiness and falling asleep at work to his PCP. This consultation example is provided to illustrate usual care in the PCBH model.

The case study will follow an initial consultation using the five A's model mentioned before (i.e., assess, advise, agree, assist, arrange; Whitlock, 2002).

Case 5.1. *The Soldier with Sleep Problems*

The BHC is asked by the PCP to develop a plan to improve sleep and assist in determining whether the soldier should be considered for sleep medication. The BHC begins the same-day encounter with an introduction to behavioral health consultation services, verifies the referral question, and briefly reviews the ISI and STOP-Bang Questionnaire. The screeners suggest insomnia but are not consistent with OSA. After completing a 10-minute functional *assessment,* the BHC identified that the sleep problems began after a recent prescription for allergy medication. The soldier reported drinking four to five energy drinks across the day to combat sleepiness and often has difficulty getting to sleep at night. The BHC then spends 3 minutes *advising* on the likely contributors to the soldier's sleep problems and possible first steps in combatting them. These include (1) moving allergy medication to the evenings after discussion with the PCP,

(2) cutting caffeine intake after 2 p.m., and (3) introducing relaxation techniques to reduce sleep latency in the evening. The BHC also offers a handout with additional information about improving sleep through behavior change. The soldier expressed resistance to cutting caffeine completely after 2 p.m., but after some discussion, the BHC and soldier *agreed* to reduce the total intake to two energy drinks per day, with neither consumed after 5 p.m. The BHC spends the remaining 10 minutes of the appointment *assisting* the soldier by demonstrating deep breathing and establishing a plan to practice nightly. The BHC *arranges* a follow-up in 6 weeks to evaluate progress and provide additional intervention as needed. At follow-up, the service member reports improved sleep latency and reduced daytime sleepiness. The BHC reemphasizes continued use of learned skills for sleep maintenance and suggests routine follow-up with the PCP.

Depression

Depression is one of the leading mental health diagnoses in the United States, afflicting 9.4% of Americans, with a similar prevalence in military service members (Kessler, Petukhova, Sampson, Zaslavsky, & Wittchen, 2012; Meadows et al., 2018). In a primary-care clinical sample, the rate is mirrored, meaning 1 in 10 encounters could benefit from the identification of and intervention for depressive symptoms (Meadows et al., 2018; Mitchell et al., 2010). Given the high prevalence of depression in primary care, treatment in this setting provides an ideal means to address the global readiness of the military population from a behavioral health perspective. However, primary-care teams are often ill-equipped to identify or treat behavioral health concerns; this leaves most untreated or undertreated with psychopharmacotherapy, which has limited long-term effectiveness (Karyotaki et al., 2016; Mitchell et al., 2010).

Assessment of Depression in Primary Care

The Patient Health Questionnaire-9 (PHQ-9) is the most extensively evaluated tool in the primary-care setting (El-Den, Chen, Gan, Wong, & O'Reilly, 2017). This nine-item screener can be administered in about 1 minute and provides a self-report measure targeting symptoms of major depressive disorder over the last 2 weeks (Kroenke, Spitzer, & Williams, 2001). With a maximum score of 27, the measure provides suggested severity categories ranging from *minimal* to *severe* (Kroenke et al., 2001). For a single threshold to identify clinically significant symptoms, a cutoff score of 10 provides sensitivity of 78% and specificity of 87% (Moriarty, Gilbody, McMillan, & Manea, 2015). The measure also includes an item that predicts increased risk for suicide and suicide attempts (Simon et al., 2013).

In some cases, the PHQ-2 can be administered as an ultra-brief screener and precursor to administering the entire PHQ-9 (Arroll et al., 2010). This pares down the PHQ-9 to the first two items targeting anhedonia and depressed mood (Kroenke, Spitzer, Williams, & Löwe, 2009). At a clinical cutoff score of 2 out of 6, this ultra-brief measure provides a sensitivity of 86% and specificity of 78% in a primary-care setting (Arroll et al., 2010). Other measures to consider for assessment of depression in primary care include the Beck Depression Inventory for Primary Care (BDI-PC; Steer, Cavalieri, Leonard, & Beck, 1999) and Edinburgh Postnatal Depression Scale (EPDS; Cox, Holden, & Sagovsky, 1987). In addition to measurement-based assessment, a functional assessment of mood and depressive symptoms using the mnemonic SIGECAPS (i.e., *sleep, interest, guilt, energy, concentration, appetite, psychomotor agitation/retardation,* and *suicidal ideation*) can guide strategies for intervention. As part of the assessment, determination of suicide risk can also guide appropriate level of care in accordance with established clinic policies and clinical practice guidelines (see Chapter 9, this volume).

Primary-Care Intervention for Depression

The options for empirically supported treatment of depression include a variety of pharmacotherapies as well as psychotherapeutic modalities. Pharmacotherapy in combination with psychotherapy provides protection from relapse after termination and is often an ideal treatment option for more severe populations (Karyotaki et al., 2016). As mentioned before, many do not, or cannot, access evidence-based treatment in specialty care clinics, emphasizing the importance of adapting established interventions to improve the delivery of services in primary care (Mitchell et al., 2010).

Evidence-based intervention in primary care is largely drawn from components of cognitive and behavioral interventions for depression. Specifically, patients may be provided with the tools and skills to implement a behavioral activation strategy, cognitive restructuring techniques, or problem-solving skills. BHCs also typically provide handouts with psychoeducation about the processes and symptoms of depression as well as mood trackers to improve awareness of thoughts, behaviors, and emotions. Patients may also be referred to resources such as VA Mobile's ACT Coach (a mobile app that utilizes acceptance and commitment therapy; *https:// mobile.va.gov/app/act-coach*) for additional assistance implementing interventions selected during the appointment. As with sleep, selection of an intervention should be informed by the functional assessment as well as a collaborative discussion with the patient about which strategy he or she is most motivated to try. Additionally, BHCs work closely with the primary-care team to discuss the appropriateness of pharmacotherapy, management of suicide risk, and referral to a higher level of care for individuals not showing improvement after about four appointments.

Posttraumatic Stress Disorder

Posttraumatic stress disorder (PTSD) has become a hallmark behavioral health concern associated with combat service over the last several decades. PTSD is estimated to present in at least 5% of service members postdeployment, with more than twice that prevalence rate reported in operational infantry units (Kok, Herrell, Thomas, & Hoge, 2012). In civilian primary-care patients, PTSD demonstrates a similar prevalence of approximately 6%, while veteran primary-care samples report rates 2 to 3 times higher (Prins et al., 2016). Unfortunately, the need for improved detection and treatment of PTSD in primary-care settings often results in continued symptomology and exacerbation of associated health issues (Wilson, 2007).

Assessment of PTSD

The Primary-Care PTSD Screen for DSM-5 (PC-PTSD-5; Prins et al., 2016) and the PTSD Checklist for DSM-5 (PCL-5; Weathers et al., 2013) offer brief screeners that permit enhanced detection of PTSD in primary care. The PC-PTSD-5 consists of six "yes" or "no" items, which are symptoms of PTSD as defined by the fifth edition of the *Diagnostic and Statistical Manual of Mental Disorders* (DSM-5; American Psychiatric Association, 2013). For patients endorsing three or more items, the measure provides a sensitivity of 95% and specificity of 85%, suggesting they should be further assessed for PTSD (Prins et al., 2016). The PCL-5 is a 20-item self-report measure that asks patients to rate on a 5-point scale (i.e., 0 to 4) how frequently and significantly symptoms of PTSD bothered them in the last month (Bovin et al., 2016; Weathers et al., 2013). In both civilian and military samples, the PCL-5 maintains strong test–retest reliability, internal consistency, and convergent and discriminant validity (Blevins, Weathers, Davis, Witte, & Domino, 2015; Bovin et al., 2016). For service members with a score of 33 out of 80 (sensitivity of 93%; specificity of 72%), the measure indicates clinically significant distress related to posttraumatic stress (Wortmann et al., 2016). These screeners take less than 5 minutes to complete and provide a starting place for initiating a conversation about exposure to traumatic events.

Primary-Care Intervention for PTSD

Many providers in the DoD and VA employ prolonged exposure and cognitive processing therapies as empirically supported interventions for PTSD in civilian and military populations. In fact, manualized trauma-focused psychotherapy is the first-line treatment for PTSD in the VA/DoD clinical practice guideline (U.S. Department of Veterans Affairs and Department of Defense, 2017). Although many of these manualized therapies require far more time and total appointments than what is characteristically available in primary care, a series of studies by Cigrang and colleagues (2017) have provided evidence for modified versions of prolonged exposure techniques with positive results across open trial and randomized clinical trial studies. In both cases, studies showed clinically significant reduction in symptoms after only four appointments, with lasting results at 8-week and 6-month follow-ups. Data at this time suggest that brief treatments for PTSD delivered in primary-care settings are effective, although referral for specialty behavioral health treatment may be appropriate for patients requiring more intensive interventions.

The most empirically validated modality for adapting prolonged exposure techniques is prolonged exposure for primary care, which emphasizes exposure through a written narrative of traumatic experiences; patients are provided a workbook with prompts for detailed trauma narratives, emotional processing questions, and a record of subjective units of distress (Cigrang et al., 2017). Using this format of intervention, the initial consultation is typically reserved for assessment, psychoeducation, and collaborative work with the patient to determine the appropriate level of care. Subsequent appointments outline the use of at-home, writing-based exposure, review of progress and barriers, and encouragement of opportunities for *in vivo* exposure or general behavior change that promote healthy functioning. Patients may also benefit from other models such as written exposure therapy (Marx & Sloan, 2019) or strategies that emphasize acceptance-based techniques (van Emmerik, Kamphuis, & Emmelkamp, 2008; Walser & Westrup, 2007).

Case 5.2. The Air Force Medic with PTSD

The BHC is asked by the PCP to see an Air Force master sergeant after he screened positive for potential PTSD on the PC-PTSD-5. The airman is an operating room technician with 19 years of active-duty service. He had previously deployed to Iraq, where he served as the noncommissioned officer in charge (NCOIC) of the operating room at a combat support hospital. During his deployment, he supported hundreds of surgical cases involving severe medical traumas, many of which involved limb amputations. Early on in his deployment, several of the younger operating room technicians whom he supervised became distressed with the high volume of traumatic amputation cases, especially when they had to dispose of the amputated limbs in a bin and incinerate them at the end of each duty shift. To protect his younger troops, the operating room NCOIC volunteered to assist in the most difficult surgical cases and to take responsibility for the incineration of all human remains at the end of each duty day. For the first 3 years after returning from deployment, he suffered with significant flashbacks, nightmares, and avoidance symptoms, which included not scheduling himself for any surgical cases. However, because of his concerns about stigmatization for being weak for "just doing his job" while deployed, he did not reveal his suffering to anyone, including his supervisor or his spouse. The BHC administers the PCL-5 to help confirm the diagnosis of PTSD, and then offers the options of a referral to the mental health clinic for specialty PTSD treatment or to receive brief treatment for PTSD in the primary-care clinic. The airman opts to be treated in primary care and completes four 30-minute treatment sessions of prolonged exposure for primary care including the completion of written exposure therapy exercises between treatment sessions. A PCL-5 administered during the fourth treatment session indicates that his PTSD symptoms have been reduced substantially, but are still at an elevated level. The BHC then discusses the options of continuing to work on his own with what he had learned from the primary-care PTSD treatment or a referral to the mental health clinic for specialty PTSD treatment. The airman indicates he was open to a specialty clinic referral, but states that he wants to think about it further and discuss this option with his wife.

Chronic Pain

Chronic pain is a significant problem for active-duty military members, veterans, and dependents, and most individuals with a chronic pain condition will seek treatment through primary care. The National Health Interview Survey revealed that up to 20% of all U.S. adults will experience a chronic pain problem, and 8% of adults will report "high-impact" pain (Dahlhamer et al., 2018). Assessing pain on both a clinical and epidemiological scale has gained increased attention since the designation of pain as the "fifth vital sign" more than 20 years ago (Morone & Weiner, 2013). A flurry of research evolved from this designation and highlighted the widespread scope of pain as an epidemiological concern and the extraordinary complexity of chronic pain as a clinical issue. Chronic pain conditions have various origins and presentations, making it difficult to establish a one-size-fits-all approach to pain conceptualization, assessment, and management. A comprehensive overview of the various categories of chronic pain is outside the scope of this chapter, but Table 5.2 gives a brief overview of different types of pain and related presentations. Musculoskeletal pain is the most prevalent pain condition among military service members and veterans and accounts for over one-third of all pain presentations (Bader, Giordano, McDonald, Meghani, & Polomano, 2018).

The Difficulty of Defining Chronic Pain

Pain is a subjective phenomenon, making it very difficult to assess or develop a common understanding of how pain is defined. The most widely agreed-upon definition of pain was developed by the International Association for the Study of Pain (IASP) and was recently revised to describe pain as "an unpleasant sensory and emotional experience associated with, or resembling

TABLE 5.2. Most Common Pain Presentations

Pain type	Prevalence	Clinical characteristics
Musculoskeletal pain	Up to 63% of military members seeking care through the military health system (Reif et al., 2018).	Pain in the muscles, joint, and/or connective tissue lasting longer than 3 months. Up to one-third of those with musculoskeletal pain report more than one location of pain.
Neuropathic pain	Approximately 7% of U.S. adults; more likely in middle age (Bouhassira et al., 2008).	Pain attributable to nerve damage due to disease or injury. Can be categorized as peripheral or central based on the cause.
Whole/widespread body pain (e.g., fibromyalgia)	Approximately 1% of all service members. More prevalent in women and middle age.	Pain, often accompanied by fatigue, present throughout the body. Patient may experience pain in response to nonpainful stimuli.
Headache	Up to 20% of military members based on headache type (Bader et al., 2018).	May include unilateral or bilateral head pain, neck pain, aura symptoms, and varying frequency and duration of headache episodes.

that associated with, actual or potential tissue damage" (Raja et al., 2020, p. 1). Pain can be further classified based on persistence or chronicity of pain, though definitions of persistence vary. The World Health Organization established a definition of persistent pain as pain present most days over the past 6 months (Gureje, Von Korff, Simon, & Gater, 1998), but this definition has been narrowed to pain that is present more days than not for 3 or more months (Steingrímsdóttir, Landmark, Macfarlane, & Neilsen, 2017). All variations on the definition of chronic pain agree that the factor best differentiating chronic from acute pain is that chronic pain lasts longer than expected or significantly affects an individual across multiple life domains (e.g., work, home, relationships, activities of enjoyment, spirituality, mood). When working with pain in primary care, a patient-centered definition of pain chronicity (i.e., pain has lasted long enough to have a significant impact on functioning across multiple domains) is likely the best approach.

Chronic Pain Assessment in Primary Care

Patient-reported outcomes are crucial to effective pain management, so choosing appropriate pain measures is a key part of treatment. Many different measures of pain exist, and choosing the best option for assessing pain in primary care can be difficult. The most ubiquitous and controversial pain assessment used in primary care is the Numeric Rating Scale (NRS). The NRS requires a patient to rate the intensity of his or her pain on an enumerated scale often ranging from 0 (*no pain*) to 10 (*worst possible pain*), with scores greater than 4 representative of "moderate" pain intensity and scores greater than 7 representative of "severe" pain (Boonstra et al., 2016). Despite some concerns about the reliability of a single pain rating as a pain treatment outcome, large studies find that a change of 2+ points on the NRS is clinically significant (Farrar, Young, LaMoreaux, Werth, & Poole, 2001).

Concerns about NRS validity gave rise to the development of *pain interference measures* that advance pain assessment by asking about the intensity of pain and the extent to which pain interferes with different activities in the patient's life. The National Institutes of Health Patient Reported Outcomes Measurement Information System (PROMIS) developed a brief pain interference module with strong validity and reliability in chronic pain populations that can be quickly administered in primary-care settings (Amtmann et al., 2010). The Brief Pain Inventory (Cleeland, 1989) is frequently used in primary care to measure multiple domains of pain interference. The PEG (Krebs et al., 2009) is a three-item measure often used in primary care because of its brevity and capacity to assess average *pain* intensity (P), interference with *enjoyment* of life (E), and interference with *general* activity (G).

The U.S. Army Surgeon General Pain Management Task Force Final Report (Office of the Army Surgeon General, 2010) emphasized the importance of pain assessment that accounts for the unique circumstances of military service-related pain. In response to this report, the Defense and Veterans Center for Integrative Pain Management developed the Defense and Veterans Pain Rating Scale (DVPRS; see Figure 5.1) as a brief validated measure of pain interference specific to military populations (Buckenmaier et al., 2013; Polomano et al., 2016). Each of these pain measures provides valuable information as part of baseline pain evaluation and prospective treatment outcomes assessment, and should be used as a standard and frequent part of behavioral pain management in primary care.

In addition to standardized measures, functional assessment by the BHC should gather information about contributing factors that exacerbate and ameliorate experienced pain, the functional impact on activities of daily living, and current patterns of coping when experiencing pain. In combination with standardized assessment, functional assessments can aid in prioritizing potential interventions that are personalized to meet the goals and motivations of individual patients.

Chronic Pain Comorbidities

Chronic pain is often accompanied by comorbid symptoms such as depression, PTSD, anxiety, sleep disturbance, fatigue, functional disability, stress,

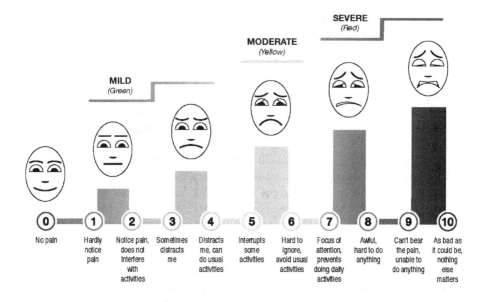

DoD/VA Pain Supplemental Questions

For clinicians to evaluate the biopsychosocial impact of pain

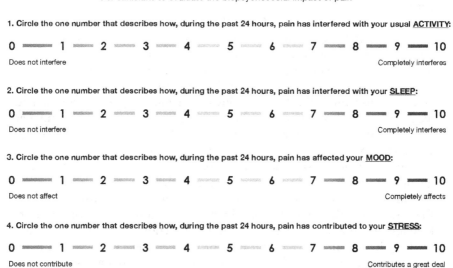

FIGURE 5.1. Defense and Veterans Pain Rating System, Version 2.0. The original scale is presented in color (see *www.va.gov/PAINMANAGEMENT/docs/DVPRS_2slides_and_references.pdf*).

and social dysfunction (Nugraha et al., 2019). All these comorbid concerns have a reciprocal impact on pain and pain management, so it is often helpful to include these as part of patient assessment and conceptualization. Posttraumatic headache disorder (McGeary et al., 2020) can make pain recalcitrant to standard of care therapies (McGeary, Moore, Vriend, Peterson, & Gatchel, 2011). Comorbid depression and anxiety can worsen pain and increase the use of opioid medication for pain management (Hooten, Shi, Gazelka, & Warner, 2011). Although insomnia is often considered a consequence of chronic pain, there is emerging evidence that patterns of disrupted sleep can increase the risk of developing chronic pain (Generaal, Vogelzanga, Penninx, & Dekker, 2017).

Chronic Pain Management Interventions

Most nonpharmacological interventions for chronic pain in primary care are rooted in cognitive and behavioral therapies (CBT) due to the accumulated body of research supporting their use and the broad spectrum of these treatments that address both chronic pain and the comorbidities that maintain and perpetuate pain (Du et al., 2017). CBT interventions such as stress management, relaxation, activity pacing, restructuring catastrophic pain cognitions, and developing healthy social support are all well-established tools for effective pain management. In 2018, the Defense Health Agency established a MHS stepped-care model of pain management including the implementation of a brief cognitive-behavioral therapy for chronic pain (BCBT-CP; Defense Health Agency, 2018). BCBT-CP is a seven-module, manualized CBT treatment program for chronic pain that was adapted from the 12-session CBT-CP program developed by the Department of Veterans Affairs (Murphy et al., 2014). CBT-CP modules and their topics are presented in Table 5.3. There is emerging evidence that outcomes associated with these modules/sessions are dose-dependent, so patients with less severe pain or less pain interference may need fewer sessions to achieve significant clinical improvement.

Telehealth Adaptions of Pain Management

There has been significant advancement in adapting behavioral pain management into military telehealth over the past 10 years (Byrne & Spevak, 2020; McGeary, McGeary, & Gatchel, 2012), and telehealth formats are now effectively being used for pain management and pain consultation. CBT programs like CBT-CP and BCBT-CP are increasingly delivered through telehealth, which allows greater accessibility to these interventions for patients who cannot travel due to pain, disability, or other health concerns (e.g., COVID-19). The Army and Navy have established specialty pain consultation for PCPs using the University of New Mexico's Project

TABLE 5.3. Cognitive-Behavioral Therapy for Chronic Pain (CBT-CP) Session Topics

Session	Topic	Content summary
1	Interview and assessment	Baseline evaluation of chronic pain
2	Treatment orientation	Education about CBT-CP
3	Assessment feedback and goal setting	Develop treatment goals based on assessment
4	Exercise and pacing	Importance of movement and planning activity
5	Relaxation training	Teach relaxation techniques for pain and stress
6	Pleasant activities 1	Identify and implement meaningful pleasant activities for coping
7	Pleasant activities 2	
8	Cognitive coping 1	Learn how thoughts affect pain and how to monitor and challenge them
9	Cognitive coping 2	
10	Sleep	Strategies for improving sleep
11	Discharge planning	Plan for flare-ups and skill review
12	Booster session	Evaluate use of skills and troubleshoot

ECHO (or TeleECHO) platform, resulting in decreased opioid prescription and better pain management outcomes (Katzman et al., 2019). CBT-based interventions delivered by telehealth show significant improvement for up to half of all patients treated, with moderate effect sizes (Rutledge et al., 2018).

Tobacco Cessation

For patients who use nicotine or tobacco, the single most important thing they can do to improve their health is to quit (Peterson, Vander Weg, & Jaén, 2011). By extension, behavioral health providers can improve the health of their patients more through evidence-based tobacco cessation than by any other brief behavioral health intervention. In most primary-care settings, nicotine and tobacco cessation refers to quitting cigarette smoking; however, in military populations, this also refers to smokeless tobacco cessation given a higher rate of smokeless tobacco use for both males and females (Peterson et al., 2007; Severson, Klein, Lichtenstein, Kaufman, & Orleans, 2005; Vander Weg, DeBon, Peterson, Mittleman, Klesges, & Relyea, 2005). In addition, with the recent proliferation of vaping, nicotine cessation also refers to electronic cigarettes (Cox, 2015).

The "Five A's" of Tobacco Cessation

The most popular evidence-based brief intervention for nicotine and tobacco cessation in medical settings is the "five A's" approach (Fiore et al., 2008; Peterson et al., 2011). The five A's include *Ask* about tobacco use, *Advise* patients to quit, *Assess* interest in quitting, *Assist* in quitting, and *Arrange* for follow-up. This brief approach can be shortened to just the first two A's, three A's, or four A's, depending on the length of time available. For example, the two A's version (i.e., Asking and Advising) can be completed in about 30 seconds. Many PCPs believe this is all the time they have available to devote to tobacco cessation. Simply asking patients about their tobacco use and then advising them to quit may seem overly simplistic; however, a large proportion of primary-care patients report that their providers have never told them they should quit (Fiore et al., 2008; Peterson et al., 2011).

Universal Screening for Nicotine and Tobacco Use

Given the apparent gap in care, the first step BHCs can take in assisting with nicotine and tobacco cessation is to assure the clinic has a universal screening program. Most health care providers are familiar with guidelines for the universal assessment of nicotine and tobacco use during every outpatient medical visit. In fact, the assessment and treatment of tobacco use is an accreditation metric for the nation's oldest and largest standards-setting and accrediting body in health care, the Joint Commission (Joint Commission, 2020). Part of the inspection process for the Joint Commission is to evaluate whether health care providers assess nicotine and tobacco use during every primary-care appointment. The initial screening for nicotine and tobacco use is often conducted by the PCP or one of the medical staff members prior to referral to the BHC; however, as part of the primary-care team, BHCs also can conduct brief screenings for nicotine and tobacco use in patients referred to them for other reasons.

Evidence-Based Interventions for Tobacco Cessation

A detailed review of evidenced-based interventions for nicotine and tobacco cessation is beyond the scope of this chapter. Specific details on tobacco cessation in primary-care settings have been previously published (Fiore et al., 2008; Hunter et al., 2017; Peterson et al., 2011). Most evidence-based interventions include a combination of behavioral, cognitive, and pharmacological approaches. Therefore, it is essential that BHCs working in primary-care settings be familiar with nicotine replacement therapy (e.g., nicotine patches, gum, lozenges) as well as prescription medications such as bupropion (Zyban) and varenicline (Chantix). In most cases, the BHC will work closely with the PCP regarding nicotine and tobacco cessation medications and then provide brief behavioral and cognitive strategies as part of the BHC visits. Additionally, BHCs should be prepared to aid with the connection to resources outside the clinic such as a telephone quitline (i.e., 1-800-QUIT-NOW) or referral to a tobacco cessation program. Quitlines provide evidence-based telehealth interventions as well as education on nicotine replacement therapy free of charge (Keller, Bailey, Koss, Baker, & Fiore, 2007).

A common challenge encountered in primary care is demotivation to engage tobacco use behaviors due to the low quit rates for many patients who are attempting to stop nicotine and tobacco use. In addressing this challenge, BHCs may work to improve the care team well-being by emphasizing the benefit of assisting even a single patient to quit successfully. Given that most individuals require multiple attempts before they quit permanently, BHCs may also help the care team to conceptualize nicotine and tobacco use as a chronic condition rather than simply a lifestyle choice. Finally, BHCs can improve the care team well-being by reducing the workload for the clinic and delivering behavior change interventions.

Weight Management

Military health systems most often define overweight and obesity using the body mass index (BMI), a height-to-weight ratio intended to estimate body fat. In the United States, two in five adults meet criteria for obesity, with growing prevalence on a global scale (Centers for Disease Control and Prevention, 2018). Even in an active-duty military population, with body composition standards and resources geared toward physical readiness, one in four individuals meets BMI criteria for obesity, and longitudinal trends show service members steadily moving into heavier categories (Rush, Leard-Mann, & Crum-Cianflone, 2016). After discharge from military service, deleterious changes in diet, sleep, and physical activity further elevate rates of weight-related health concerns in veteran populations (Bookwalter et al., 2019). Despite the pervasiveness of obesity and clear relationship to weight-related health conditions, only one in five adults with obesity receives weight-related counseling when seen in primary care (Bleich, Pickett-Blakely, & Cooper, 2011). Even when patients receive weight-related counseling, it often is not consistent with clinical guidelines for weight management (Ko et al., 2008). This may be partly attributable to weight stigma, which can create health disparity as providers discount obesity as an avoidable risk (Phelan et al., 2015). Although obesity is the result of a caloric surplus, the factors that impact the basic equation are a far more complicated interaction of cultural, behavioral, social, metabolic, physiologic, and genetic factors that are not completely understood (Sharma, 2003).

Functional Assessment for Overweight and Obesity

As mentioned above, BMI provides one of the quickest and most frequently used measures for identifying patients in need of weight-loss interventions in primary care. However, identifying weight as a health concern is not the end of a good assessment. Part of working with a medical team is understanding the patient's medical history sufficiently to help guide conversations about weight-related medical conditions such as diabetes, hypertension, or cardiovascular health concerns. Equally important is identifying the patient's existing knowledge, motivation for behavior change, and weight-related goals. To develop a personalized intervention with the greatest chance of successful implementation, a functional assessment also should include an understanding of previous weight-loss attempts, dietary habits, eating behaviors, and physical activity. A cursory review for disordered eating behaviors also may identify other areas of clinical concern.

Intervention for Overweight and Obesity

A combined report by the American College of Cardiology, the American Heart Association, and the Obesity Society recommends aiming for a 5% to 10% weight reduction in 6 months for clinically meaningful change (Jensen et al., 2014). Weight loss requires an energy deficit resulting from a restriction of calorie intake and engagement in physical activity. To address health–behavior changes related to weight loss, clinical guidelines suggest engagement in at least 14 individual or group specialty behavioral health appointments across 6 months; for some, pharmacotherapy also may be appropriate (Jensen et al., 2014). Although treatment in primary care cannot support such intensive behavioral interventions, integration with the medical team can aid in fostering a holistic biopsychosocial approach. Additionally, initial data on weight management in PCBH suggest a positive impact on weight loss (Sadock, Auerbach, Rybarczyk, & Aggarwal, 2013).

In the PCBH model, successful weight management can be optimized by assisting the patient with three things: (1) a clear goal for weight loss consistent with the aforementioned 5% to 10% weight reduction in 6 months, (2) education on healthy dietary planning and eating behaviors, and (3) a behavior-change plan that encompasses both calorie restriction and increased physical activity. With the aid of handouts to capture critical educational information and guided discussion about feasible changes, a personalized behavior-change plan realistically can be established in one to two appointments (Hunter et al., 2017). Once a plan is established, follow-up is arranged, as necessary, to provide continued support, as additional strategies likely will be necessary for overcoming obstacles to weight maintenance. For example, initial weight loss is best predicted by calorie restriction, but sustained weight management after meeting the weight-loss goal is largely reliant on physical activity with regular weight monitoring (Stubbs & Lavin, 2013). In some ways, weight management may deviate from the typical maximum of four appointments with the BHC; however, treatment of obesity is similar to chronic disease management and benefits from long-term follow-up with the patient's medical home.

SUMMARY

Behavioral health services have been delivered in primary care since long before the introduction of specialized providers. Since 2000, military primary-care clinics have made efforts to improve these services by integrating psychologists as part of the primary-care team (Hunter & Peterson, 2001). Currently, psychologists and social workers are integrated into primary-care clinics across the MHS, delivering specialized behavioral health consultation using the PCBH model. Providing services as a BHC requires ethical considerations, clinical competencies, and a training curriculum that are unique from many of their specialty behavioral health counterparts. These differences serve to provide a stepped-care model in which delivering evidence-based interventions for behavioral health concerns, enhancing health behaviors, and managing disease processes are routine parts of the primary-care experience.

REFERENCES

American Psychiatric Association. (2013). *Diagnostic and statistical manual of mental disorders* (5th ed.). Arlington, VA: Author.

American Psychological Association. (2017). *Ethical principles of psychologists and code of conduct*. Retrieved from *www.apa.org/ethics/code*.

Amtmann, D., Cook, K. F., Jensen, M. P., Chen, W. H., Choi, S., Revicki, D., et al. (2010). Development of a PROMIS item bank to measure pain interference. *Pain, 150*(1), 173–182.

Archer, J., Bower, P., Gilbody, S., Lovell, K., Richards, D., Gask, L., et al. (2012). Collaborative care for depression and anxiety problems. *Cochrane Database of Systematic Reviews*. Retrieved from *https://doi.org/10.1002/14651858.CD006525.*

Arroll, B., Goodyear-Smith, F., Crengle, S., Gunn, J., Kerse, N., Fishman, T., et al. (2010). Validation of PHQ-2 and PHQ-9 to screen for major depression in the primary care population. *Annals of Family Medicine, 8*(4), 348–353.

Bader, C. E., Giordano, N. A., McDonald, C. C., Meghani, S. H., & Polomano, R. C. (2018). Musculoskeletal pain and headache in the active duty military population: An integrative review. *Worldviews on Evidence-Based Nursing, 15*(4), 264–271.

Bastien, C. H., Vallières, A., & Morin, C. M. (2001). Validation of the Insomnia Severity Index as an outcome measure for insomnia research. *Sleep Medicine, 2*(4), 297–307.

Bleich, S. N., Pickett-Blakely, O., & Cooper, L. A. (2011). Physician practice patterns of obesity diagnosis and weight-related counseling. *Patient Education and Counseling, 82*(1), 123–129.

Blevins, C. A., Weathers, F. W., Davis, M. T., Witte, T. K., & Domino, J. L. (2015). The Posttraumatic Stress Disorder Checklist for DSM-5 (PCL-5): Development and initial psychometric evaluation. *Journal of Traumatic Stress, 28*(6), 489–498.

Bookwalter, D. B., Porter, B., Jacobson, I. G., Kong, S. Y., Littman, A. J., Rull, R. P., et al. (2019). Healthy behaviors and incidence of overweight and obesity in military veterans. *Annals of Epidemiology, 39,* 26–32.

Boonstra, A. M., Stewart, R. E., Köke, A. J., Oosterwijk, R. F., Swaan, J. L., Schreurs, K. M., et al. (2016). Cut-off points for mild, moderate, and severe pain on the numeric rating scale for pain in patients with chronic musculoskeletal pain: Variability and influence of sex and catastrophizing. *Frontiers in Psychology, 7,* Article 1466.

Bouhassira, D., Lantéri-Minet, M., Attal, N., Laurent, B., & Touboul, C. (2008). Prevalence of chronic pain with neuropathic characteristics in the general population. *Pain, 136*(3), 380–387.

Bovin, M. J., Marx, B. P., Weathers, F. W., Gallagher, M. W., Rodriguez, P., Schnurr, P. P., et al. (2016). Psychometric properties of the PTSD Checklist for diagnostic and statistical manual of mental disorders–fifth edition (PCL-5) in veterans. *Psychological Assessment, 28*(11), 1379–1391.

Bryan, C. J., Blount, T., Kanzler, K. A., Morrow, C. E., Corso, K. A., Corso, M. A., et al. (2014). Reliability and normative data for the Behavioral Health Measure (BHM) in primary care behavioral health settings. *Families, Systems, & Health, 32*(1), 89–100.

Buckenmaier, C. C., III, Galloway, K. T., Polomano, R. C., McDuffie, M., Kwon, N., & Gallagher, R. M. (2013). Preliminary validation of the Defense and Veterans Pain Rating Scale (DVPRS) in a military population. *Pain Medicine, 14*(1), 110–123.

Buysse, D. J., Germain, A., Moul, D. E., Franzen, P. L., Brar, L. K., Fletcher, M. E., et al. (2011). Efficacy of brief behavioral treatment for chronic insomnia in older adults. *Archives of Internal Medicine, 171*(10), 887–895.

Byrne, T., & Spevak, C. (2020). The use of telepain for chronic pain in the U.S. Armed Forces: Patient experience from Walter Reed National Military Medical Center. *Military Medicine, 185*(5–6), e632–e637.

Centers for Disease Control and Prevention. (2014). *Annual number and percent distribution of ambulatory care visits by setting type according to diagnosis group, United States 2009–2010.* Retrieved from *www.cdc.gov/nchs/data/ahcd/combined_tables/2009–2010_combined_web_table01.pdf.*

Centers for Disease Control and Prevention. (2018). *Defining adult overweight and obesity.* Retrieved from *www.cdc.gov/obesity/adult/defining.html.*

Chung, F., Yegneswaran, B., Liao, P., Chung, S. A., Vairavanathan, S., Islam, S., et al. (2008). STOP Questionnaire: A tool to screen patients for obstructive sleep apnea. *Anesthesiology, 108*(5), 812–821.

Cigrang, J. A., Rauch, S. A., Mintz, J., Brundige, A. R., Mitchell, J. A., Najera, E., et al. (2017). Moving effective treatment for posttraumatic stress disorder to primary care: A randomized controlled trial with active duty military. *Families, Systems, & Health, 35*(4), 450–462.

Cleeland, C. S. (1989). Measurement of pain by subjective report. *Advances in Pain Research and Therapy, 12,* 391–403.

Collins, C., Hewson, D. L., Munger, R., & Wade, T. (2010). *Evolving models of behavioral health integration in primary care.* Milbank Memorial Fund. Retrieved from *www.milbank.org/publications/evolving-models-of-behavioral-health-integration-in-primary-care.*

Cox, B. (2015). Can the research community respond adequately to the health risks of vaping? *Addiction, 110*(11), 1708–1709.

Cox, J. L., Holden, J. M., & Sagovsky, R. (1987). Detection of postnatal depression. *British Journal of Psychiatry, 150*(6), 782–786.

Dahlhamer, J., Lucas, J., Zelaya, C., Nahin, R., Mackey, S., DeBar, L., et al. (2018). Prevalence of chronic pain and high-impact chronic pain among adults— United States, 2016. *Morbidity and Mortality Weekly Report, 67*(36), 1001– 1006.

Defense Health Agency. (2018, June 8). *Procedural instruction 6025.04: Pain management and opioid safety in the Military Health System.* Retrieved from *https://health.mil/Reference-Center/Policies/2018/06/08/DHA-PI-6025–04-Pain-Management-and-Opioid-Safety-in-the-MHS.*

Defense Health Agency. (2020, January 6). *2018 stakeholder report.* Retrieved from *https://health.mil/Reference-Center/Reports/2020/01/06/Defense-Health-Agency-2018-Stakeholder-Report.*

Department of Veterans Affairs and Department of Defense. (2017). *VA/DoD clinical practice guideline for management of post-traumatic stress disorder and acute stress disorder.* Retrieved from *www.healthquality.va.gov/guidelines/MH/ptsd/VADoDPTSDCPGFinal012418.pdf.*

Dobmeyer, A. C. (2013). Primary care behavioral health: Ethical issues in military settings. *Families, Systems, & Health, 31*(1), 60–68.

Dobmeyer, A. C., Hunter, C. L., Corso, M. L., Nielsen, M. K., Corso, K. A., Polizzi, N. C., et al. (2016). Primary care behavioral health provider yraining: Systematic development and implementation in a large medical system. *Journal of Clinical Psychology in Medical Settings, 23*(3), 207–224.

Du, S., Hu, L., Dong, J., Xu, G., Chen, X., Jin, S., et al. (2017). Self-management program for chronic low back pain: A systematic review and meta-analysis. *Patient Education and Counseling, 100*(1), 37–49.

El-Den, S., Chen, T. F., Gan, M. Y. L., Wong, M. E., & O'Reilly, C. L. (2017). The psychometric properties of depression screening tools in primary healthcare settings: A systematic review. *Journal of Affective Disorders, 225,* 503–522.

Engel, C. C., Kroenke, K., & Katon, W. J. (1994). Mental health services in Army primary care: The need for a collaborative health care agenda. *Military Medicine, 159*(3), 203–209.

Falloon, K., Elley, C. R., Fernando, A., Lee, A. C., & Arroll, B. (2015). Simplified sleep restriction for insomnia in general practice: A randomised controlled trial. *British Journal of General Practice, 65*(637), e508–e515.

Farrar, J. T., Young, J. P., Jr., LaMoreaux, L., Werth, J. L., & Poole, R. M. (2001). Clinical importance of changes in chronic pain intensity measured on an 11-point numerical pain rating scale. *Pain, 94*(2), 149–158.

Fernando, A., III, Arroll, B., & Falloon, K. (2013). A double-blind randomised controlled study of a brief intervention of bedtime restriction for adult patients with primary insomnia. *Journal of Primary Health Care, 5*(1), 5–10.

Fiore, M. C., Jaén, C. R., Baker, T. B., Bailay, W. C., Benowitz, N. L., Curry, S. J., et al. (2008). *Treating tobacco use and dependence: 2008 update* (Clinical Practice Guideline, AHRQ Publication No. 08–0050–1). Washington, DC: U.S. Department of Health and Human Services, Public Health Service.

Gagnon, C., Bélanger, L., Ivers, H., & Morin, C. M. (2013). Validation of the insomnia severity index in primary care. *Journal of the American Board of Family Medicine, 26*(6), 701–710.

Gehrman, P., Seelig, A. D., Jacobson, I. G., Boyko, E. J., Hooper, T. I., Gackstetter, G. D., et al. (2013). Predeployment sleep duration and insomnia symptoms as risk factors for new-onset mental health disorders following military deployment. *Sleep, 36*(7), 1009–1018.

Generaal, E., Vogelzanga, N., Penninx, B. W., & Dekker, J. (2017). Insomnia, sleep duration, depressive symptoms, and the onset of chronic multisite musculoskeletal pain. *Sleep, 40*(1), Article zsw030.

Goodie, J. L., Isler, W. C., Hunter, C. L., & Peterson, A. L. (2009). Using behavioral health consultants to treat insomnia in primary care: A clinical case series. *Journal of Clinical Psychology, 65*(3), 294–304.

Goodie, J. L., Kanzler, K. E., Hunter, C. L., Glotfelter, M. A., & Bodart, J. J. (2013). Ethical and effectiveness considerations with primary care behavioral health research in the medical home. *Families, Systems, & Health, 31*(1), 86–95.

Gureje, O., Von Korff, M., Simon, G. E., & Gater, R. (1998). Persistent pain and well-being: A World Health Organization study in primary care. *Journal of the American Medical Association, 280*(2), 147–151.

Hooten, W. M., Shi, Y., Gazelka, H. M., & Warner, D. O. (2011). The effects of depression and smoking on pain severity and opioid use in patients with chronic pain. *Pain, 152*(1), 223–229.

Hunter, C. L. &, Goodie, J. L. (2012). Behavioral health in the Department of Defense patient-centered medical home: History, finance, policy, work force development, and evaluation. *Translational Behavior Medicine, 2*(3), 355–363.

Hunter, C. L., Goodie, J. L., Dobmeyer, A. C., & Dorrance, K. A. (2014). Tipping points in the Department of Defense's experience with psychologists in primary care. *American Psychologist, 69*(4), 388–398.

Hunter, C. L., Goodie, J. L., Oordt, M. S., & Dobmeyer, A. C. (2017). *Integrated behavioral health in primary care: Step-by-step guidance for assessment and intervention* (2nd ed.). Washington, DC: American Psychological Association.

Hunter, C. L., & Peterson, A. L. (2001). Primary care training at Wilford Hall Medical Center. *Behavior Therapist, 24*(10), 220–222.

Isler, W. C., Peterson, A. L., & Isler, D. (2005). Behavioral treatment of insomnia in primary care settings. In L. James & R. Folen (Eds.), *The primary care consultant: The next frontier for psychologists in hospitals and clinics* (pp. 121–151). Washington, DC: American Psychological Association.

Jensen, M. D., Ryan, D. H., Apovian, C. M., Ard, J. D., Comuzzie, A. G., Donato, K. A., et al. (2014). 2013 AHA/ACC/TOS guideline for the management of overweight and obesity in adults: A report of the American College of Cardiology/American Heart Association Task Force on Practice Guidelines and the Obesity Society. *Journal of the American College of Cardiology, 63*(25B), 2985–3023.

Joint Commission. (2020). *Tobacco treatment chart abstracted measures used by the Joint Commission.* Retrieved from *www.jointcommission*.org/*measurement/measures/tobacco-treatment.*

Kanzler, K. E., Goodie, J. L., Hunter, C. L., Glotfelter, M. A., & Bodart, J. J. (2013). From colleague to patient: Ethical challenges in integrated primary care. *Families, Systems, & Health, 31*(1), 41–48.

Karyotaki, E., Smit, Y., Henningsen, K. H., Huibers, M. J. H., Robays, J., De Beurs, D., et al. (2016). Combining pharmacotherapy and psychotherapy or monotherapy for major depression? A meta-analysis on the long-term effects. *Journal of Affective Disorders, 194,* 144–152.

Katzman, J. G., Qualls, C. R., Satterfield, W. A., Kistin, M., Hofmann, K., Greenberg, N., et al. (2019). Army and Navy ECHO pain telementoring improves clinician opioid prescribing for military patients: An observational cohort study. *Journal of General Internal Medicine, 34*(3), 387–395.

Kearney, L. K., Dollar, K. M., Beehler, G. P., Goldstein, W. R., Grasso, J. R., Wray, L. O., et al. (2019). Creation and implementation of a national interprofessional integrated primary care competency training program: Preliminary findings and lessons learned. *Training and Education in Professional Psychology, 14*(3), 219–227.

Keller, P. A., Bailey, L. A., Koss, K. J., Baker, T. B., & Fiore, M. C. (2007). Organization, financing, promotion, and cost of U.S. quitlines, 2004. *American Journal of Preventive Medicine, 32*(1), 32–37.

Kessler, R. C., Petukhova, M., Sampson, N. A., Zaslavsky, A. M., & Wittchen, H.-U. (2012). Twelve-month and lifetime prevalence and lifetime morbid risk of anxiety and mood disorders in the United States. *International Journal of Methods in Psychiatric Research, 21*(3), 169–184.

Kessler, R., & Stafford, D. (2008). Primary care is the de facto mental health system. In R. Kessler & D. Stafford (Eds.), *Collaborative medicine case studies: Evidence in practice* (pp. 9–21). New York: Springer Science.

Ko, J. Y., Brown, D. R., Galuska, D. A., Zhang, J., Blanck, H. M., & Ainsworth, B. E. (2008). Weight loss advice U.S. obese adults receive from health care professionals. *Preventive Medicine, 47*(6), 587–592.

Kok, B. C., Herrell, R. K., Thomas, J. L., & Hoge, C. W. (2012). Posttraumatic stress disorder associated with combat service in Iraq or Afghanistan: Reconciling prevalence differences between studies. *Journal of Nervous and Mental Disease, 200*(5), 444–450.

Krebs, E. E., Lorenz, K. A., Bair, M. J., Damush, T. M., Wu, J., Sutherland, J. M., et al. (2009). Development and initial validation of the PEG, a three-item scale assessing pain intensity and interference. *Journal of General Internal Medicine, 24*(6), 733–738.

Kroenke, K., Spitzer, R. L., & Williams, J. B. W. (2001). The PHQ-9: Validity of a brief depression severity measure. *Journal of General Internal Medicine, 16*(9), 606–613.

Kroenke, K., Spitzer, R. L., Williams, J. B., & Löwe, B. (2009). An ultra-brief screening scale for anxiety and depression: The PHQ–4. *Psychosomatics, 50*(6), 613–621.

Larkin, K. T., Bridges, A. J., Fields, S. A., & Vogel, M. E. (2016). Acquiring competencies in integrated behavioral health care in doctoral, internship, and postdoctoral programs. *Training and Education in Professional Psychology, 10*(1), 14–23.

Marx, B. P., & Sloan, D. M. (2019) *Written exposure therapy for PTSD: A brief treatment approach for mental health providers.* Washington, DC: American Psychological Association.

McDaniel, S. H., Grus, C. L., Cubic, B. A., Hunter, C. L., Kearney, L. K., Schuman, C. C., et al. (2014). Competencies for psychology practice in primary care. *American Psychologist, 69*(4), 409–429.

McGeary, D. D., McGeary, C. A., & Gatchel, R. J. (2012). A comprehensive review of telehealth for pain management: Where we are and the way ahead. *Pain Practice, 12*(7), 570–577.

McGeary, D., Moore, M., Vriend, C. A., Peterson, A. L., & Gatchel, R. J. (2011). The evaluation and treatment of comorbid pain and PTSD in a military setting: An overview. *Journal of Clinical Psychology in Medical Settings, 18,* 155–163.

McGeary, D. D., Resick, P., Penzien, D. B., Eapen, B. C., Jaramillo, C., McGeary, C. A., et al. (2020). Reason to doubt the ICHD-3 7-day inclusion criterion for mild TBI-related posttraumatic headache: A nested cohort study. *Cephalalgia, 40*(11), 1155–1167.

Meadows, S. O., Engel, R. C., Collins, R. B., Beckman, R. L., Cefalu, M., Hawes-Dawson, J., et al. (2018). *2015 Department of Defense Health Related Behaviors Survey (HRBS).* Santa Monica, CA: RAND Corporation. Retrieved from *www.rand.org/pubs/research_reports/RR1695.html.*

Mitchell, A. J., Rao, S., & Vaze, A. (2010). Do primary care physicians have particular difficulty identifying late-life depression? A meta-analysis stratified by age. *Psychotherapy and Psychosomatics, 79*(5), 285–294.

Moriarty, A. S., Gilbody, S., McMillan, D., & Manea, L. (2015). Screening and case finding for major depressive disorder using the Patient Health Questionnaire (PHQ-9): A meta-analysis. *General Hospital Psychiatry, 37*(6), 567–576.

Morone, N. E., & Weiner, D. K. (2013). Pain as the fifth vital sign: Exposing the vital need for pain education. *Clinical Therapeutics, 35*(11), 1728–1732.

Moyer, V. A. (2013). Screening and behavioral counseling interventions in primary care to reduce alcohol misuse: U.S. Preventive Services Task Force recommendation statement. *Annals of Internal Medicine, 159*(3), 210–218.

Murphy, J. L., McKellar, J. D., Raffa, S. D., Clark, M. E., Kerns, R. D., & Karlin, B. E. (2014). *Cognitive behavioral therapy for chronic pain among veterans: Therapist manual.* Washington, DC: U.S. Department of Veterans Affairs. Retrieved from *www.va.gov/PAINMANAGEMENT/docs/CBT-CP_Therapist_Manual.pdf.*

Mysliwiec, V., McGraw, L., Pierce, R., Smith, P., Trapp, B., & Roth, B. J. (2013). Sleep disorders and associated medical comorbidities in active duty military personnel. *Sleep, 36*(2), 167–174.

Netzer, N. C., Stoohs, R. A., Netzer, C. M., Clark, K., & Strohl, K. P. (1999).

Using the Berlin Questionnaire to identify patients at risk for the sleep apnea syndrome. *Annals of Internal Medicine, 131*(7), 485–491.

Nugraha, B., Gutenbrunner, C., Barke, A., Karst, M., Schiller, J., Schäfer, P., et al. (2019). The IASP classification of chronic pain for ICD-11: Functioning properties of chronic pain. *Pain, 160*(1), 88–94.

Office of the Army Surgeon General (2010). *Pain Management Task Force—Final report.* Retrieved from *www.dvcipm.org/site/assets/files/1070/pain-task-force-final-report-may-2010.pdf.*

Peterson, A. L. (2018). I don't know where we're going, but I sure know where we've been: Continuing the journey of empirically supported treatments in primary care. *Clinical Psychology: Science and Practice, 25*(3), Article e12245.

Peterson, A. L., Severson, H. H., Andrews, J. A., Gott, S. P., Cigrang, J. A., Gordon, J. S., et al. (2007). Smokeless tobacco use in military personnel. *Military Medicine, 172*(12), 1300–1305.

Peterson, A. L., Vander Weg, M. W., & Jaén, C. R. (2011). *Nicotine and tobacco dependence.* Newburyport, MA: Hogrefe & Huber.

Phelan, S. M., Burgess, D. J., Yeazel, M. W., Hellerstedt, W. L., Griffin, J. M., & van Ryn, M. (2015). Impact of weight bias and stigma on quality of care and outcomes for patients with obesity. *Obesity Reviews, 16*(4), 319–326.

Polomano, R. C., Galloway, K. T., Kent, M. L., Brandon-Edwards, H., Kwon, K. N., Morales, C., et al. (2016). Psychometric testing of the Defense and Veterans Pain Rating Scale (DVPRS): A new pain scale for military population. *Pain Medicine, 17*(8), 1505–1519.

Prins, A., Bovin, M. J., Smolenski, D. J., Marx, B. P., Kimerling, R., Jenkins-Guarnieri, M. A., et al. (2016). The Primary Care PTSD Screen for DSM-5 (PC-PTSD-5): Development and evaluation within a veteran primary care sample. *Journal of General Internal Medicine, 31*(10), 1206–1211.

Raja, S. N., Carr, D. B., Cohen, M., Finnerup, N. B., Flor, H., Gibson, S., et al. (2020). The revised International Association for the Study of Pain definition of pain: Concepts, challenges, and compromises. *Pain, 161*(9), 1976–1982.

Ram, S., Seirawan, H., Kumar, S. K., & Clark, G. T. (2010). Prevalence and impact of sleep disorders and sleep habits in the United States. *Sleep and Breathing, 14*(1), 63–70.

Reif, S., Adams, R. S., Ritter, G. A., Williams, T. V., & Larson, M. J. (2018). Prevalence of pain diagnoses and burden of pain among active duty soldiers, FY2012. *Military Medicine, 183*(9–10), e330–e337.

Reiter J. T., Dobmeyer A. C., & Hunter C. L. (2018). The Primary Care Behavioral Health (PCBH) Model: An overview and operational definition. *Journal of Clinical Psychology in Medical Settings, 25*(2), 109–126.

Riemann, D., & Perlis, M. L. (2009). The treatments of chronic insomnia: A review of benzodiazepine receptor agonists and psychological and behavioral therapies. *Sleep Medicine Reviews, 13*(3), 205–214.

Runyan, C. N., Carter-Henry, S., & Ogbeide, S. (2018). Ethical challenges unique to the Primary Care Behavioral Health (PCBH) Model. *Journal of Clinical Psychology in Medical Settings, 25*(2), 224–236.

Runyan, C. N., Robinson, P., & Gould, D. A. (2013). Ethical issues facing providers in collaborative primary care settings: Do current guidelines suffice to guide the future of team based primary care? *Families, Systems, & Health, 31*(1), 1–8.

Rush, T., LeardMann, C. A., & Crum-Cianflone, N. F. (2016). Obesity and associated adverse health outcomes among U.S. military members and veterans: Findings from the Millennium Cohort Study. *Obesity, 24*(7), 1582–1589.

Rutledge, T., Atkinson, J. H., Holloway, R., Chircop-Rollick, T., D'Andrea, J., Garfin, S. R., et al. (2018). Randomized controlled trial of nurse-delivered cognitive-behavioral therapy versus supportive psychotherapy telehealth interventions for chronic back pain. *Journal of Pain, 19*(9), 1033–1039.

Sadock, E., Auerbach, S. M., Rybarczyk, B., & Aggarwal, A. (2013). Evaluation of integrated psychological services in a university-based primary care clinic. *Journal of Clinical Psychology in Medical Settings, 21*(1), 19–32.

Severson, H. H., Klein, K., Lichtenstein, E., Kaufman, N., & Orleans, C. T. (2005). Smokeless tobacco use among professional baseball players: Survey results, 1998 to 2003. *Tobacco Control, 14*(1), 31–36.

Sharma, A. M. (2003). Obesity and cardiovascular risk. *Growth Hormone & IGF Research, 13*(Suppl.), S10–S17.

Simon, G. E., Rutter, C. M., Peterson, D., Oliver, M., Whiteside, U., Operskalski, B., et al. (2013). Does response on the PHQ-9 depression questionnaire predict subsequent suicide attempt or suicide death? *Psychiatric Services, 64*(12), 1195–1202.

Steer, R. A., Cavalieri, T. A., Leonard, D. M., & Beck, A. T. (1999). Use of the Beck Depression Inventory for Primary Care to screen for major depression disorders. *General Hospital Psychiatry, 21*(2), 106–111.

Steingrímsdóttir, Ó. A., Landmark, T., Macfarlane, G. J., & Nielsen, C. S. (2017). Defining chronic pain in epidemiological studies: A systematic review and meta-analysis. *Pain, 158*(11), 2092–2107.

Strosahl, K. D. (2005). Training behavioral health and primary care providers for integrated care: A core competencies approach. In W. T. O'Donohue, M. R. Byrd, N. A. Cummings, & D. A. Henderson (Eds.), *Behavioral integrative care: Treatments that work in the primary care setting* (pp. 15–52). New York: Brunner-Routledge.

Strosahl, K. D., & Sobel, D. (1996). Behavioral health and the medical cost offset effect: Current status, key concepts and future applications. *HMO Practitioner, 10*(4), 156–162.

Stubbs, R., & Lavin, J. (2013). The challenges of implementing behaviour changes that lead to sustained weight management. *Nutrition Bulletin, 38*(1), 5–22.

Troxel, W. M., Germain, A., & Buysse, D. J. (2012). Clinical management of insomnia with brief behavioral treatment (BBTI). *Behavioral Sleep Medicine, 10*(4), 266–279.

Vander Weg, M. W., DeBon, M., Peterson, A. L., Mittleman, D., Klesges, R. C., & Relyea, G. E. (2005). Prevalence and correlates of smokeless tobacco use among female military recruits. *Nicotine & Tobacco Research, 7*(3), 431–441.

van Emmerik, A. A., Kamphuis, J. H., & Emmelkamp, P. M. (2008). Treating acute stress disorder and posttraumatic stress disorder with cognitive behavioral therapy or structured writing therapy: A randomized controlled trial. *Psychotherapy and Psychosomatics, 77*(2), 93–100.

Walser, R. D., & Westrup, D. (2007). *Acceptance and commitment therapy for the treatment of post-traumatic stress disorder and trauma-related problems: A practitioner's guide to using mindfulness and acceptance strategies.* Oakland, CA: New Harbinger.

Weathers, F. W., Litz, B. T., Keane, T. M., Palmieri, P. A., Marx, B. P., & Schnurr, P. P. (2013). *The PTSD Checklist for DSM–5 (PCL-5)*. Washington, DC: U.S. Department of Veterans Affairs, National Center for PTSD. Retrieved from *www.ptsd.va.gov/professional/assessment/adult-sr/ptsd-checklist.asp*.

Whitlock, E. P., Orleans, C. T., Pender, N., & Allan, J. (2002). Evaluating primary care behavioral counseling interventions: An evidence-based approach. *American Journal of Preventive Medicine, 22*(4), 267–284.

Williams, J. I., Bishop, F. M., Hennen, B. K., & Johnson, T. W. (1974). The teaching of behavioural sciences in the family medicine residency programs in Canada and in the United States. *Social Science and Medicine, 8*(11–12), 565–574.

Wilson, J. F. (2007). Posttraumatic stress disorder needs to be recognized in primary care. *Annals of Internal Medicine. 146*(8), 617–620.

Wortmann, J. H., Jordan, A. H., Weathers, F. W., Resick, P. A., Dondanville, K. A., Hall-Clark, B., et al. (2016). Psychometric analysis of the PTSD Checklist-5 (PCL-5) among treatment-seeking military service members. *Psychological Assessment, 28*(11), 1392–1403.

CHAPTER 6

Managing Military-Specific Concussion for the General Practitioner

Heather G. Belanger, Patrick Armistead-Jehle,
Jessica Parker, Sara M. Lippa, and Eveline F. Yao

Traumatic brain injury (TBI) has become the focus of considerable clinical and research efforts in both the Department of Defense (DoD) and the Department of Veterans Affairs (VA) due to the prolonged nature of conflicts in Iraq and Afghanistan, the frequent use of explosive devices, and attention by the media. According to the Defense and Veterans Brain Injury Center (DVBIC[1]; 2021), between 2000 and 2019, there were approximately 414,000 active-duty military service members who sustained a TBI. The vast majority (80–95%) of TBIs were classified as mild (mTBI) or, more colloquially, concussion. The terms mTBI and concussion are typically used interchangeably. Systemwide concussion screening programs within DoD and VA have led to an increasing focus on identification, assessment, and treatment. This, in turn, has led to an increasing need for clinical expertise and evaluations related to concussion. This chapter will focus on military-specific concussion, with a basic introduction to identification, assessment, and management, including when a referral is appropriate. It is geared toward the general psychologist practitioner who undoubtedly has seen an increase in concussion-related complaints in recent years.

Despite the attention given to brain injuries sustained in the combat theater, documented concussions more frequently occur in garrison. Service members routinely engage in physically demanding training and operational activities that increases their risk. Additionally, the majority of service

---

[1] DVBIC is now called TBICoE (TBI Center of Excellence).

members are men between 18 to 24 years of age, and this particular demographic carries a higher risk for concussion via motor vehicle accidents and sporting events, independent of military service. Even with the significant reduction of service members deployed overseas in support of combat, TBI and concussion will continue to be a condition of interest in the military.

CONCUSSION BASICS

A concussion occurs when an external force impacts the brain, disrupting its functioning. VA and DoD clinical practice guidelines (CPGs) define a concussion as a brain injury with normal structural neuroimaging and up to 24 hours' alteration of consciousness (AOC), up to a day of posttraumatic amnesia (PTA), or up to 30 minutes of loss of consciousness (LOC) (Department of Veterans Affairs and Department of Defense, 2016). It is important to distinguish concussions from moderate, severe, and penetrating TBIs, which generally have longer duration of LOC, PTA, AOC; may have abnormal structural neuroimaging; and often result in different prognostic recovery trajectories and outcomes.

Objective neuropsychological testing reveals a reduction in cognitive functioning across most domains in the acute phase of concussion that generally returns to baseline within 3 months of injury (Belanger, Tate, & Vanderploeg, 2018). Other factors, including psychiatric symptoms, use of benzodiazepines, litigation, and invalid responses, can impact neuropsychological test scores with relatively large deleterious effects (Iverson, 2005). Sleep disturbance, pain, substance abuse, social support, coping abilities, beliefs about concussion, and expectations for recovery may also impact cognitive performance and other outcomes (Belanger et al., 2018). Therefore, identification, treatment, and management of these and other potential comorbidities and contributing factors are clearly important.

A number of physical or somatic (e.g., headaches, fatigue, nausea/vomiting), cognitive (e.g., attention, memory, processing speed), vestibular (e.g., balance, dizziness, vertigo, nausea/vomiting), and affective (e.g., depressed mood, anxiety, irritability, psychiatric disorders) symptoms may occur immediately following a concussion. These symptoms may resolve within hours (Iverson, 2005), but generally last no longer than 3 months if there are no other contributing factors (McCrea, 2008). When postconcussion symptoms linger, diagnostic criteria for postconcussional syndrome per the *International Statistical Classification of Disease and Related Health*, Tenth Edition (ICD-10; World Health Organization, 1992) may be met. It is notable that the diagnosis of postconcussion disorder was removed in the fifth edition of the *Diagnostic and Statistical Manual of Mental Disorders* (DSM-5; American Psychiatric Association, 2013). This may be due to the fact that these post-event symptoms do not tend to change together over time, as is typical for a syndrome (Belanger et al., 2018). Postconcussion symptoms are nonspecific, making the diagnosis more challenging as these symptoms are common in patients with bodily injuries but without concussion (Meares et al., 2011), psychiatric disorders (Donnell, Kim, Silva, & Vanderploeg, 2012), and even healthy college students (Wang, Chan, & Deng, 2006). It has been suggested that if symptoms persist for several months in multiple domains resulting in functional impairment, the term postconcussion syndrome not be used. Rather, *persistent symptoms that occur after a concussion* is recommended as this allows for acknowledgment that multiple factors have played a role in maintaining and/or propagating these symptoms (Silva & Kay, 2013).

Psychiatric disorders, most commonly depression, anxiety, and post-traumatic stress disorder (PTSD), are more prevalent following concussion than in the general population. Depression is the most common psychiatric diagnosis following TBI and may be the result of premorbid risk factors, psychological reaction to the injury and related psychosocial factors, and/or neurological dysfunction (Belanger et al., 2018). Post-injury depression (Iverson et al., 2017), anxiety (Silverberg et al., 2015), combat stress (Kennedy et al., 2012), and PTSD (Hoge et al., 2008) have all been clearly linked to worse outcomes. Importantly, premorbid psychological disorders increase the likelihood of psychiatric diagnosis following concussion (Belanger et al., 2018). Indeed, pre-injury mental health has been implicated as one of the most important factors in recovery from concussion (Iverson et al., 2017; Silverberg et al., 2015).

In contrast to psychiatric, medical, and psychosocial factors, neuroimaging findings tend not to play a significant role in concussion recovery (Lange, Yeh, Brickell, Lippa, & French, 2019). Magnetic resonance imaging (MRI) scans may reveal white matter hyperintensities (i.e., abnormal changes seen in the white matter of the brain) in patients with a history of concussion. At times, patients may focus on these white matter hyperintensities as a sign of lasting brain damage from their injury. However, white matter hyperintensities are nonspecific, and can also result from normal aging (Lindemer, Greve, Fischl, Augustinack, & Salat, 2017) or other conditions to include migraines (Aradi et al., 2013). In a study of 152 active-duty service members (Tate et al., 2017), the presence of white matter hyperintensities was not significantly different between participants with concussion (41%), orthopedic injuries only (49%), and PTSD only (29%). Therefore, the presence of white matter hyperintensities cannot be used as diagnostic criteria for postconcussive complications. Additionally, white matter hyperintensities were not increased in patients diagnosed with post-concussion syndrome compared to controls without a history of concussion (Panwar, Hsu, Tator, & Mikulis, 2020) and generally have not been found to be related to postconcussive symptom severity (Clark et al., 2016; Tate et al., 2017). In contrast, lesions found with susceptibility weighted imaging, or microbleeds, have been shown to be relatively specific to TBI, though they are not necessarily correlated with worse symptom reporting or cognitive functioning in concussed patients (Tate et al., 2017). Diffusion tensor imaging (DTI) has shown alterations in white matter integrity following concussion that correlate to objective cognitive performance as well as subjective symptoms, though these findings are not universal across studies (Asken, DeKosky, Clugston, Jaffee, & Bauer, 2018). DTI is not currently used clinically.

BLAST VERSUS NON-BLAST TBI

TBIs have historically been associated with blunt force trauma. Prolonged conflicts in Afghanistan and Iraq have featured frequent use of improvised explosive devices (IED), explosively formed penetrator (EFP) rockets, and mortars, and as such, the phenomenon of blast-force trauma has gained increased attention. As alluded to above, the majority of military-related TBIs occur in garrison and stem from causes similar to nonmilitary injuries (i.e., MVAs and blows to the head with falls, hits, or assaults); however, the majority of combat-related TBIs involve blast-related forces (DVBIC, 2020; Owens et al., 2008). For instance, Owens and colleagues (2008) report that an explosive mechanism accounted for 81% of all injuries in Iraq and Afghanistan, while gunshot wounds accounted for 19%. The authors note that this is the highest percentage of explosive injuries in any U.S. conflict.

Blast injuries are not a unitary insult, but rather encompass up to five separate types of injuries incurred either directly or indirectly from a blast. These consist of the following: (1) primary injury from the pressure wave; (2) possible secondary injury from blunt or penetrating trauma (i.e., fragments of debris propelled by the explosion); (3) tertiary translation force injuries (e.g., being forced to the ground or against an adjacent object from the blast); (4) quarternary heat and burn injuries; and (5) quinary indirect injures such as chemical exposure or hypoxia.

Non-combat-related blast injuries from breacher training have also become the focus of increased research attention (Carr, Polejaeva, et al., 2015; Carr, Stone, et al., 2016; Tate et al., 2013). There is mounting concern (by service members, the medical community, and legislators) that repeated low-level blast exposures, which do not result in subsequent LOC, PTA, or even AOC, could lead to physiological disruption. These types of experiences have been termed subconcussive injuries.

Research surrounding blast-related TBIs has focused predominantly on two areas: (1) the possibility of unique physiological disruptions subsequent to blast exposure and (2) whether or not there are functional outcomes that differ from blunt force TBI. With regard to the former, research findings suggesting neuroanatomical disruption from blast are varied. For instance, Ivanov et al. (2017) concluded that combat veterans with blast exposure but no TBI compared to combat veterans with a remote history of blast-related TBI had poorer white matter integrity on DTI, particularly in the left cingulum. Newsome et al. (2016) demonstrated that combat veterans with a history of blast-related TBI had compromised functional connectivity in the globus pallidus relative to demographically similar veterans with no history of TBI or blast exposure. In a case series, Martindale and colleagues (2018) found changes in white matter hyperintensities related to severity of blast exposure. Shively et al. (2016) found that blast exposure produced unique brain lesions in postmortem veterans with histories of blast exposure. More specifically, blast-exposed brains had prominent astroglial scarring at neuroanatomical boundary zones between tissue and fluid and between gray and white matter junctions. Mu and colleagues (2017) conducted a review of imaging in blast-related mTBI and found a number of studies revealed decreased cortical thickness and decreased thalamus and amygdala volume, as well as white matter tract abnormalities (including the corpus callosum and superior longitudinal fasciculus). However, the Mu et al. study also noted that clear variations across study designs and methods precluded the formulation of salient conclusions regarding the pathomechanisms of blast-related TBI.

Research to identify any potentially different functional outcomes between blast and non-blast-related TBIs has also been conducted. While the current data indicate that there may be unique aspects of brain disruption associated with blast injury, several studies have suggested that functional outcomes are generally similar to non-blast injuries. After covarying for psychiatric symptoms, Lange et al. (2012) reported no additive effect of a blast plus blunt force trauma injury over a blunt force trauma injury alone on various cognitive measures. Belanger et al. (2009) and Cooper et al. (2012) found similar nonsignificant differences across cognitive measures when comparing blast and non-blast-related groups. Moreover, the previously mentioned Ivanov et al. (2017) study, which demonstrated diminished left cingulum white matter integrity in blast-injured combat veterans, failed to show any relationship between blast exposure and standardized cognitive measures. Belanger and colleagues (2010) found no differences between blast and non-blast TBI groups in a sample of veterans more than a month post-injury, save a higher degree of hearing complaints in the blast group. To this end, outside of possible hearing issues, there appear to be no functional differences between blast and non-blast TBIs outlined in the current literature. Finally, the available literature indicates that low-level blast exposure is associated with biological markers of neurological dysfunction and deficiencies in aspects of cognition (Carr et al., 2016; Tate et al., 2013). However, these deficiencies resolved within 2 weeks following the last blast exposure (Tate et al., 2013). This literature, however, is incomplete and continues to develop (see Belanger et al., 2020, for a review).

CHRONIC TRAUMATIC ENCEPHALOPATHY

One issue that has garnered significant media attention on concussion, largely related to professional sports, is chronic traumatic encephalopathy (CTE), hypothesized to be secondary to repetitive blunt force head trauma and to represent a distinct neurodegenerative condition that leads to long-term cognitive, neurological, and neurobehavioral problems (McKee et al., 2009). The prevalence, cause, and clinical criteria for CTE are unknown, yet recent media reports suggest otherwise. Public awareness about repetitive brain trauma is positive from a preventive perspective, but tends to create the impression that more is known about CTE than is actually the case. It is therefore imperative that clinical providers be educated about CTE as to best inform patients and avoid perpetuating misinformation.

Pathologically, recently proposed preliminary consensus criteria for CTE include the pathognomonic presence of an accumulation of abnormal p-tau in neurons, astrocytes, and cell processes around small vessels in an irregular pattern at the depths of the cortical sulci (McKee et al., 2016). However, the sensitivity and specificity of these criteria are unknown. In addition, there are no current clinical diagnostic criteria for CTE, and the proposed clinical features are broad. These clinical symptoms are highly variable and nonspecific to CTE pathology, and include diverse disorders and symptoms including depression, anxiety, PTSD, alcohol/substance abuse/dependence, dysarthria, dysphagia, gaze disturbance, chronic pain, anabolic steroid use, coronary artery disease, headaches, suicide, aggression, dementia, poor impulse control, gait instability/parkinsonism, ocular deficits, cognitive difficulties, paranoid ideations, poor insight, disinhibition, inappropriate sexual behavior, apathy, and risk taking (Mez, Stern, & McKee, 2013; Omalu et al., 2011; Stern et al., 2013). Proposed clinical subtypes based on symptom presentation and onset have not been validated, and there are no operational clinical diagnostic criteria for these proposed subtypes. Overall, more systematic, prospective, and longitudinal research is needed to determine the risk of CTE and whether there is an association between repetitive head impacts or concussion and CTE.

For providers, Belanger et al. (2020) provide a three-phased schematic approach for intervening with individuals who have repetitive head impact and/or concussion histories and are concerned about CTE. This approach includes (1) assessment and education, (2) targeted interventions for specific symptoms and comorbidities (e.g., sleep disturbance, headache, depression), and (3) psychotherapy to address mental health concerns (see Case 6.1 that follows later in this chapter). This specific strategy also applies to management of concussion writ large (see below for specific clinical recommendations).

RELEVANT MILITARY INSTRUCTIONS AND GUIDELINES

The DoD has generated a number of publications that inform the military's approach to concussion management (Table 6.1). In 2004, the VA and DoD partnered to establish an Evidenced Based Practice Working Group (EBPWG) to develop CPGs, informing physical medicine and behavioral health care among their respective populations. The Management of Concussion-mTBI CPG was first published in 2009. It has been revised several times since its initial release, with the most recent version published in February 2016 (Department of Veterans Affairs and Department of Defense, 2016). Originally intended to assist primary-care providers with the diagnosis, assessment, treatment, and follow-up of mTBI patients, the CPG was utilized across health care disciplines and shaped the standard of care for physical and behavioral health providers alike. In addition to the comprehensive Management of Concussion-mTBI CPG, the accompanying mTBI Clinician Summary, Patient Summary, and Pocket Card CPG tools are also available for provider and patient use (Department of Veterans Affairs and Department of Defense, 2021).

The Management of Concussion-mTBI CPG (Department of Veterans Affairs and Department of Defense, 2021) includes a discussion of 23 evidence-based recommendations for the diagnosis and assessment, co-occurring conditions, treatment, and setting of care for mTBI management, several of which pertain specifically to cognitive symptoms and are subsequently reviewed. Particularly relevant to psychologists, the review concluded that post-mTBI cognitive symptoms tend to resolve within hours to days following an injury, and there is an absence of a clear relationship between self-report and cognitive assessment findings 30 days postconcussion. The CPG provides a "strong against" recommendation for neuropsychological testing within 30 days following a concussion (Recommendation 4). For patients with a concussion history who continue to report cognitive symptoms 30 days or more postconcussion and are refractory to treatment, the CPG posits a "weak for" recommendation for administration of a structured cognitive assessment to determine functional limitations and assist with treatment planning (Recommendation 17). For patients identified via postdeployment screening or who present for care with complaints possibly associated with a concussion, the CPG provides a "strong against" recommendation for comprehensive neuropsychological testing (including the Automated Neuropsychological Assessment Metrics, Neurocognitive Assessment Tool, or Immediate Post-Concussion Assessment and Cognitive Testing) for routine diagnostic and treatment purposes (Recommendation 5), based on insufficient evidence in the literature for doing so.

With regard to managing postconcussive cognitive symptoms, the CPG (Department of Veterans Affairs and Department of Defense, 2021) offers a "weak for" recommendation for referral to cognitive rehabilitation with a mTBI rehabilitation therapist for patients with a history of mTBI presenting with treatment refractory cognitive complaints 30 to 90 days post-event. However, prolonged therapy, in the absence of symptom improvement, has a "strong against" recommendation (Recommendation 18). The CPG Working Group noted that treatment specialists must consider comorbid and pre-existing conditions (to include psychological diagnoses) as these may reduce cognitive functioning. The use of medication, supplements, nutraceuticals, or herbal medicine is also not recommended for treating cognitive complaints associated with concussion (Recommendation 19) due to the lack of demonstrated evidence and potential harmful effects in this population.

Two algorithms, Module A: Initial Presentation and Module B: Management of Symptoms Persisting > 7 Days (Figures 6.1 and 6.2), provide clinicians with a diagnostic and therapeutic decision-making framework for assessing service members at critical junctures. As providers progress through the clinical decision-making algorithms, they may utilize the specific and detailed symptom evaluation and management recommendations provided in the CPG to guide treatment planning and referrals.

In addition to the CPG, the DoD released several TBI instruction memorandums, to include guidance on mTBI management in a deployed setting and TBI neuropsychological assessment. As with all DoD instructions, the services follow DoD guidance and ensure that subsequent service-specific policies created align with DoD instruction.

DoD Policy Guidance for Management of mTBI/Concussion in the Deployed Setting (Department of Defense Instruction 6490.11; Department of Defense, 2019) established that DoD components will identify, track, and ensure evaluation and treatment of service members exposed to potentially concussive events, and those with medically documented concussions will be managed in accordance with the DoD clinical practice theater guidelines and documented in the service member's electronic health record. Commanders or their designated representatives will report exposure and assessment of all service members, using an Injury/Evaluation/Distance (I.E.D) Checklist, who were, at minimum, involved in a vehicle blast/collision/rollover event, within 50 meters of a blast radius; experienced a direct blow to the head or loss of consciousness; or were exposed to more than one blast event. The I.E.D. Checklist assesses for bodily harm (I/Injury), concussion-related symptoms such as vomiting and dizziness (E/Evaluation), and proximity to the blast (D/Distance). Service members involved in a potentially concussive event or who respond "yes" to any of the I.E.D. Checklist questions or demonstrate listed symptoms post-injury should be referred for medical evaluation. Medical guidance, in accordance with DVBIC guidance (2019), emphasizes post-event rest periods. These guidelines inform medical providers and encourage command support for a required 24-hour rest period after a potentially concussive

A. Module A: Initial Presentation (>7 Days Post-injury)

1 Person injured with head trauma resulting in alteration or loss of consciousness

2 Urgent/emergent conditions identified? (See sidebar 1) — Yes →

No

4 Evaluate for severity of TBI based on history (See sidebar 2)

3 Refer for emergency evaluation and treatment

5 Is the severity moderate or severe TBI? — Yes →

No

6 Consult with TBI specialist; Exit Algorithm

7 Diagnosis of concussion/mTBI: Are symptoms present? (See sidebar 3) — Yes →

9 Is person currently deployed on military or combat operation? — Yes →

10 **Follow** DoD Policy guidance for management of mTBI/concussion in the deployed setting

No (from 7)

8
- Provide education and access to information regarding concussion/mTBI (See section on educational resources)
- Provide usual care
- Follow-up as indicated

No (from 9)

11 **Go to Algorithm B** Management of Symptoms Persisting >7 days

Sidebar 1: Indicators for Immediate Referral

1. Progressively declining level of consciousness
2. Progressively declining neurological exam
3. Pupillary asymmetry
4. Seizures
5. Repeated vomiting
6. Neurological deficit: motor or sensory
7. Double vision
8. Worsening headache
9. Cannot recognize people or disoriented to place
10. Slurred speech
11. Unusual behavior

Sidebar 2: Classification of TBI Severity
(If a patient meets criteria in more than one category of severity, the higher severity level is assigned)

Criteria	Mild	Moderate	Severe
Structural imaging, see Recommendation 3	Normal	Normal or abnormal	Normal or abnormal
Loss of Consciousness (LOC)	0-30 min	>30 min and <24 hours	>24 hours
Alteration of consciousness/ mental state (AOC)*	up to 24 hours	>24 hours; severity based on other criteria	
Posttraumatic amnesia (PTA)	0-1 day	>1 and <7 days	>7 days
Glasgow Coma Scale (GCS) (best available score in first 24 hours)**	13-15	9-12	<9

Sidebar 3: Possible Post-mTBI Related Symptoms***

Physical Symptoms:
Headache, dizziness, balance disorders, nausea, fatigue, sleep disturbance, blurred vision, sensitivity to light, hearing difficulties/loss, tinnitus, sensitivity to noise, seizure, transient neurological abnormalities, numbness, tingling

Cognitive Symptoms:
Problems with attention, concentration, memory, speed of processing, judgment, executive control

Behavior/Emotional Symptoms:
Depression, anxiety, agitation, irritability, impulsivity, aggression

*Alteration of mental status must be immediately related to the trauma to the head. Typical symptoms would be: looking and feeling dazed and uncertain of what is happening, confusion, difficulty thinking clearly or responding appropriately to mental status questions, and being unable to describe events immediately before or after the trauma event.
**In April 2015, the DoD released a memorandum recommending against the use of GCS scores to diagnose TBI. See the memorandum for additional information.
***Symptoms that may develop within 30 days post injury.

FIGURE 6.1. VA/DOD Clinical Practice Guideline for Management of Concussion/ Mild Traumatic Brain Injury: Version 2.0. Module A: initial presentation (> 7 days post-injury). Public domain. Department of Veterans Affairs and Department of Defense (2021).

B. Module B: Management of Symptoms Persisting >7 days

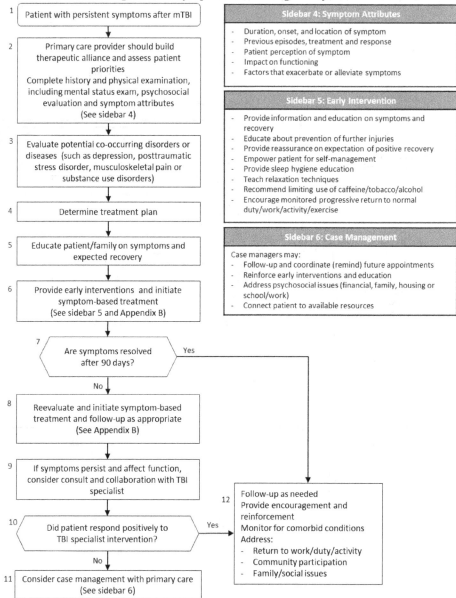

FIGURE 6.2. VA/DOD Clinical Practice Guideline for Management of Concussion/ Mild Traumatic Brain Injury: Version 2.0. Module B: management of symptoms persisting > 7 days. Public domain. Department of Veterans Affairs and Department of Defense (2021).

event. Service members diagnosed with a first concussive event must have a minimum 24-hour rest period unless clinical evaluation indicates a longer period is necessary. Service members diagnosed with two concussive events in a 12-month period should delay returning to duty 7 days following symptom resolution. A history of three diagnosed concussions over a 12-month period delays returning to duty until a recurrent concussion evaluation has been completed. Commanders have the latitude to impose longer recovery periods in consultation with medical personnel. Similar guidelines for recovery based on number of previous concussions have also been mandated for the garrison environment.

Specific to mTBI neuropsychological assessment practices, DoD Instruction 6490.13 (March 2017), *Comprehensive Policy on Traumatic Brain Injury-Related Neurocognitive Assessments by the Military Services,* designated the Army as the Military Health System (MHS) lead for testing and determined that all service members and DoD civilians across the deployment cycle will undergo computerized neurocognitive assessment. The current DoD designated neurocognitive assessment tool is the Automated Neuropsychological Assessment Metrics (ANAM). A predeployment baseline ANAM is administered within 12 months prior to deployment. Per instruction and in accordance with DVBIC guidelines, post-injury assessment is completed after a diagnosed concussion, comparing baseline and post-injury results to inform return to duty decisions. Of note, neurocognitive assessment measures, such as the ANAM, are not to be used as stand-alone diagnostic tools. Service members endorsing head injury-related questions on the Post-Deployment Health Assessment are referred for additional evaluation and potential neurocognitive test administration. Service-level programs may establish additional guidance that incorporates the aforementioned core testing elements. As an example, in 2019, U.S. Special Operations Command (SOCOM) instituted a new brain health policy (USSOCOM Policy Memorandum 19-01) mandating the establishment of a baseline cognitive assessment followed by periodic cognitive assessments using ANAM, documentation of historical symptoms and exposure baseline with periodic updates, and a requirement for at-risk operators to wear blast gauges in relevant training and deployment settings to capture overt and subconcussive repetitive blast exposures. In addition, a working group was formed to evaluate ongoing brain health efforts and current science, and to adapt to changing requirements of the force. This brain health policy only applies to those personnel working within the SOCOM enterprise.

MILITARY-SPECIFIC ASSESSMENT TOOLS

While many of the neuropsychological measures employed in the civilian sector to evaluate and treat TBI are applicable in military settings, there are

TABLE 6.1. Military Concussion Instructions and Guidelines

Instruction	Title	Purpose	Population
DoD/VA clinical practice guidelines (CPG)	*The Management of Concussion-Mild Traumatic Brain Injury*[a]	Assists providers in managing patients with a history of mTBI via a review of evidence-based recommendations for diagnosis and assessment, co-occurring conditions, treatment, and setting of care.	Applies to adults eligible for care in the VHA and DoD health care systems
DoDI 6490.11	*DoD Policy Guidance for Management of Mild Traumatic Brain Injury/ Concussion in the Deployed Setting*	Establishes the identification, tracking, evaluation, and treatment of service members exposed to potentially concussive events, and those with medically documented concussions are managed in accordance with DoD clinical practice theater guidelines and are documented in the electronic medical record.	Applies to the military departments
DoDI 6490.13	*Comprehensive Policy on Traumatic Brain Injury-Related Neurocognitive Assessments by the Military Services*	Establishes the use of computerized neurocognitive assessment (ANAM4) across the deployment cycle (predeployment, post-injury, and postdeployment) with service members and DoD civilians.	Applies to military departments and the Coast Guard when it is a service in the Department of Homeland Security by agreement with that department
USSOCOM Policy Memorandum 19-01	*Comprehensive Strategy for Special Operations Forces Warfighter Brain Health*	Establishes baseline cognitive assessment, periodic ANAM cognitive testing, documentation of historical symptoms and exposure baseline with periodic updates, and a requirement for at-risk operators to wear blast gauges in relevant training and deployment settings to record overt and subconcussive repetitive blast exposures.	Applies to personnel in the SOCOM enterprise

[a]CPG update in progress at the time of this chapter's publication.

some measures that may be exclusive to a military context. One such measure is the ANAM, which is a collection of computer-based assessments, initially developed by the DoD, designed to measure attention, concentration, reaction time, memory, processing speed, and decision making. As stated earlier, ANAM is mandated for use in the military to establish a predeployment baseline unique to each service member. Subsequent administrations can then be compared during or after deployment to establish any intra-individual differences potentially due to concussive injury (Department of Defense Instruction 6490.13; Department of Defense, 2017). An ANAM Performance Validity Index was derived from the accuracy and response time (RT) discrepancies of four subtests (i.e., Matching to Sample, Simple RT, Procedural RT, and Code Substitution Learning). Cutoff scores of ≥ 10 maximized sensitivity/specificity (0.68/0.90) in an outpatient setting (Roebuck-Spencer, Vincent, Gilliland, Johnson, & Cooper, 2013). USSOCOM's brain health policy (2019) requires a periodic reassessment using the ANAM Version 4 Military Expanded (ANAM4 MilExp), which includes an additional three subtests that tap visual cognitive, executive functioning, and memory abilities.

Another tool used almost exclusively by the military is the Military Acute Concussion Evaluation (MACE) that is not intended to be a neuropsychological measure, but rather a quick and easy screener to detect concussion and mental status in the immediate setting (e.g., on the battlefield or sports field) (McCrea et al., 2014). The MACE was updated to MACE 2 (DVBIC, 2018) in 2018. MACE 2 is made up of four parts: (1) a history component that records information on the injury event (mechanism of injury, acute characteristics, postconcussive symptoms, etc.); (2) a brief neurological exam; (3) a cognitive screening called the Standardized Assessment of Concussion (SAC; McCrea, Randolph, & Kelly, 2000); and (5) Vestibular/Ocular-Motor Screening (VOMS). The SAC assesses orientation, immediate memory, concentration, and delayed recall and has a total score of 30. Preliminary data suggest that the VOMS improves diagnosis of concussion, as well as prediction of recovery (Mucha et al., 2014).

CLINICAL MANAGEMENT OF CONCUSSION

Management of concussion is highly dependent on two factors: (1) time since injury and (2) specific symptomatology. In the first 24 hours of injury, cognitive and physical rest is strongly indicated. Symptoms during this time are expected, but should be aided by rest. After 24 hours, the patient should begin to engage in a graded return to activities. DVBIC has published a six stage progressive recovery process: Stage 1: Rest—only basic activities of daily living; Stage 2: Light Routine Activity—walking, stretching, simple cognitive activities; Stage 3: Light Occupation-Oriented Activity—brisk walk, lift objects less than 20 pounds; Stage 4: Moderate Activity—light resistance training, jogging; Stage 5: Intensive Activity—normal routine and exercise, return to driving; Stage 6: Unrestricted Activity—return to pre-injury activities. For those who are not asymptomatic after 24 hours, the service member is progressed to the next stage only when activities can be completed without exacerbation of symptoms at the current stage.

At a minimum, the service member spends 24 hours at each stage with an expectation that within several days to a few weeks, concussive symptoms will resolve and normal activities can be resumed.

During staged recovery, symptom specific treatments can be provided. These might include over-the-counter medications for headaches or prescription medication for dizziness. Most often, this care will be overseen by a primary-care provider or specialist with concussion-specific training (e.g., neurologist or neuropsychologist). However, patients may already be engaged with BH- or behavioral health–specific care, especially by primary-care behavioral health consultants (BHCs; see Chapter 5, this volume). In such cases, the BHC assists with behavioral interventions for symptoms like insomnia or headache pain. BHCs also educate patients about expectations for recovery and, in turn, work to minimize potential iatrogenic effects or misattribution of symptoms. As noted above, during the immediate (0–7 days) and acute periods of concussion management, extended psychological or cognitive testing is not recommended. However, brief self-report measures of concussive symptoms, for example, the Neurobehavioral Symptom Inventory (Cicerone & Kalmar, 1995), can be useful in tracking symptoms. Moreover, brief cognitive test batteries that focus on domains likely impacted by concussion (i.e., processing speed, reaction time, attention, and memory) can also be useful in tracking recovery. Commonly, these measures are administered via computer, for example, the Immediate Post-Concussion Assessment and Cognitive Testing (ImPACT; Lovell, 2015) and the Automated Neuropsychological Assessment Metrics (ANAM; Kane, Roebuck-Spencer, Short, Kabat, & Wilken, 2007).

Frequently, mental health providers in both primary care and in specialty clinics will see patients with a remote history of concussion. In many cases, these patients will have one or more comorbid conditions that include dysregulated sleep (e.g., insomnia or a breathing-related sleep disorder), chronic pain, psychological diagnoses (e.g., depression, anxiety, PTSD), fatigue, and/or substance use disorders. Treating these patients can be complex, but success hinges on accurate diagnoses so that appropriate interventions can be engaged. Given the nonspecific nature of concussive symptoms, this can be a challenging endeavor. First, mental health treatment for any comorbid psychological diagnoses can substantially improve overall functioning. Formal psychological testing, via instruments like the Personality Assessment Inventory (PAI; Morey, 1997) or the Minnesota Multiphasic Personality Inventory (MMPI-2/RF/MMPI-3; Ben-Porath & Tellegen, 2008/2011/2020), can assist with differential diagnosis, as well as the potential identification of symptom overreport and somatization. Next, behavioral interventions for pain management (in particular, headache management) are of utility in improving outcomes. Finally, where insomnia exists, the employment of cognitive-behavioral therapy for insomnia (CBT-I) can greatly improve sleep (Trauer, Qian, Doyle, Rajaratnam, &

Cunnington, 2015), which in turn may improve mood, pain, and cognition (Beetar, Guilmette, & Sparadeo, 1996; Bloomfield, Espie, & Evans, 2010; Chaput, Giguere, Chauny, Denis, & Lavigne, 2009; Waldron-Perrine et al., 2012).

Patients with a history of concussion will often present with cognitive complaints, such as poor memory, slower processing speed, and inattention. As with many concussion-related symptoms, cognitive complaints are nonspecific to mTBI and can result from a range of etiologies. Cognitive screening measures commonly employed in primary-care settings, such as the Folstein Mini Mental Status Exam (Folstein, Folstein, & McHugh, 1975) or Montreal Cognitive Assessment (MoCA; Nasreddine et al., 2005), have low ceilings and thus may be limited in terms of sensitivity for patients with a history of concussion. As noted above, several computerized measures have been devised for use with concussed patients. However, deficits on these measures are not necessarily specific to concussion, in particular in those with a remote history of concussion. The same is true of more formal cognitive testing. To this end, screening for cognitive deficits could be completed by nonneuropsychologists; however, care must be taken in interpreting test results, as deficits do not necessarily suggest residual neurological dysfunction. If such screening is undertaken, given the high base rates of invalid cognitive testing in service members and veterans with a history of TBI (Denning & Shura, 2019), validity testing should be included. The training and experience of the psychologist engaging in the test administration and interpretation should dictate the measures administered; however, some cognitive screening instruments include embedded validity tests. The Repeatable Battery for the Assessment of Neuropsychological Status (RBANS; Randolph, 1998), for example, has a handful of embedded performance validity tests (PVTs). While such measures can provide additional data to assist with case conceptualization, it is of note that embedded PVTs lack sensitivity relative to stand-alone PVTs (Armistead-Jehle & Hansen, 2011; Miele, Gunner, Lynch, & McCaffrey, 2012). Therefore, these measures may erroneously classify invalid data as valid. Patients with a remote history of concussion who demonstrate exceptionally low scores on cognitive screening measures should be referred to a neuropsychologist for a more thorough evaluation, informing case-conceptualization and treatment.

Clearly, treatment of pre- and postconcussion psychiatric symptoms is paramount. Some mental health providers unfamiliar with concussion may worry that they are unqualified to provide treatment to patients with history of concussion; however, this is not the case. Therapy should not be withheld or delayed because the patient has experienced a concussion. If therapy begins more than 3 months after the most recent concussion, there is likely no need for any alterations/modifications to therapy. If therapy is conducted in the acute phase of recovery, it is possible that minor modifications for reduced attention, processing speed, and memory (such as having the patient rephrase important information and repeating it as necessary, writing down important points/homework assignments) would be beneficial.

In addition to interventions targeting psychological comorbidities, early psychoeducation regarding concussion has been shown to be beneficial for recovery (Belanger et al., 2018). This may help the patient manage expectations, both normalizing immediate symptoms, as well as indicating that a complete recovery is anticipated (Kennedy, 2020). Psychoeducation is especially important given media portrayals of TBI, concussion, and chronic traumatic encephalopathy (CTE), and a gradual resumption of activities and physical exercise as tolerated (Silverberg & Iverson, 2013) should be emphasized. Although rest has historically been prescribed for concussion, extensive rest ("cocoon therapy") has not proven beneficial, and, in fact, an early and graded return to activity (to include aerobic activity) is associated with faster recovery (De Kruijk et al., 2002; DiFazio, Silverberg, Kirkwood, Bernier, & Iverson, 2016; Lawrence, Richards, Comper, & Hutchison, 2018; Thomas, Apps, Hoffmann, McCrea, & Hammeke, 2015). Additionally, it is recommended that the term *concussion* be used with patients to reduce potential for iatrogenesis (Hoge, Goldberg, & Castro, 2009). Though the terms mTBI and concussion are generally used interchangeably, mTBI is perceived by patients to be more severe (Sullivan, Edmed, & Kempe, 2014) and result in worse outcomes than concussion (Weber & Edwards, 2010).

ILLUSTRATIVE CASE EXAMPLES

In order to allow for practice in integrating the information presented in this chapter, what follows are two case examples to provide a context to concussions sustained in the military environment. In the first case, the service member's presentation is affected by misattribution of symptoms and the need for psychological health care. In the second, the concussion is discovered by the mental health provider following routine psychological health screening.

Case 6.1. The Soldier Who Is Concerned That He Has CTE

The specialist (SPC) is a 25-year-old male who is seeing his mental health provider for mild depressive symptoms, having been referred by his primary-care provider. He previously sustained a concussion in training 13 months ago, falling during a training exercise and striking his head against a metal pole. He was reportedly dazed and a bit confused for several minutes but did not lose consciousness. The medic evaluated him and diagnosed him with concussion (MACE 2 Positive; Cognitive Results = 23/30). A CT scan was negative. He suffered with headaches and mild dizziness for a few days, but was gradually able to return to training. He did not experience any subsequent symptoms. His medical history is notable for another concussion when he was playing football in middle school (no loss of consciousness, no lasting symptoms, no hospitalization) and one prior depressive episode at age 20 that was successfully treated with psychotherapy. He began having difficulty with depressed mood a few months ago, following separation from his wife. He is now experiencing insomnia and is binge-drinking on the weekends. He has been experiencing memory problems recently and is concerned that he has CTE given his history of concussions. His memory problems began several months ago in the form of forgetting where he was going while driving, difficulty remembering his schedule at work, and difficulty focusing. The initial findings suggest the presence of significant depressive symptoms on a screening tool. The SPC attributes his cognitive and mood difficulties to his prior concussions. He is very concerned that he is at the beginning stages of CTE. He saw the headlines about former NFL players having CTE at autopsy and believes that, like the football players, his concussion may be most likely cause of his recent decline.

This type of referral is very common in DoD and VA settings. This case illustrates common conundrums in treating individuals with a history of past concussion(s). Let's examine some of the factors of this case:

- The SPC experienced the expected gradual recovery following his concussion. If he had been tested soon after his injury, he likely would have demonstrated some mild decline in his cognitive performance, but the long-term prognosis following an uncomplicated concussion with normal neuroimaging is favorable, with full cognitive recovery.
- His memory complaints surfaced after separation from his wife, along with the onset of his depressive symptoms.
- He has a prior history of depression. Pre-injury mental health has been implicated as one of the most important factors in recovery from concussion.
- CTE can only be diagnosed postmortem; there are no current clinical diagnostic criteria for CTE and his history of two concussions with full recovery does not support a serious neurological diagnosis.

Because of the specialist's concerns, he was referred to both neurology and the mental health clinic. Neurological evaluation was negative; the neurologist did not feel that his symptoms were the result of a concussion. During his initial evaluation in the mental health clinic, he endorsed significant depressive symptoms, insomnia, and memory problems. He has no history of legal or prior substance problems, but has recently been binge-drinking on weekends. His provider was concerned that his drinking may be complicating the clinical picture—possibly exacerbating sleep issues and indirectly exacerbating memory complaints, and suggesting poor coping.

After a thorough assessment, his mental health provider believed the specialist did not quite meet the criteria for a major depressive episode, but he was certainly at risk. His prior successful experience with psychotherapy was a strength. The provider decided against referring for additional workup for the concussion or memory complaints, due to her hypothesis that treating the other mental health issues, as well as instilling more adaptive coping strategies, would likely mitigate them. After providing a brief education about CTE, the provider suggested short-term, focused psychotherapy and note-taking during psychotherapy to circumvent reported memory issues. The initial agreed upon goals were the development of more adaptive coping strategies and cognitive-behavioral therapy for insomnia. The SPC successfully completed therapy, used his chain of command to assist him with his divorce, and experienced full symptom remission. He was retained in the military, fit for full duty. Let's now turn to a case of acute concussion.

Case 6.2. The Soldier Who Sucked It Up

The Army Staff Sergeant (SSG) is a 30-year-old 31B (pronounced 31-Bravo; i.e., military police) who has been assigned to an airborne unit for the past 2 years. She presented to the primary-care clinic in the course of a routine annual evaluation. On one of her mandatory psychological screening instruments, she endorsed significant difficulty concentrating and was referred to a same-day appointment with the BHC (see Chapter 5, this volume). On questioning, she revealed that 5 days ago, she was engaged in airborne training and experienced a difficult landing. She stated that she "blacked out" for a few seconds and felt confused for several minutes. After she "shook out the cobwebs," she made it to the rally point. She stated that she did not report her symptoms or see a medic because "I wasn't bleeding or blind and besides another soldier busted up his leg pretty bad and the medics were busy." She developed a headache that has continued and is notably exacerbated by morning physical training with her unit. She also acknowledged a sense of vertigo when working out, as well as increased distractibility and a feeling of fogginess while at work. Finally, she noted that she is unusually fatigued by mid-afternoon, which is problematic because her unit is preparing for an inspection and she is working 10- to 12-hour days.

Given the military culture that values self-reliance, toughness, and a unit-first mentality, and where "manning up" and "sucking it up" are expected, the SSG's decision to avoid medical care is not uncommon. Let's examine some facts of this case:

- The SSG struck her head during airborne activities and experienced a subsequent brief period of either posttraumatic amnesia or lost consciousness followed by several moments of altered consciousness.
- She experienced various somatic and cognitive symptoms after this injury that continue without improvement.
- The SSG continues to engage in usual work activities to include physical training and has not been evaluated by a medical provider for her injury or symptoms.

The BHC re-referred the SSG back to the primary-care physician for confirmation of the concussion diagnosis, appropriate treatment, and duty limitations. No further psychological health assessment or care was indicated.

CONCLUSIONS

The contributions of behavioral health providers in the concussion management process are crucial. While neurological assessment and care may be needed in the acute and postacute concussion phases, psychological care, particularly for those individuals with ongoing symptoms, is important given the nonspecific nature of these symptoms and the prevalence of comorbid psychiatric disorders. Psychological care includes psychoeducation (particularly important in the immediate and acute periods), monitoring of both cognitive and psychological symptoms, treatment of depression and anxiety symptoms, sleep and pain interventions, and monitoring patients in order to facilitate referrals to necessary specialists (e.g., sleep specialist, neuropsychologist). There is no evidence that a history of concussion(s) interferes with empirically valid psychological treatments. The most important thing a provider can do is to remain educated on the typical recovery patterns following concussion in order to provide accurate education to patients and not cause unintended iatrogenic effects with misinformation.

REFERENCES

American Psychiatric Association. (2013). *Diagnostic and statistical manual of mental disorders* (5th ed.). Arlington, VA: Author.
Aradi, M., Schwarcz, A., Perlaki, G., Orsi, G., Kovacs, N., Trauninger, A., et al. (2013). Quantitative MRI studies of chronic brain white matter hyperintensities in migraine patients. *Headache, 53*(5), 752–763.
Armistead-Jehle, P., & Hansen, C. L. (2011). Comparison of the Repeatable Battery for the Assessment of Neuropsychological Status Effort Index and standalone symptom validity tests in a military sample. *Archives of Clinical Neuropsychology, 26*(7), 592–601.

Asken, B. M., DeKosky, S. T., Clugston, J. R., Jaffee, M. S., & Bauer, R. M. (2018). Diffusion tensor imaging (DTI) findings in adult civilian, military, and sport-related mild traumatic brain injury (mTBI): A systematic critical review. *Brain Imaging & Behavior, 12*(2), 585–612.

Beetar, J. T., Guilmette, T. J., & Sparadeo, F. R. (1996). Sleep and pain complaints in symptomatic traumatic brain injury and neurologic populations. *Archives of Physical Medicine & Rehabilitation, 77*(12), 1298–1302.

Belanger, H. G., Kretzmer, T., Vanderploeg, R., & French, L. M. (2010). Symptom complaints following combat-related TBI: Relationship to TBI severity and PTSD. *Journal of the International Neuropsychological Society, 16*(1), 194–199.

Belanger, H. G., Kretzmer, T., Yoash-Gantz, R., Pickett, T., & Tupler, L. A. (2009). Cognitive sequelae of blast-related versus other mechanisms of brain trauma. *Journal of the International Neuropsychological Society, 15*(1), 1–8.

Belanger, H. G., Tate, D. F., & Vanderploeg, R. D. (2018). Concussion and mild traumatic brain injury. In J. E. Morgan & J. H. Ricker (Eds.), *Textbook of clinical neuropsychology* (2nd ed., pp. 411–448). New York: Routledge.

Belanger, H. G., Wortzel, H. S., Vanderploeg, R. D., & Cooper, D. B. (2020). A model for intervening with veterans and service members who are concerned about developing chronic traumatic encephalopathy (CTE). *Clinical Neuropsychologist, 34*(6), 1105–1123.

Ben-Porath, Y. S., & Tellegen, A. (2008/2011/2020). *MMPI-2-RF (Minnesota Multiphasic Personality Inventory-2-Restructured Form): Manual for administration, scoring, and interpretation*. Minneapolis: University of Minnesota Press

Bloomfield, I. L., Espie, C. A., & Evans, J. J. (2010). Do sleep difficulties exacerbate deficits in sustained attention following traumatic brain injury? *Journal of the International Neuropsychological Society, 16*(1), 17–25.

Carr, W., Polejaeva, E., Grome, A., Crandall, B., LaValle, C., Eonta, S. E., et al. (2015). Relation of repeated low-level blast exposure with symptomology similar to concussion. *Journal of Head Trauma Rehabilitation, 30*(1), 47–55.

Carr, W., Stone, J. R., Walilko, T., Young, L. A., Snook, T. L., Paggi, M. E., et al. (2016). Repeated low-level blast exposure: A descriptive human subjects study. *Military Medicine, 181*(5 Suppl.), 28–39.

Chaput, G., Giguere, J. F., Chauny, J. M., Denis, R., & Lavigne, G. (2009). Relationship among subjective sleep complaints, headaches, and mood alterations following a mild traumatic brain injury. *Sleep Medicine, 10*(7), 713–716.

Cicerone, K. D., & Kalmar, K. (1995). Persistent post-concussive syndrome: Structure of subjective complaints after mild traumatic brain injury. *Journal of Head Trauma Rehabilitation, 10*, 1–17.

Clark, A. L., Sorg, S. F., Schiehser, D. M., Luc, N., Bondi, M. W., Sanderson, M., et al. (2016). Deep white matter hyperintensities affect verbal memory independent of PTSD symptoms in veterans with mild traumatic brain injury. *Brain Injury, 30*(7), 864–871.

Cooper, D. B., Chau, P. M., Armistead-Jehle, P., Vanderploeg, R. D., & Bowles, A. O. (2012). Relationship between mechanism of injury and neurocognitive functioning in OEF/OIF service members with mild traumatic brain injuries. *Military Medicine, 177*(10), 1157–1160.

De Kruijk, J. R., Leffers, P., Menheere, P. P., Meerhoff, S., Rutten, J., & Twijnstra, A. (2002). Prediction of post-traumatic complaints after mild traumatic brain injury: Early symptoms and biochemical markers. *Journal of Neurology, Neurosurgery and Psychiatry, 73*(6), 727–732.

Defense and Veterans Brain Injury Center (DVBIC). (2018). *Military Acute Concussion Evaluation 2* (MACE 2). Retrieved from *https://dvbic.dcoe.mil/material/military-acute-concussion-evaluation-2-mace-2*.

Defense and Veterans Brain Injury Center. (2019). *Concussion management tool*. Retrieved from *https://dvbic.dcoe.mil/material/concussion-management-tool*.

Defense and Veterans Brain Injury Center. (2020). *TBI and the military*. Retrieved from *https://dvbic.dcoe.mil/tbi-military*.

Defense and Veterans Brain Injury Center. (2021). Management and rehabilitation of post-acute mild traumatic brain injury (mTBI). Retrieved February 7, 2021, from *healthquality.va.gov/guidelines/Rehab/mtbi*.

Department of Veterans Affairs and Department of Defense. (2021). *VA/DOD clinical practice guideline for management of concussion/mild traumatic brain injury* (Version 2.0). Retrieved from *www.healthquality.va.gov/guidelines/Rehab/mtbi/mTBICPGFullCPG50821816.pdf*.

Denning, J. H., & Shura, R. D. (2019). Cost of malingering mild traumatic brain injury-related cognitive deficits during compensation and pension evaluations in the Veterans Benefits Administration. *Applied Neuropsychology Adult, 26*(1), 1–16.

Department of Defense. (2017, March). *Comprehensive policy on traumatic brain injury-related neurocognitive assessments by the military service* (Department of Defense Instruction 6490.13). Retrieved from *www.esd.whs.mil/Portals/54/Documents/DD/issuances/dodi/649013p.pdf*.

Department of Defense. (2019). *DoD policy for management of mild traumatic brain injury/concussion in the deployed setting* (Department of Defense Instruction 6490.11). Retrieved from *www.esd.whs.mil/Portals/54/Documents/DD/issuances/dodi/649011p.pdf*.

DiFazio, M., Silverberg, N. D., Kirkwood, M. W., Bernier, R., & Iverson, G. L. (2016). Prolonged activity restriction after concussion: Are we worsening outcomes? *Clinical Pediatrics (Phila), 55*(5), 443–451.

Donnell, A. J., Kim, M. S., Silva, M. A., & Vanderploeg, R. D. (2012). Incidence of postconcussion symptoms in psychiatric diagnostic groups, mild traumatic brain injury, and comorbid conditions. *Clinical Neuropsychologist, 26*(7), 1092–1101.

Folstein, M. F., Folstein, S. E., & McHugh, P. R. (1975). "Mini-mental status": A practical method for grading the cognitive state of patients for the clinician. *Journal of Psychiatric Research, 12*(3), 189–198.

Hoge, C. W., Goldberg, H. M., & Castro, C. A. (2009). Care of war veterans with mild traumatic brain injury–flawed perspectives. *New England Journal of Medicine, 360*(16), 1588–1591.

Hoge, C. W., McGurk, D., Thomas, J. L., Cox, A. L., Engel, C. C., & Castro, C. A. (2008). Mild traumatic brain injury in U.S. soldiers returning from Iraq. *New England Journal of Medicine, 358*(5), 453–463.

Ivanov, I., Fernandez, C., Mitsis, E. M., Dickstein, D. L., Wong, E., Tang, C. Y., et al. (2017). Blast exposure, white matter integrity, and cognitive function in Iraq and Afghanistan combat veterans. *Frontiers in Neurology, 8*, 127.

Iverson, G. L. (2005). Outcome from mild traumatic brain injury. *Current Opinions in Psychiatry, 18*(3), 301–317.

Iverson, G. L., Gardner, A. J., Terry, D. P., Ponsford, J. L., Sills, A. K., Broshek, D. K., et al. (2017). Predictors of clinical recovery from concussion: A systematic review. *British Journal of Sports Medicine, 51*(12), 941–948.

Kane, R. L., Roebuck-Spencer, T., Short, P., Kabat, M., & Wilken, J. (2007). Identifying and monitoring cognitive deficits in clinical populations using Automated Neuropsychological Assessment Metrics (ANAM) tests. *Archives of Clinical Neuropsychology, 22*(Suppl. 1), S115–S126.

Kennedy, C. H., Porter Evans, J., Chee, S., Moore, J. L., Barth, J. T., & Stuessi, K. A. (2012). Return to combat duty after concussive blast injury. *Archives of Clinical Neuropsychology, 27*(8), 817–827.

Lange, R. T., Pancholi, S., Brickell, T. A., Sakura, S., Bhagwat, A., Merritt, V., et al. (2012). Neuropsychological outcome from blast versus non-blast: Mild traumatic brain injury in U.S. military service members. *Journal of the International Neuropsychological Society, 18*(3), 595–605.

Lange, R. T., Yeh, P. H., Brickell, T. A., Lippa, S. M., & French, L. M. (2019). Postconcussion symptom reporting is not associated with diffusion tensor imaging findings in the subacute to chronic phase of recovery in military service members following mild traumatic brain injury. *Journal of Clinical and Experimental Neuropsychology, 41*(5), 497–511.

Lawrence, D. W., Richards, D., Comper, P., & Hutchison, M. G. (2018). Earlier time to aerobic exercise is associated with faster recovery following acute sport concussion. *PLoS One, 13*(4), e0196062.

Lindemer, E. R., Greve, D. N., Fischl, B. R., Augustinack, J. C., & Salat, D. H. (2017). Regional staging of white matter signal abnormalities in aging and Alzheimer's disease. *Neuroimage Clinical, 14,* 156–165.

Lovell, M. R. (2015). *ImPACT test administration and interpretation manual.* Retrieved from *www.impacttest.com.*

Martindale, S. L., Rowland, J. A., Shura, R. D., & Taber, K. H. (2018). Longitudinal changes in neuroimaging and neuropsychiatric status of post-deployment veterans: A CENC pilot study. *Brain Injury, 32*(10), 1208–1216.

McCrea, M. (2008). Acute symptoms and symptom recovery. In *Mild traumatic brain injury and postconcussion syndrome* (pp. 85–96). New York: Oxford University Press.

McCrea, M., Guskiewicz, K., Doncevic, S., Helmick, K., Kennedy, J., Boyd, C., et al. (2014). Day of injury cognitive performance on the Military Acute Concussion Evaluation (MACE) by U.S. military service members in OEF/OIF. *Military Medicine, 179*(9), 990–997.

McCrea, M., Randolph, C., & Kelly, J. P. (2000). *The Standardized Assessment of Concussion (SAC): Manual for administration, scoring and interpretation.* Waukesha, WI: CNS.

McKee, A. C., Cairns, N. J., Dickson, D. W., Folkerth, R. D., Keene, C. D., Litvan, I., et al. (2016). The first NINDS/NIBIB consensus meeting to define neuropathological criteria for the diagnosis of chronic traumatic encephalopathy. *Acta Neuropathologica, 131*(1), 75–86.

McKee, A. C., Cantu, R. C., Nowinski, C. J., Hedley-Whyte, E. T., Gavett, B. E., Budson, A. E., et al. (2009). Chronic traumatic encephalopathy in athletes: Progressive tauopathy after repetitive head injury. *Journal of Neuropathology and Experimental Neurology, 68*(7), 709–735.

Meares, S., Shores, E. A., Taylor, A. J., Batchelor, J., Bryant, R. A., Baguley, I. J., et al. (2011). The prospective course of postconcussion syndrome: The role of mild traumatic brain injury. *Neuropsychology, 25*(4), 454–465.

Mez, J., Stern, R. A., & McKee, A. C. (2013). Chronic traumatic encephalopathy: Where are we and where are we going? *Current Neurology and Neuroscience Reports, 13*(12), 407.

Miele, A. S., Gunner, J. H., Lynch, J. K., & McCaffrey, R. J. (2012). Are embedded validity indices equivalent to free-standing symptom validity tests? *Archives of Clinical Neuropsychology, 27*(1), 10–22.

Morey, L. C. (1997). *The Personality Assessment Screener (professional manual)*. Lutz, FL: Psychological Assessment Resources.

Mu, W., Catenaccio, E., & Lipton, M. L. (2017). Neuroimaging in blast-related mild traumatic brain injury. *Journal of Head Trauma Rehabilitation, 32*(1), 55–69.

Mucha, A., Collins, M. W., Elbin, R. J., Furman, J. M., Troutman-Enseki, C., DeWolf, R. M., et al. (2014). A Brief Vestibular/Ocular Motor Screening (VOMS) assessment to evaluate concussions: Preliminary findings. *American Journal of Sports Medicine, 42*(10), 2479–2486.

Nasreddine, Z. S., Phillips, N. A., Bédirian, V., Charbonneau, S., Whitehead, V., Collin, I., et al. (2005). The Montreal Cognitive Assessment, MoCA: A brief screening tool for mild cognitive impairment. *Journal of the American Geriatric Society, 53*(4), 695–699.

Newsome, M. R., Mayer, A. R., Lin, X., Troyanskaya, M., Jackson, G. R., Scheibel, R. S., et al. (2016). Chronic effects of blast-related TBI on subcortical functional connectivity in veterans. *Journal of the International Neuropsychological Society, 22*(6), 631–642.

Omalu, B., Hammers, J. L., Bailes, J., Hamilton, R. L., Kamboh, M. I., Webster, G., et al. (2011). Chronic traumatic encephalopathy in an Iraqi war veteran with posttraumatic stress disorder who committed suicide. *Neurosurgical Focus, 31*(5), E3.

Owens, B. D., Kragh, J. F., Jr., Wenke, J. C., Macaitis, J., Wade, C. E., & Holcomb, J. B. (2008). Combat wounds in operation Iraqi Freedom and operation Enduring Freedom. *Journal of Trauma, 64*(2), 295–299.

Panwar, J., Hsu, C. C., Tator, C. H., & Mikulis, D. (2020). Magnetic resonance imaging criteria for post-concussion syndrome: A study of 127 post-concussion syndrome patients. *Journal of Neurotrauma, 37*(10), 1190–1196.

Randolph, C. (1998). *Repeatable battery for the assessment of neuropsychological status*. San Antonio, TX: The Psychological Corporation.

Roebuck-Spencer, T. M., Vincent, A. S., Gilliland, K., Johnson, D. R., & Cooper, D. B. (2013). Initial clinical validation of an embedded performance validity measure within the automated neuropsychological metrics (ANAM). *Archives of Clinical Neuropsychology, 28*(7), 700–710.

Shively, S. B., Horkayne-Szakaly, I., Jones, R. V., Kelly, J. P., Armstrong, R. C., & Perl, D. P. (2016). Characterisation of interface astroglial scarring in the human brain after blast exposure: A post-mortem case series. *Lancet Neurology, 15*(9), 944–953.

Silva, M. A., & Kay, T. (2013). Persistent symptoms after a concussion. In N. D. Zasler, R. D. Arciniegas, R. D. Vanderploeg, & M. S. Jaffee (Eds.),

Management of adults with traumatic brain injury (pp. 475–500). Washington, DC: American Psychiatric Association.

Silverberg, N. D., Gardner, A. J., Brubacher, J. R., Panenka, W. J., Li, J. J., & Iverson, G. L. (2015). Systematic review of multivariable prognostic models for mild traumatic brain injury. *Journal of Neurotrauma, 32*(8), 517–526.

Silverberg, N. D., & Iverson, G. L. (2013). Is rest after concussion "the best medicine?": Recommendations for activity resumption following concussion in athletes, civilians, and military service members. *Journal of Head Trauma Rehabilitation, 28*(4), 250–259.

Stern, R. A., Daneshvar, D. H., Baugh, C. M., Seichepine, D. R., Montenigro, P. H., Riley, D. O., et al. (2013). Clinical presentation of chronic traumatic encephalopathy. *Neurology, 81*(13), 1122–1129.

Sullivan, K. A., Edmed, S. L., & Kempe, C. (2014). The effect of injury diagnosis on illness perceptions and expected postconcussion syndrome and post-traumatic stress disorder symptoms. *Journal of Head Trauma Rehabilitation, 29*(1), 54–64.

Tate, C. M., Wang, K. K., Eonta, S., Zhang, Y., Carr, W., Tortella, F. C., et al. (2013). Serum brain biomarker level, neurocognitive performance, and self-reported symptom changes in soldiers repeatedly exposed to low-level blast: A breacher pilot study. *Journal of Neurotrauma, 30*(19), 1620–1630.

Tate, D. F., Gusman, M., Kini, J., Reid, M., Velez, C. S., Drennon, A. M., et al. (2017). Susceptibility weighted imaging and white matter abnormality findings in service members with persistent cognitive symptoms following mild traumatic brain injury. *Military Medicine, 182*(3), e1651–e1658.

Thomas, D. G., Apps, J. N., Hoffmann, R. G., McCrea, M., & Hammeke, T. (2015). Benefits of strict rest after acute concussion: A randomized controlled trial. *Pediatrics, 135*(2), 213–223.

Trauer, J. M., Qian, M. Y., Doyle, J. S., Rajaratnam, S. M., & Cunnington, D. (2015). Cognitive behavioral therapy for chronic insomnia: A systematic review and meta-analysis. *Annals of Internal Medicine, 163*(3), 191–204.

U.S. Special Operations Command. (2019). *Comprehensive strategy for Special Operations Forces warfighter brain health* (Policy Memorandum 19-01). Tampa, FL: USSOCOM.

Waldron-Perrine, B., McGuire, A. P., Spencer, R. J., Drag, L. L., Pangilinan, P. H., & Bieliauskas, L. A. (2012). The influence of sleep and mood on cognitive functioning among veterans being evaluated for mild traumatic brain injury. *Military Medicine, 177*(11), 1293–1301.

Wang, Y., Chan, R. C., & Deng, Y. (2006). Examination of postconcussion-like symptoms in healthy university students: relationships to subjective and objective neuropsychological function performance. *Archives of Clinical Neuropsychology, 21*(4), 339–347.

Weber, M., & Edwards, M. G. (2010). The effect of brain injury terminology on university athletes' expected outcome from injury, familiarity and actual symptom report. *Brain Injury, 24*(11), 1364–1371.

World Health Organization. (1992). *International statistical classification of diesases and related health problems* (10th ed.). Geneva, Switzerland: Author.

CHAPTER 7

Substance Use Disorder Services and Gambling Treatment in the Military

Tim Hoyt, Christopher J. Spevak, John A. Hodgson,
William A. McDonald, and Revonda Grayson

In 1740, Admiral Edward Vernon of the Royal Navy directed that sailors in the West Indies fleet be given a daily ration of a half-pint of rum diluted with water. This diluted beverage was named "grog" by the sailors, after the waterproof grogram cloak worn by Admiral Vernon (Pack, 1983). The admiral's intent was to minimize the harmful effects of drinking straight liquor on the health and behavior of sailors under his charge. The American Navy, patterned after its British predecessors, continued the practice and even formalized it through congressional legislation in 1794, marking the first formal substance abuse prevention effort in the U.S. military. The rationing of grog remained in effect until 1862, when it was abolished by a general order, although alcohol on U.S. Navy vessels was not banned entirely until 1914 (Sobocinski, 2004).

Periods of conflict pose significant risk for problematic substance use, and risk may increase significantly when low operational tempo allows service members "spare time" in which to misuse substances (Jones, 1995). During the Texas Revolution, entire battalions were rendered combat ineffective due to hangovers from regular and excessive consumption of whiskey (Austerman, 2010). During the Civil War, alcohol and opium commonly were available, and were the primary medications used in field medicine and amputations (Lewy, 2014). In a sample of Civil War veterans from Indiana, 22.4% were treated for alcoholism and 5.2% were addicted to chloral hydrate, cocaine, morphine, or opium (Dean, 1997). Historically, the worst substance problems were evident in the Vietnam War: In 1971, a survey of U.S. service members returning from Southeast Asia showed that 92% had used alcohol while serving in Vietnam, 69% had used marijuana, 43% had used heroin, and 25% had used amphetamines (Robins, Hetzer, & Davis, 1975). By July 1972, one of eight medical evacuations of soldiers from Vietnam was due to a positive urine drug screen (Camp, 2015). In contrast, U.S. forces' exposure to alcohol during the first Persian Gulf War was minimal, in part because of the relatively short duration of the war, but mainly because Muslim tradition forbids the consumption of alcohol and Saudi Arabia prohibited its importation (Quilter, 1993). Under these environmental conditions, alcohol was more difficult to acquire, and many alcohol-related problems were reduced substantially during this conflict (Gunby, 1991).

The same prohibitions against alcohol—known as General Order 1—have been present for the more recent wars in Iraq and Afghanistan. Nonetheless, studies conducted in the combat environment show that between 6.8% and 8% of service members reported using alcohol while deployed and between 1.4 and 2.6% reported using illegal drugs (U.S. Army Medical Command, 2006, 2008). In addition, 3.8% of service members reported "huffing" or using inhalants such as compressed air, fuels, or paint to get high (U.S. Army Medical Command, 2008). Based on a 2007 inspection, illegal drugs and alcohol were typically procured through contractors, third-country nationals, local nationals, coalition forces from other nations, and mail from home (Kaner et al., 2007). Approximately 1.7% of service members tested positive for illegal drugs immediately after returning from deployment in Iraq or Afghanistan (Larson, Mohr, Jeffery, Adams, & Wilson, 2016). Furthermore, meta-analysis of studies since the Gulf War shows that military personnel who have deployed are consistently at greater risk for alcohol and substance use disorders (SUDs) compared to those who do not deploy (Kelsall et al., 2015).

In the past decade, the military also has faced a significant increase in the use of "designer drugs" or synthetics, including substituted cathinones (bath salts), synthetic cannabinoids (spice), and other hallucinogens (Weaver, Hopper, & Gunderson, 2015). The initial appeal of these drugs was that they could not be detected on the standard urine drug screen panel used by the military (Craig & Loeffler, 2014). These drugs were typically purchased over the counter in smoke shops, marketed as "plant food" or "incense" with specific instructions that the compounds are "not for human consumption" (Lenz et al., 2013). Most of these compounds were not added formally to the Controlled Substances Act until 2012 (Brantley, 2012). In one sample of treatment-seeking service members, 11% reported using synthetics in the last 90 days (Walker et al., 2014). Because these substances are not well regulated, so the exact contents of any given sample are not precisely known, clinical symptom presentations are wide-ranging, including instances of psychosis requiring hospitalization for more than a week (Loeffler, Hurst, Penn, & Yung, 2012). As a result, significant medical management is frequently required to stabilize patients using these drugs (e.g., Craig & Loeffler, 2014; Weaver et al., 2015), as exhibited by the following case.

Case 7.1. The Marine Who Used Bath Salts

In the early hours of a Saturday, the military police were called to the local Marine Corps barracks about a lance corporal (LCpl). When they arrived, several Marines reported that the LCpl had been extremely agitated, but in a trance, and had attempted to push another service member out of a sealed window. Suspecting drug use, the police took the LCpl to the emergency department at the local military treatment facility. When the toxicology screen came back negative, he was admitted to the inpatient psychiatric ward due to delirium and disinhibition. Two days later, he reported to the attending psychiatrist that he had been using "red dove," a synthetic cathinone (bath salts) that he had purchased from another Marine.

Since 1980, the Department of Defense (DoD) has conducted a series of periodic studies on service member health trends, known as the Health Related Behavior Survey (HRBS). These studies have included surveillance of substance use trends and their impact on military readiness. Data on illegal drug use show a significant decline from 36% of service member reporting any drug use in the past year in 1980 to 0.7% in 2015 (Burt, Biegel, Carnes, & Farley, 1980; Meadows et al., 2018). Throughout this time, marijuana use has accounted for the vast majority of reported illegal drug use. The overall decline in drug use by military members since the 1980s is largely attributable to the military's zero-tolerance policy for illicit drug use (Bray, Marsden, Herbold, & Peterson, 1992). Beginning in 2005, prescription drug misuse was included in the HRBS, with a high point of 11% past-year misuse identified in the 2008 survey, and a rate of 4.1% identified in the 2015 survey (Bray et al., 2009; Meadows et al., 2018). Prescription pain relievers were the most likely to be misused, followed by prescription sedatives. Misuse of prescription drugs was highest among senior enlisted personnel, and there were no differences in misuse of prescription drugs between men and women (Meadows et al., 2018).

Whereas illicit drug use rates have generally decreased, rates of problematic alcohol use in the military have remained higher than in comparable civilian samples (Meadows et al., 2018). Between 1998 and 2008, there was a significant increase in binge-drinking (defined as 5 or more drinks on a single occasion at least once in in the past 30 days) by service members, with rates increasing from 35 to 47% of service members (Bray et al., 2009). This rate decreased to 30% by 2015 (Meadows et al., 2018).

Using scores from the Alcohol Use Disorders Identification Test (AUDIT; Saunders, Aasland, Babor, De la Fuente, & Grant, 1993; see Figure 7.1), 33% of service members received a score of 8 or more, indicating hazardous drinking (scores of 8–15), harmful drinking (scores of 16–19), or possible dependence (scores of 20 or more) in 2008 (Bray et al., 2009). By 2015, this overall rate had increased to 35% (Meadows et al., 2018). Problematic alcohol use rates are consistently higher in the military among men (36%) compared to women (31.3%); hazardous drinking is highest in the Marine Corps (48.6%) and lowest in the Air Force (26.1%; Meadows et al., 2018). In line with these findings, 68.2% of service members believe that the military culture is supportive of drinking alcohol, and 42.4% of service members indicate that military supervisors do not discourage alcohol use (Meadows et al., 2018). Problematic alcohol use also has a direct impact on military readiness, with 8% reporting serious consequences related to drinking alcohol in the past year, such as occupational problems, arrests, fights, causing an accident, or a low-performance rating (Meadows et al., 2018).

The costs associated with alcohol misuse are numerous. A study of health care costs for high alcohol consumption among beneficiaries conservatively estimated the annual cost to the program to be approximately $1.2 billion (Dall et al., 2007), with a breakdown of $425 million in increased medical costs and $745 million in reduced readiness (Harwood, Zhang, Dall, Olaiya, & Fagan, 2009). Alcohol problems also affect mission readiness in a variety of ways. Service members who are heavy drinkers (five or more drinks at least once per week) are more likely than nondrinkers and light drinkers to be late to work, to leave work early, to exhibit decreased job performance, and to suffer on-the-job injuries (Fisher, Hoffman, Austin-Lane, & Kao, 2000). An estimated 10,400 active-duty service members are unable to deploy each year because of drinking, and another 2,200 are separated from service each year because of alcohol problems. These early separations cost the DoD about $108 million annually, and missed deployments resulting from alcohol problems cost the DoD $510 million per year (Harwood et al., 2009). At least 26.6% of military suicide deaths in 2018 involved alcohol (Tucker, Smolenski, & Kennedy, 2020). In 2018, 62% of sexual assaults perpetrated against women in the military and 49% of sexual assaults perpetrated against men in the military involved alcohol (Sexual Assault Prevention and Response Office, 2019). Problem drinking by service members significantly increases risk for intimate partner violence (Sparrow, Kwan, Howard, Fear, & MacManus, 2017). Between 42% and 56% of moderate to heavy alcohol users in the military report driving after drinking (Brown, Bray, & Hartzell, 2010). Problematic alcohol use is also a risk factor for injury, with between 28% and 30% of service members endorsing problematic alcohol use on the AUDIT after having a subsequent medical encounter for injuries such as fractures, dislocations, concussion,

Patient's name _____

Because alcohol use can affect your health and can interfere with certain medications and treatments, it is important that we ask some questions about your use of alcohol. Your answers will remain confidential, so please be honest. Place an X in one box that best describes your answer to each question.

Questions	0	1	2	3	4	Item Score
	Never	Monthly less	2–4 times a month	2–3 times a week	4 or more times a week	
1. How often do you have a drink containing alcohol?						
	1 or 2	3 or 4	5 or 6	7 to 9	10 or more	
2. How many drinks containing alcohol do you have on a typical day when you are drinking?						
	Never	Less than monthly	Monthly	Weekly	Daily or almost daily	
3. How often do you have six or more drinks on one occasion?						
4. How often during the last year have you found that you were not able to stop drinking once you had started?						
5. How often during the last year have you failed to do what was normally expected of you because of drinking?						
6. How often during the last year have you needed a first drink in the morning to get yourself going after a heavy drinking session?						
7. How often during the last year have you had a feeling of guilt or remorse after drinking?						
8. How often during the last year have you been unable to remember what happened the night before because of your drinking?						
	No		Yes, but not in the last year		Yes, during the last year	
9. Have you or someone else been injured because of your drinking?						
10. Has a relative, friend, doctor, other health care worker been concerned about your drinking or suggested you cut down?						
					Total	

FIGURE 7.1. The Alcohol Use Disorders Identification Test: Self-report version. From Saunders et al. (1993). Public domain.

or burns (Hurt, 2015). Whereas quantifying the negative impact of substance abuse on the military is relatively simple, addressing the problem is
complicated.

Military members face a great deal of stress not typically encountered
by the civilian population, such as loss of personal freedom, deployment
to dangerous or austere areas, frequent moves, and separation from family (Campbell & Nobel, 2009). The military lifestyle itself is considered a
contributing factor to abusive levels of alcohol use (Ames, Cunradi, Moore,
& Stern, 2007; Ong & Joseph, 2008). This high level of stress is associated
with increased high-risk behaviors such as heavy episodic drinking during
off-duty hours, particularly after combat or on return home from a deployment (Brady, Credé, Harms, Bachrach, & Lester, 2019). Overall, military
personnel who have deployed are at greater risk for alcohol and substance
use disorders than those who do not deploy (Kelsall et al., 2015). Research
consistently demonstrates that certain subgroups of military personnel are
at increased risk of significant alcohol problems, including U.S. Marines
(Woodruff, Hurtado, & Simon-Arndt, 2018) and Special Operations
Forces (Skipper, Forsten, Kim, Wilk, & Hoge, 2014). From a demographic
perspective, the military faces particular challenges because a majority of
personnel are young adult males, a population considered at elevated risk
for substance abuse problems. One 5-year longitudinal study found that
75% of U.S. Navy recruits used alcohol prior to enlistment and 31% had
used illegal drugs (Ames, Cunradi, & Moore, 2002). In fact, teens who
engage in binge-drinking show a greater propensity to enlist in the military
after high school (Barry et al., 2013).

Although substance-related problems continue among uniformed
personnel, significant attention has been given to reducing their impact
across the military community. This chapter addresses the widespread prevention efforts under way throughout the military (e.g., zero tolerance of
illicit drug use, alcohol deglamorization campaigns, random urinalysis,
and mandatory education), early intervention services (e.g., alcohol screenings and intense education), the components of a comprehensive evaluation
of a possible substance or gambling disorder, treatment options available
for active-duty service members who experience these problems, and the
comorbidity of SUDs and posttraumatic stress disorder (PTSD).

PREVENTION AND EDUCATIONAL SERVICES

Many early prevention efforts in the military focused on punishment for
offenses. Alcohol-related incidents were the primary cause for 80% of U.S.
Navy floggings until the practice was abolished in 1850 (Mateczun, 1995).
Before 1970, chronic alcohol and drug problems were generally met with
legal punishment and discharge from the service (Prugh, 1975). In 1970,

Congress stipulated that efforts be directed toward treatment and reha-bilitation rather than automatic punishment and discharge (Baker, 1972). Another significant event in the 1970s was the development of an office to focus on the prevention of drug abuse, which was created in response to significant increases in drug- and alcohol-dependent military personnel in Vietnam (Prugh, 1975). In 1971, the U.S. Army began urine testing for opiates upon the completion of Vietnam tours and quickly added routine, unannounced testing for opiates, barbiturates, and amphetamines (Zin-berg, 1972). Those service members who screened positive were required to undergo supervised detoxification and a brief treatment program before returning to the United States. There was briefly an effort to establish a 3-week drug rehabilitation program at an Army airfield in Vietnam for deployed service members (Joseph, 1974). Beginning in the 1980s, mili-tary programs became increasingly standardized, including mandates for prevention training for 100% of new military members, annual training required for all troops, and expanded random urine drug testing that have continued until today (Department of Defense, 1980, 1985, 2014).

Whereas each military branch manages its own prevention programs, they all share the same basic objectives of promoting mission readiness and the health and wellness of troops through the prevention of substance abuse (Sirratt, Ozanian, & Fraenkner, 2012). Prevention efforts throughout the military can be conceptualized through a tiered prevention–intervention model (Witkiewitz & Estrada, 2011). The first tier of this model is univer-sal prevention, with efforts targeted toward the entire population of service members. One example of such a program is the DoD "Own Your Limits" campaign (*www.ownyourlimits.org*). This campaign promotes respon-sible drinking among service members, provides education resources about problematic alcohol use, and includes tools for calculating standard drinks and blood alcohol concentration. Another example is delivering alcohol risk education courses to all service members during certain phases of ini-tial entry training. One such program—the Alcohol Misconduct Preven-tion Program at Lackland Air Force Base—delivered a 1-hour brief alcohol intervention to all trainees, and was associated with significant reductions in alcohol-related incidents over a 12-month period following implementa-tion (Klesges et al., 2013). Interestingly, this program also showed cost avoidance of over $9,000 for every alcohol-related incident (ARI) prevented by this initiative (Li et al., 2017). Targeted primary prevention efforts with young service members have significant potential to reduce future alcohol use disorders (Fink et al., 2016). Interventions to reduce problematic drink-ing behavior also may occur at the military installation level. For example, a base-wide policy restricting nighttime sales of alcohol at one installation coincided with significantly reduced overall rates of citations for driving under the influence or driving while intoxicated (Grattan, Mengistu, Bull-ock, Santo, & Jackson, 2019). In a similar vein, the military is addressing the use of tobacco with Internet and other media-based resources. In 2007, the military launched a multimedia tobacco cessation campaign called YouCanQuit2 (*www.ycq2.org*). This program offers step-by-step processes for quitting smoking, a live chat resource, self-assessment tools, and stories from other service members who present real-life strategies for quitting tobacco (Lin et al., 2018).

The second tier of the prevention–intervention model is selective prevention; it focuses on specific groups of service members identified as being at higher risk for developing SUDs (Witkiewitz & Estrada, 2011). In the military setting, these interventions are typically education-based programs, and are recommended at the first sign that an individual is making unwise decisions about alcohol use. The trigger for a referral to an early intervention program is usually an ARI, for example, an arrest for drunk and disorderly conduct, underage drinking, or drunk driving. Generally, a single alcohol-related incident or concerns of the command about an individual's pattern of alcohol use will result in referral to an early intervention program. Courses usually involve 15 to 20 hours of training and discussion related to improving awareness about the effects of alcohol on the body and brain, identifying risky situations, and making positive choices for responsible drinking (see Schmid et al., 2017). The primary goals are to promote responsible drinking, prevent further alcohol-related incidents, and prevent the development of clinical and psychosocial substance abuse problems. Indeed, even single-session interventions that focus on normative alcohol use feedback and motivation for change can reduce alcohol use by service members and decrease the likelihood of subsequent alcohol use disorder diagnoses (Walker et al., 2017). Similar Web-based adaptations of these educational programs also have been developed for service members, with participants in programs such as Drinker's Check-Up (*https://checkupandchoices.com*) showing significant improvements in levels of drinking, frequency of heavy drinking, and reductions in peak blood alcohol concentration (Pemberton et al., 2011). When early education interventions are not successful in deterring problematic alcohol and drug use, then the third tier of the prevention–intervention model is appropriate, involving indicated prevention through formal assessment of substance abuse problems (Witkiewitz & Estrada, 2011).

REFERRAL AND ASSESSMENT SERVICES

Diagnostic evaluations to determine the presence of SUDs generally occur in several stages: referral, screening, and comprehensive evaluation. Although service members are encouraged to self-refer if they believe that they may have an alcohol problem, the most common referral route for a screening is an ARI or concern on the part of command leadership (Ong & Jóseph, 2008). For the most part, alcohol screening and intervention services are considered commander's programs, or resources that senior leaders can use to ensure that their troops get needed help. Command-level advisors on drug and alcohol issues across the services include Navy Drug and Alcohol Program Advisors (DAPA), Substance Abuse Control Officers (SACO) in the Marine Corps, the Army Substance Abuse Program (ASAP), and the Air Force Alcohol and Drug Abuse Prevention and Treatment program (ADAPT). Table 7.1 provides the various regulations for substance abuse evaluations for each branch of the military. Some of the most common reasons for command referrals are illegal civil or military behavior involving drugs or alcohol, intimate partner violence involving alcohol, or driving under the influence or while intoxicated (Ong & Joseph, 2008). Given that various levels of the chain of command are involved in processing documentation related to an ARI, there is limited confidentiality in drug and alcohol misuse referrals (Hoyt, 2013). Nonetheless, efforts to promote self-referral to alcohol treatment through increased confidentiality have been successfully piloted (Gibbs & Rae Olmsted, 2011), creating limited exceptions in which voluntary clinical services related to alcohol can be made available without command notification in certain situations (e.g., Department of the Air Force, 2018a; Department of the Army, 2020).

Primary-care physicians play a key role in the screening and diagnosis of alcohol-related problems. Several steps can be helpful in this setting (Fiellin, Reid, & O'Connor, 2000): (1) Inquire about current and past alcohol use with all patients, including any family history of substance-related problems; (2) for individuals identified as "drinkers," obtain enough detailed information to differentiate between moderate and heavy drinkers; (3) use standard screening questionnaires such as CAGE (e.g., Have you ever felt the need to *cut* down on drinking? Have you ever felt *a*nnoyed by criticism of your drinking? Have you ever had *g*uilty feelings about your drinking? Have you ever taken a morning *e*ye opener?); (4) based on information from Steps 1–3, ask more specific questions to determine whether criteria for an alcohol use disorder are met and to assess for evidence of any medical, psychiatric, or behavioral complications associated with excessive drinking and/or other substance use. In their review of 22 studies, Kaner et al. (2007) found that general practitioners can help patients alter patterns of harmful drinking with brief interventions, including feedback on alcohol use and dangers, identification of high-risk situations for drinking and coping strategies, increased motivation, and the development of a personal plan to reduce drinking. Research with veteran samples showed that such brief interventions can significantly reduce problematic drinking for up to 6 months (Wigham et al., 2017). Such assessments also can be integrated

TABLE 7.1. Substance-Related Instructions by Branch of Service

Instruction	Air Force	Army	Coast Guard	Marine Corps	Navy
Alcohol rehabilitation failure	AFI 44-121; AFI 36-3208 Chapter 10	AR 600-85; AR 635-200	COMDTINST M1000.4	MCO 1900.16 CH 2	MILPERSMAN article 1910-152
Substance use disorders; Chapter 4	AFI 44-121	AR 600-85 Chapter 4	COMDTINST M1000.10A	MCO 5300.17A	SECNAVINST 5300.28F
Aviation personnel	AFI 44-121	AR 600-85 Chapter 4	COMDTINST M6410.3A	MANMED Chapter 15 Section IV	MANMED Chapter 15 Section IV
Submarine and nuclear weapon personnel	AFMAN 13-501	AR 50-5	No specific instruction.	SECNAVINST 5510.35D	SECNAVINST 5510.35D
Substance use and security clearances	AFMAN 16-1405	AR 380-67	COMDTINST M5520.12C	SECNAVINST 5510.30C	SECNAVINST 5510.30C
Substance abuse prevention and control; OPNAVINST 5350.4D	AFI 44-121 Chapter 3	AR 600-85 Chapter 2	COMDTINST M6320.5	MCO 5300.17A MCO1700.22G	SECNAVINST 5300.28F
Standards for provision of substance-related disorder treatment services; BUMEDINST 5353.4B	AFI 44-121 Chapter 3	SUDCC Operations Manual	COMDTINST M6320.5	MCO 5300.17A	BUMEDINST 5353.4B

Note. AFI, Air Force Instruction; AR, Army Regulation; BUMEDINST, Department of the Navy, Bureau of Medicine and Surgery Instruction; COMDTINST, United States Coast Guard, Commandant Instruction; MCO, Marine Corps Order; MILPERSMAN, Navy Military Personnel Manual; OPNAVINST, Chief of Naval Operations Instruction; SECNAVINST, Secretary of the Navy Instruction; SUDCC, Substance Use Disorder Clinical Care. Full reference entries for the specific publications noted in this table are listed in the References under the "U.S. Department of . . ." citations.

into postdeployment screening to identify emerging alcohol-related problems (e.g., Larson et al., 2014).

Navy flight surgeons are taught during their initial aeromedical training to employ the SBIRT (Screening, Brief Intervention and Referral to Treatment) approach in their practice of aviation medicine (Babor et al., 2007; Babor & Higgins-Biddle, 2000). In addition to the CAGE, they are also instructed in the use of the Alcohol Use Disorders Identification Test (AUDIT); the Alcohol Use Disorders Identification Test-Consumption (AUDIT-C), consisting of only the 3 alcohol consumption items from the full 10-item AUDIT (Bush, Kivlahan, McDonell, Fihn, & Bradley, 1998); and quantity/frequency questions, including the single-item alcohol pre-screening question ("On any single occasion during the past 3 months, have you had more than 5 drinks containing alcohol?") recommended by the National Institute on Alcohol Abuse and Alcoholism (Taj, Devara-Sales, & Vinson, 1998). The student flight surgeons also receive experiential training in brief interventions using motivational interviewing techniques (Miller & Rollnick, 2002) and guidance on referral to treatment when indicated.

It is also common for substance problems to be detected by emergency room physicians (e.g., when patients present after fights or accidents while intoxicated), mental health providers (e.g., diagnoses made during outpatient evaluation or while on the inpatient mental health unit), and internists (e.g., patients admitted for detoxification). A strong collaboration with these areas of medical treatment facilities is important and can lead to an increase in referrals and earlier detection of problems (e.g., Fernandez, Hartman, & Olshaker, 2006). Storer (2003) noted significant benefits to brief inpatient interventions in both preventing repeat alcohol-related hospitalizations to Naval Medical Center Portsmouth, as well as reducing the length of stay of individuals who were readmitted.

Once a referral is made, the active-duty member undergoes an outpatient or inpatient substance abuse screening. Screenings focus mainly on the extent of the alcohol or drug use. Substance-related diagnoses are based on criteria established by the fifth edition of the *Diagnostic and Statistical Manual of Mental Disorders* (DSM-5; American Psychiatric Association, 2013). If DSM-5 criteria are met for a SUD, a provisional diagnosis is made by the screener and the individual is referred for a more comprehensive evaluation. The majority of referrals are for single ARIs (Ong & Joseph, 2008). Many of these one-time incident referrals do not result in diagnostic criteria being met for a SUD. Although some service members not meeting diagnostic criteria are returned to their commands with recommendations for "no action," most are recommended for early intervention education programs conducted by service-specific prevention personnel, as discussed (Schmid et al., 2017). The following case is a typical depiction of a service member and a one-time incident.

Case 7.2. The Underage Drinker

The airman first class (A1C) was a 20-year-old service member in the Air Force with 1 year of service. He came to the attention of his command when he showed up at morning formation still smelling of alcohol from heavy drinking with other service members the night before. When given a command-initiated breathalyzer test that morning, his blood alcohol concentration was still above the legal limit. Due to the breathalyzer finding and underage drinking, the A1C was referred to the ADAPT program. The ADAPT assessment did not formally diagnose him with an alcohol use disorder, but recommended that he enroll in alcohol brief counseling with an enlisted certified alcohol and drug abuse counselor to address this alcohol-related incident. The command reduced him in rank to airman as a result of his misconduct, and he showed good engagement with the educational program.

A word of caution is offered here about both the overdiagnosis and the underdiagnosis of alcohol use disorders among military personnel. Some clinicians strictly adhere to DSM-5 criteria for alcohol use disorder and will sometimes make the diagnosis based on two alcohol-related incidents that occur within a 12-month period regardless of their severity. A common example might involve a 19- or 20-year-old service member who is referred for evaluation because he or she has had two underage drinking incidents (involving one or two beers) but no accompanying behavioral problem such as fighting or disorderly conduct. This type of individual might be better served by an early intervention approach rather than alcohol treatment if the infraction is attributable to simple rule breaking rather than a bona fide SUD. On the other hand, too strict an interpretation of the 12-month temporal cluster criterion may mean that service members with recurrent episodes of clinically significant abusive drinking that spans several years could be underdiagnosed because their incidents do not fall within the stipulated 12-month time frame. Thus, a service member with four DUIs at 18-month intervals across several duty stations could conceivably be found to not meet the diagnostic criteria for an alcohol use disorder even though his or her continuing pattern of problematic drinking is undeniable. These service members may seek "geographic cures," as the documentation of incidents from one command sometimes does not arrive at the next duty station. A reasonable application of flexibility to the diagnostic criteria should allow diagnosis of alcohol use disorder in such cases because maladaptive drinking patterns have been found to be persistent over significant time periods. The use of the DSM-5 residual category of unspecified alcohol use disorder is sometimes helpful in this regard, as it "applies to presentations in which symptoms characteristic of an alcohol-related disorder that cause clinically significant distress or impairment in social, occupational, or other important areas of functioning predominate but do not meet the full criteria for any specific alcohol-related disorder" (DSM-5; American Psychiatric Association, 2013).

LEVELS OF TREATMENT

Service members who meet criteria for a SUD during a screening then undergo a comprehensive evaluation to determine an appropriate treatment plan. This evaluation typically covers topics addressed in a traditional psychological evaluation as well as an in-depth exploration of the onset of substance use, changes in use over time, current use, triggers to maladaptive use, availability of a support system, current stressors, and coping strategies (e.g., Hawkins, Grossbard, Benbow, Nacev, & Kivlahan, 2012). Diagnostic information is integrated with treatment placement criteria from the American Society of Addiction Medicine (ASAM; Mee-Lee, 2013) to determine the appropriate level of care (for an evaluation example, see Appendix 7.1 at the end of the chapter). ASAM placement criteria establish guidelines for outpatient treatment, intensive outpatient treatment, residential treatment, and medically managed intensive inpatient treatment such as detoxification, all of which are available through military medical treatment facilities (Bollinger & Waters, 2018). Patient placement decisions are based on assessment of various dimensions, including acute intoxication/withdrawal risk, medical conditions, coexisting psychological diagnoses, treatment acceptance and resistance, relapse potential, and the recovery environment (Defense Health Agency, 2019). Integration of diagnostic and placement criteria in the treatment of substance abuse problems requires a thorough knowledge of withdrawal symptoms, evaluation procedures, and comorbidities of substance abuse problems with other mental health and medical conditions (Hawkins et al., 2012).

In general, a diagnosis of mild alcohol use disorder warrants outpatient treatment (ASAM Level 1), although an individual considered to be at heightened risk (e.g., multiple alcohol-related incidents and severe psychosocial problems) could be placed in a more intensive level of treatment. In the same vein, a diagnosis of moderate alcohol use disorder generally warrants intensive outpatient treatment (Level 2), and a diagnosis of severe alcohol use disorder warrants residential treatment (Level 3). Exceptions to this rule might include those who previously completed treatment for alcohol use disorder and were able to remain sober for a significant period of time, but then had a brief relapse. If such individuals want to stay sober and demonstrate singular motivation to follow a recovery plan, they may be best served by a time-limited period of outpatient (OP) treatment or a revision of their after-care plan to include increased attendance in Alcoholics Anonymous (AA) meetings, developing and following a relapse prevention plan, and/or establishing environmental changes that support an abstinence-based lifestyle. The length of OP treatment differs among the services, ranging from weekly meetings for 2–3 months to daily sessions for about 2 weeks (Bollinger & Waters, 2018). OP treatment typically focuses on substance education, stress management, and boosting coping strategies. It is considered appropriate for individuals who are exhibiting problematic alcohol or drug use and who may be developing a more serious substance problem, but who have not yet demonstrated signs of dependence. In some ways, OP is an extension of early intervention in that the emphasis is on education, alternative activities to drinking or other substance use, and the development of more adaptive behaviors and stress management techniques (Schmid et al., 2017). In OP, however, members attend individual therapy, receive an introduction to AA or comparable mutual-support programs, and are integrated into group therapy with individuals with varying levels of severity of substance abuse.

Intensive outpatient (IOP) treatment is appropriate for those individuals with significant alcohol or drug problems that can be effectively treated in an outpatient environment (McCarty et al., 2014). Given the level of military structure, this model is the most frequently used because there are significant command supports in place for abstinence and alternative activities (see Institute of Medicine, 2013; Hoyt et al., 2018). IOP generally lasts 2–3 weeks and focuses on the same areas as OP, but it provides more in-depth education, increased individual and group therapy, and an emphasis on regular attendance at 12-Step meetings. Residential treatment is available for individuals who need that higher level of structure in order to remain abstinent during the treatment program or who have comorbid disorders that require additional medical and/or mental health support. One such residential program is a 22-bed inpatient center established in 2009 at Dwight D. Eisenhower Army Medical Center to cover all branches of the military. This program includes daily physical training, 12-Step groups, life skills, recreational therapy, and CBT for addiction behavior (Mooney et al., 2014).

A treatment modality often used across outpatient, intensive outpatient, and inpatient/residential treatment programs for SUDs is medication-assisted treatment (MAT). MAT is the use of medications, in combination with counseling and behavioral therapies, to provide a "whole-patient" approach to the treatment of SUDs. Medications used for MAT are evidence-based treatment options and do not just substitute one drug for another (Connery, 2015). Research shows that a combination of medication and psychotherapy can successfully treat and maintain recovery as well as prevent or reduce opioid overdose (Klein & Seppala, 2019). MAT is primarily used for the treatment of addiction to opioids such as heroin and prescription opioids. MAT normalizes brain chemistry, blocks the euphoric effects of alcohol and opioids, relieves physiological cravings, and normalizes body functions without the negative and euphoric effects of the substance used (Connery, 2015).

MAT has proved to be clinically effective and to significantly reduce the need for inpatient detoxification services (Kenney, Bailey, Anderson, & Stein, 2017). While the ultimate goal of MAT is sustained recovery, this treatment approach also has been shown to improve patient survival, increase retention in treatment, decrease illicit opioid use and other criminal activity among people with SUDs, increase patients' ability to gain and maintain employment, and improve birth outcomes among women who have SUDs and are pregnant (Bailey, Herman, & Stein, 2013). Research also shows that these medications and therapies can contribute to lowering a person's risk of contracting HIV or hepatitis C by reducing the potential for relapse (Schranz, Barrett, Hurt, Malvestutto, & Miller, 2018).

Clinical practice guidelines (U.S. Department of Veterans Affairs and Department of Defense, 2015) recommend three medications for the treatment of opioid use disorders (OUDs): buprenorphine, methadone, and naltrexone. These medications are used to treat addiction to short-acting opioids such as heroin, morphine, and codeine, as well as semi-synthetic opioids like oxycodone and hydrocodone (Rosenberg, Bilka, Wilson, & Spevak, 2018). These MAT medications generally have been shown to be safe for long-term (months to years) maintenance (Oesterle, Thusius, Rummans, & Gold, 2019). Federal policies specify treatment delivery settings for the use of certain MAT (see Priest et al., 2019). Methadone is a full agonist at the mu opioid receptor that is prescribed and dispensed by a federally licensed opioid treatment facility (OTP). It is important to note that methadone is not prescribed for the treatment of OUD outside of a federal OTP. In contrast, physicians in office-based treatment (OBT) settings may prescribe buprenorphine, increasing the availability of MAT in primary-care and specialty settings (Priest et al., 2019). Naltrexone is used as both a once daily pill and as a monthly long-acting injectable agent. The choice of MAT for OUD is driven by patient-specific characteristics and needs, to include access and costs. Multiple drug-to-drug interactions have to be taken into account, such as increased sedation with psychotropic medications (Connery, 2015). Finally, naloxone is recommended to prevent opioid overdose by reversing the toxic effects of the overdose (see Oliva et al., 2017).

There are currently three FDA-approved amethystic medications to support abstinence from drinking in patients with alcohol use disorders: disulfiram, naltrexone, and acamprosate. Several other medications have been found to be helpful in off-label use in these patients.

A word of caution: MAT may not be appropriate for certain patients in safety-sensitive occupations, such as pilots, air traffic controllers, UAV operators, and other special duty personnel. Before considering the use of these drugs in such patients, it is advisable to consult with the patient's flight surgeon or other cognizant operational medical officer for guidance about community-specific limitations. Patients requiring this level of treatment are restricted from deployment and many specialty duties by policy. U.S. Central Command (USCENTCOM, 2020) specifically prohibits personnel from deploying if pharmacotherapy for SUD or AUD is required for maintenance of these conditions. Furthermore, service members undergoing formal treatment using MAT must have completed treatment successfully—with a demonstrated period of stability lasting at least 12 months—before they can be medically cleared for deployment (USCENTCOM, 2020). Parallel requirements govern deployment restrictions to other areas of the globe, including U.S. Indo-Pacific Command (USINDOPACOM, 2020) and U.S. Africa Command (USAFRICOM, 2019). Whereas the military is supportive of these service members receiving needed treatment, this level of treatment is incompatible with military service in austere environments.

PTSD AND SUDs

Given exposure to combat and traumatic incidents associated with training exercises, peacekeeping missions, and humanitarian relief, the military population as a group is thought to be at a particularly high risk of developing PTSD and other mental health disorders (see also Chapter 4, this volume). Meta-analysis indicates that rates of PTSD among veterans of Operation Iraqi Freedom (OIF) and Operation Enduring Freedom (OEF) range from 1.4 to 60% in individual studies, with an overall prevalence estimate of 23% (Fulton et al., 2015). PTSD and SUDs commonly occur in conjunction with one another among service members and veterans (Dworkin, Bergman, Walton, Walker, & Kaysen, 2018). Veterans report regular use of substances to manage PTSD symptoms (Ruzek, 2003), and 75% of Vietnam veterans who met the criteria for PTSD following their military service also met the criteria for SUDs (Jacobsen, Southwick, & Kosten, 2001). Among OIF and OEF veterans diagnosed with alcohol or other substance use disorders, a national study showed that 63–76% also were diagnosed with PTSD (Seal et al., 2011). In fact, alcohol as a coping mechanism among veterans is the primary factor that accounts for the relationship between PTSD symptoms and alcohol-related problems, such as hazardous drinking (McDevitt-Murphy, Luciano, Tripp, & Eddinger, 2017; Miller, Pederson, & Marshall, 2017).

A number of factors may exacerbate the likelihood of comorbid PTSD and SUD diagnoses. In a study that surveyed 1,120 soldiers returning from Iraq, of the 1,080 soldiers who responded to alcohol-related questions, 25% screened positive for alcohol misuse 3–4 months after returning home, and those who screened positive had significantly more combat experiences than those who screened negative (Wilk et al., 2010). Similarly, in another postdeployment sample, 27% of service members screened positive for alcohol misuse, with the highest rates among those with the greatest combat exposure (Santiago et al., 2010). Externalizing personality factors among veterans with PTSD also may increase the risk for alcohol and substance use disorders (Rielage, Hoyt, & Renshaw, 2010; Boland, Rielage, & Hoyt, 2018). The combination of PTSD and SUD also may significantly increase suicide risk. Nationally representative samples of veterans show significantly increased risk of both PTSD and suicide behavior among those with a lifetime history of alcohol use disorder (Fuehrlein et al., 2016). A large nationwide survey of veterans with PTSD showed that the comorbid presence of a SUD significantly increased risk of self-directed violence and death by suicide (Ronzitti et al., 2019). Alcohol use disorders and other mental health disorders also may have a bidirectional relationship. A study of newly enlisted service members showed that mental health diagnoses prior to enlistment significantly predicted the onset of alcohol use disorders, but also that prior alcohol use disorders significantly predicted subsequent mental health diagnoses (Stein et al., 2017).

Individuals with co-occurring PTSD and SUD typically have more intensive treatment needs from an addictions-services perspective compared to addicted individuals with no PTSD component (e.g., Bernhardt, 2009; Korte et al., 2017). Individuals with co-occurring SUDs and PTSD tend to have worse treatment outcomes overall, including more psychiatric, medical, legal, and social problems, and tend to relapse sooner than those with just one of these disorders (McCauley, Killeen, Gros, Brady, & Back, 2012). PTSD treatment has been shown to reduce not only immediate but also long-term risk of SUD relapse if provided during the transitional period beginning soon after discharge from inpatient SUD treatment and during the long-term recovery period (Ford, Russo, & Mallon, 2007). In the recent past, the assumed interventional model for treating comorbid PTSD and SUD was that trauma-focused treatment could not be initiated until SUD problems had been resolved (see van Dam, Vedel, Ehring, & Emmelkamp, 2012). More recently, integrative treatments have been studied that combine treatment for PTSD and SUD. A randomized clinical trial of combined naltrexone and exposure-based treatment showed no exacerbation of alcohol use disorder symptoms as a result of trauma-focused treatment (Foa et al., 2013). Another example is Seeking Safety, a trauma-focused treatment that also emphasizes harm reduction in SUD and has shown positive treatment effects among service members (Najavits, Lande, Gragnani, Isenstein, & Schmidtz, 2016). Secondary analysis from clinical trials of exposure-based treatment furthermore shows no difference in treatment response based on whether or not service members with PTSD also exhibited problematic alcohol use (Dondanville et al., 2019).

Due to the frequent co-occurrence of PTSD and SUD, screening for PTSD and related treatment should be integrated into military substance abuse assessments and programs. A recommended screening instrument, the PTSD Checklist for DSM-5 (PCL-5; Blevins et al., 2015; see Figure 7.2) can be easily integrated into the existing questionnaires that are completed by every military member as a part of the substance use evaluation process. The PCL-5 is in the public domain and has been validated among military samples (Wortmann et al., 2016). The need not only for PTSD screenings but also for concurrent treatment for both disorders has been recognized by some providers, and some military substance abuse programs include integrated treatment of PTSD within that realm. However, treatment integration remains at the discretion of individual facilities and is not standardized throughout the services. Given the high rates of traumatic exposure reported by veterans of combat operations in Afghanistan and Iraq, integrated treatment will be a crucial step forward for today's active-duty population.

TREATMENT OF GAMBLING DISORDER IN THE MILITARY

With 77% of the U.S. population participating in gambling each year, the rate of gambling disorder is approximately 2.4% (Welte, Barnes, Tidwell, Hoffman, & Wieczorek, 2015). Population studies also show significant rates of comorbidity with pathological gambling, with 73% also having an alcohol use disorder and 38% also having a drug use disorder (Petry, Stinson, & Grant, 2005). Gambling problems are also no stranger to the military. General George Washington issued orders against his soldiers and officers participating in gambling (Washington, 1776). The most recent population-based study of problematic gambling in service members was conducted in 2002 (Bray et al., 2003). This survey indicated that the lifetime prevalence of gambling-related problems among service members is approximately 6.3%, with 1.2% reporting pathological gambling. Specific to each military branch, lifetime rates of pathological gambling are 0.7% in the Air Force, 1.4% in the Army, 1.4% in the Marine Corps, and 1.5% in the Navy. The highest rates of pathological gambling were reported among heavy alcohol drinkers (5.1%). Consistent findings were identified in a subsequent sample (Weis & Manos, 2007).

One study of treatment for pathological gambling among service members shows a typical profile (Kennedy, Cook, Poole, Brunson, & Jones, 2005). Participants in this program were 33 years old on average, typically ranking between grades E-4 and E-6. The mean reported debt per individual was $11,407.35, with a standard deviation of $17,746.26. The average reported financial losses from gambling per individual were $24,154.41, with a standard deviation of $33,125.22. Of the 25 active-duty members referred for treatment in this program, 21 were retained in the military and four were court-martialed and subsequently discharged for crimes related

Patient's Name: _____

Instructions: Below is a list of problems that people sometimes have in response to a very stressful experience. Please read each problem carefully; put an X in the box to indicate how much you have been bothered by that problem in the past month.

In the past month, how much were you bothered by:	Not at all (0)	A little bit (1)	Moderately (2)	Quite a bit (3)	Extremely (4)
1. Repeated, disturbing, and unwanted memories of the stressful experience?					
2. Repeated, disturbing dreams of the stressful experience?					
3. Suddenly feeling or acting as if the stressful experience were actually happening again (as if you were actually back there reliving it)?					
4. Feeling very upset when something reminded you of the stressful experience?					
5. Having strong physical reactions when something reminded you of the stressful experience (e.g., heart pounding, trouble breathing, sweating)?					
6. Avoiding memories, thoughts, or feelings related to the stressful experience?					
7. Avoiding external reminders of the stressful experience (e.g., people, places, conversations, activities, objects, or situations)?					
8. Trouble remembering important parts of the stressful experience?					
9. Having strong negative beliefs about yourself, other people, or the world (e.g., having thoughts such as: I am bad, there is something seriously wrong with me, no one can be trusted, the world is completely dangerous)?					
10. Blaming yourself or someone else for the stressful experience or what happened after it?					
11. Having strong negative feelings such as fear, horror, anger, guilt, or shame?					
12. Loss of interest in activities that you used to enjoy?					
13. Feeling distant or cut off from other people?					
14. Trouble experiencing positive feelings (e.g., being unable to feel happiness or have loving feelings for people close to you)?					
15. Irritable behavior, angry outbursts, or acting aggressively?					
16. Taking too many risks or doing things that could cause you harm?					
17. Being "super-alert" or watchful or on guard?					
18. Feeling jumpy or easily startled?					
19. Having difficulty concentrating?					
20. Trouble falling or staying asleep?					
Total:					

FIGURE 7.2. PTSD Checklist for DSM-5 (Weathers et al., 2013).

to their gambling. The following depicts a typical example of how service members with a gambling problem may be identified.

Case 7.3. The Soldier with Gambling Debts

The company officer, an Army Captain, received a late-night phone call from a local collection agency about one of his Staff Sergeants (SSG). Over the course of several months, the SSG had taken out several payday loans but was behind on the payments; the collection agency requested garnishment of her military wages in order to cover these payments. When the Captain confronted the SSG about this incident, she reluctantly admitted that she had been spending a lot of time at the local casino on the weekend, and had taken out the loans to cover gambling losses. The Captain consulted with providers at the Army Substance Use Disorder Clinical Care (SUDCC) program, and command referred the SSG for an assessment. This assessment revealed that she had struggled for some time with a gambling disorder, as well as a moderate alcohol use disorder. The SSG was enrolled in an intensive outpatient program to address these issues.

Rates of problematic gambling may differentially affect certain groups within the military. A large study of recruits in Air Force basic training showed that 10.4% of these service members participated in gambling weekly or more often, with 6.2% reporting gambling-related problems and 1.9% reporting likely pathological gambling (Steenbergh, Whelan, Meyers, Kiesges, & De Bon, 2008). A study of National Guard members showed that 13% of those surveyed participated in gambling weekly or more often, with 7.7% reporting lifetime potential problematic gambling (Gallaway et al., 2019). Alcohol use disorders also significantly increase rates of pathological gambling among veterans (Edens & Rosenheck, 2012).

Despite these identified rates, medical record data show that only a small percentage (.03%) of service members seek treatment for gambling disorder (U.S. Government Accountability Office, 2017). Although specialized programs for gambling disorders had been established at some Navy bases (e.g., Kennedy et al., 2005), these programs were closed due to low referral rates (Tiron, 2007). Treatment for problematic gambling behavior now is reportedly integrated into routine outpatient treatment in service-specific addictions programs (U.S. Government Accountability Office, 2017). Army and Air Force regulations specifically detail the inclusion of gambling disorder treatment in these programs (Department of the Air Force, 2018a; Department of the Army, 2020). Military policy regarding confidentiality in cases of pathological gambling differs from that of SUDs. Whereas substance abuse has to be reported to a command, a gambling problem per se does not (e.g., Department of the Air Force, 2018a). Most pathological gambling cases encountered by military psychologists involve addictive behaviors associated with legal activities such as slot machines and casino games. Unless a service member who seeks help for pathological gambling presents with suicidality, maintains a security clearance (see Chapter 14 for a discussion of security clearances and pathological gambling), or another issue that requires mandatory reporting, he or she will enjoy a greater degree of confidentiality than substance patients and can thus self-refer with less worry of stigma, career damage, and similar impediments.

General population studies show that there are a number of other negative sequelae associated with gambling disorders (Rash, Weinstock, & Van Patten, 2016). Gambling disorders significantly increase the risk of suicide (Karlsson & Håkansson, 2018). Overall comorbidity rate estimates for individuals with lifetime gambling disorder and at least one other mental health diagnosis exceed 90% (Bischof et al., 2013; Kessler et al., 2008). A review of the literature shows average comorbidity rate estimates with gambling disorder of 58% with SUD, 38% with mood disorders, and 37% with anxiety disorders (Lorains, Cowlishaw, & Thomas, 2011). Longitudinal models suggest that the relationship between gambling disorders and other mental health diagnoses is bidirectional, such that risk of comorbidity increases regardless of which condition is first identified (Dussault, Brendgen, Vitaro, Wanner, & Tremblay, 2011). Veterans who report frequent gambling are at greater risk for homelessness (Harris, Kintzle, Wenzel, & Castro, 2017).

The treatment of pathological gambling has many similarities to that of other addictions as well as some differences. The evaluation of the pathological gambler cannot be a brief screen, as is done for a preliminary substance abuse evaluation. Because of the severity and frequency of suicidality, as well as other comorbid mental health issues and SUDs, a full psychological evaluation or, at a minimum, a suicide risk assessment must be provided. For a sample gambling evaluation, see Appendix 7.2 at the end of the chapter. The majority of cognitive-behavioral treatments (CBTs) for addiction can be readily applied to gambling behavior with good treatment outcomes (Gooding & Tarrier, 2009; Pallesen, Mitsem, Kvale, Johnson, & Molde, 2005). Studies have shown that 12-Step programs (Petry, 2005), cognitive-behavioral interventions (Champine & Petry, 2010), and motivational approaches (Yakovenko, Quigley, Hemmelgarn, Hodgins, & Ronksley, 2015) all are effective treatments for addressing gambling disorder. Interventions that include family members—such as community reinforcement and family training (CRAFT)—also may be a crucial component of ensuring that gains during treatment can be integrated into the service member's life (e.g., Nayoski & Hodgins, 2016). Clinics may also consider integrating treatment with services for financial counseling, spousal education, marital counseling, and emergent suicide risk assessments (Kennedy et al., 2005).

SUMMARY

Although SUDs continue to be a problem in the military, each service provides a comprehensive range of services, from prevention programs to progressively intensive levels of treatment. Early intervention is provided at the first indication of a possible problem, and excellent treatment options exist and are available to any military member who needs them. The military environment provides significant social support to military members with substance problems and state-of-the-art treatment for all members. Although substance abuse and pathological gambling are very difficult to treat in any arena, military members have an array of educational and treatment options that support readiness and recovery.

REFERENCES

American Psychiatric Association. (2013). *Diagnostic and statistical manual of mental disorders* (5th ed.). Arlington, VA: Author.

Ames, G. M., Cunradi, C. B., & Moore, R. S. (2002). Alcohol, tobacco, and drug use among young adults prior to entering the military. *Prevention Science, 3,* 135–144.

Ames, G. M., Cunradi, C. B., Moore, R. S., & Stern, R. (2007). Military culture and drinking behavior among U.S. Navy careerists. *Journal of Studies on Alcohol and Drugs, 68,* 336–344.

Austerman, W. R. (2010). Aguardiente at the Alamo: Alcohol abuse and the Texas war for independence, 1835–1836. *United States Army Medical Department Journal, PB 8–10 (4/5/6),* 72–80.

Babor, T. F., & Higgins-Biddle, J. C. (2000). Alcohol screening and brief intervention: Dissemination strategies for medical practice and public health. *Addiction, 95,* 677–686.

Babor, T. F., McRee, B. G., Kassebaum, P. A., Grimaldi, P. L., Ahmed, K., & Bray, J. (2007). Screening, Brief Intervention, and Referral to Treatment (SBIRT): Toward a public health approach to the management of substance abuse. *Substance Abuse, 28*(3), 7–30.

Bailey, G. L., Herman, D. S., & Stein, M. D. (2013). Perceived relapse risk and desire for medication assisted treatment among persons seeking inpatient opiate detoxification. *Journal of Substance Abuse Treatment, 45*(3), 302–305.

Baker, S. L. (1972). Present status of the drug abuse counteroffensive in the Armed Forces. *Bulletin of the New York Academy of Medicine, 48*(5), 719–732.

Barry, A. E., Stellefson, M. L., Hanik, B., Tennant, B. L., Whiteman, S. D., Varnes, J., et al. (2013). Examining the association between binge drinking and propensity to join the military. *Military Medicine, 178*(1), 37–42.

Bernhardt, A. (2009). Rising to the challenge of treating OEF/OIF veterans with co-occurring PTSD and substance abuse. *Smith College Studies in Social Work, 79*(3–4), 344–367.

Bischof, A., Meyer, C., Bischof, G., Kastirke, N., John, U., & Rumpf, H. J. (2013). Comorbid Axis I-disorders among subjects with pathological, problem, or at-risk gambling recruited from the general population in Germany: Results of the PAGE study. *Psychiatry Research, 210*(3), 1065–1070.

Blevins, C. A., Weathers, F. W., Davis, M. T., Witte, T. K., & Domino, J. L. (2015). The Posttraumatic Stress Disorder Checklist for DSM-5 (PCL-5): Development and initial psychometric evaluation. *Journal of Traumatic Stress, 28*(6), 489–498.

Boland, M., Rielage, J. K., & Hoyt, T. (2018). The power of negative mood in predicting posttraumatic stress disorder and alcohol abuse comorbidity. *Psychological Trauma: Theory, Research, Practice, and Policy, 10*, 572–575.

Bollinger, J. W., & Waters, A. J. (2018). Substance use treatment programs in the active duty U.S. military: A narrative review. *Military Psychology, 30*(1), 1–9.

Brady, L. L., Credé, M., Harms, P. D., Bachrach, D. G., & Lester, P. B. (2019). Meta-analysis of risk factors for substance abuse in the U.S. military. *Military Psychology, 31*(6), 450–461.

Brantley, C. L. (2012, April). Spice, bath salts, salvia divinorum, and huffing: A judge advocate's guide to disposing of designer drug cases in the military. *The Army Lawyer*, DA PAM 27–50–467, 15–25.

Bray, R. M., Hourani, L. L., Rae, K. L., Dever, J. A., Brown, J. M., Vincus, A. A., et al. (2003). *2002 Department of Defense survey of health related behaviors among military personnel*. Research Triangle Park, NC: RTI International.

Bray, R. M., Marsden, M. E., Herbold, J. R., & Peterson, M. R. (1992). Progress toward eliminating drug and alcohol abuse among U.S. military personnel. *Armed Forces & Society, 18*(4), 476–496.

Bray, R. M., Pemberton, M. R., Hourani, L. L., Witt, M., Rae Olmstead, K. L., Brown, J. N., et al. (2009). *2008 Department of Defense survey of health related behaviors among active duty military personnel*. New York: RTI International.

Brown, J. M., Bray, R. M., & Hartzell, M. C. (2010). A comparison of alcohol use and related problems among women and men in the military. *Military Medicine, 175*, 101–107.

Burt, M. R., Biegel, M. M., Carnes, Y., & Farley, E. C. (1980). *Worldwide survey of nonmedical drug use and alcohol use among military personnel: 1980*. Bethesda, MD: Burt Associates.

Bush, K., Kivlahan, D. R., McDonell, M. B., Fihn, S. D., & Bradley, K. A. (1998). The AUDIT alcohol consumption questions (AUDIT-C): An effective brief screening test for problem drinking. *Archives of Internal Medicine, 158*(16), 1789–1795.

Camp, N. M. (2015). *U.S. Army psychiatry in the Vietnam War: New challenges in extended counterinsurgency warfare*. Washington, DC: Borden Institute.

Campbell, D. J., & Nobel, O. B. Y. (2009). Occupational stressors in military service: A review and framework. *Military Psychology, 21*(Suppl. 2), S47–S67.

Champine, R. B., & Petry, N. M. (2010). Pathological gamblers respond equally well to cognitive-behavioral therapy regardless of other mental health treatment status. *The American Journal on Addictions, 19*(6), 550–556.

Connery, H. S. (2015). Medication-assisted treatment of opioid use disorder: Review of the evidence and future directions. *Harvard Review of Psychiatry, 23*(2), 63–75.

Craig, C. L., & Loeffler, G. H. (2014). The ketamine analog methoxetamine: A new designer drug to threaten military readiness. *Military Medicine, 179*(10), 1149–1157.

Dall, T. M., Zhang, Y., Chen, Y. J., Askarinam Wagner, R. C., Hogan, P. F., Fagan, N. K., et al. (2007). Cost associated with being overweight and with obesity, high alcohol consumption, and tobacco use within the military health system's TRICARE Prime-enrolled population. *American Journal of Health Promotion, 22,* 120–139.

Dean, E. T. (1997). *Shook over hell: Post-traumatic stress, Vietnam, and the Civil War.* Cambridge, MA: Harvard University Press.

Defense Health Agency. (2019). *Management of problematic substance use by DoD personnel* (Defense Health Agency Procedural Instruction 6025.15). Falls Church, VA: Author.

Department of the Air Force. (2004). *Administrative separation of airmen* (Air Force Instruction 36–3208). Arlington, VA: Author.

Department of the Air Force. (2018a). *Alcohol and Drug Abuse Prevention and Treatment (ADAPT) program* (Air Force Instruction 44–121). Arlington, VA: Author.

Department of the Air Force. (2018b). *Nuclear weapons personnel reliability program* (Air Force Manual 13–501). Arlington, VA: Author.

Department of the Air Force. (2018c). *Air Force personnel security program* (Air Force Manual 16–1405). Arlington, VA: Author.

Department of the Army. (2014). *Personnel security program* (Army Regulation 380–67). Arlington, VA: Author.

Department of the Army. (2016). *Active duty enlisted administrative separations* (Army Regulation 635–200). Arlington, VA: Author.

Department of the Army. (2018). *Nuclear surety* (Army Regulation 50–5). Arlington, VA: Author.

Department of the Army. (2020). *The Army Substance Abuse Program* (Army Regulation 600–85). Arlington, VA: Author.

Department of Defense. (1980). *Alcohol and drug abuse by DoD personnel* (Department of Defense Directive 1010.4). Arlington, VA: Author.

Department of Defense. (1985). *Rehabilitation and referral services for alcohol and drug offenders* (Department of Defense Instruction 1010.6). Arlington, VA: Author.

Department of Defense. (2014). *Problematic substance use by DoD personnel* (Department of Defense Instruction 1010.04). Arlington, VA: Author.

Department of the Navy. (2009a). *Separation by reason of alcohol rehabilitation failure or multiple driving under the influence/driving while intoxicated* (MILPERSMAN 1910–152). Arlington, VA: Author.

Department of the Navy. (2009b). Navy alcohol and drug abuse prevention and control (OPNAVINST 5350.4D). Arlington, VA: Author.

Department of the Navy. (2015a). *Alcoholic beverage control in the Marine Corps* (Marine Corps Order 1700.22G). Arlington, VA: Author.

Department of the Navy. (2015b). *Standards for provision of substance related disorder treatment services* (BUMED Instruction 5353.4B). Arlington, VA: Author.

Department of the Navy. (2018a). *Marine Corps substance abuse program* (Marine Corps Order 5300.17A). Arlington, VA: Author.

Department of the Navy. (2018b). *Manual of the Medical Department* (MANMED; NAVMED P-117). Arlington, VA: Author.

Department of the Navy. (2019a). *Separation and retirement manual* (Marine Corps Order 1900.16 CH 2). Arlington, VA: Author.

Department of the Navy. (2019b). *Department of the Navy nuclear weapons personnel reliability program* (SECNAVINST 5510.35D). Arlington, VA: Author.

Department of the Navy. (2019c). *Military substance abuse prevention and control* (SECNAVINST 5300.28F). Arlington, VA: Author.

Department of the Navy. (2020). *Department of the Navy personnel security program* (SECNAVINST 5510.30C). Arlington, VA: Author.

Department of Veterans Affairs & Department of Defense (2015). *VA/DoD clinical practice guideline for the management of substance use disorders.* Retrieved from *www.healthquality.va.gov/guidelines/mh/sud.*

Dondanville, K. A., Wachen, J. S., Hale, W. J., Mintz, J., Roache, J. D., Carson, C., et al. (2019). Examination of treatment effects on hazardous drinking among service members with posttraumatic stress disorder. *Journal of Traumatic Stress, 32*(2), 310–316.

Dussault, F., Brendgen, M., Vitaro, F., Wanner, B., & Tremblay, R. E. (2011). Longitudinal links between impulsivity, gambling problems and depressive symptoms: A transactional model from adolescence to early adulthood. *Journal of Child Psychology and Psychiatry, 52*(2), 130–138.

Dworkin, E. R., Bergman, H. E., Walton, T. O., Walker, D. D., & Kaysen, D. L. (2018). Co-occurring post-traumatic stress disorder and alcohol use disorder in U.S. military and veteran populations. *Alcohol Research: Current Reviews, 39*(2), 161–169.

Edens, E. L., & Rosenheck, R. A. (2012). Rates and correlates of pathological gambling among VA mental health service users. *Journal of Gambling Studies, 28*(1), 1–11.

Fernandez, W. G., Hartman, R., & Olshaker, J. (2006). Brief interventions to reduce harmful alcohol use among military personnel: Lessons learned from the civilian experience. *Military Medicine, 171*(6), 538–543.

Fiellin, D. A., Reid, M. C., & O'Connor, P. G. (2000). Screening for alcohol problems in primary care: A systematic review. *Archives of Internal Medicine, 160*(13), 1977–1989.

Fink, D. S., Gallaway, M. S., Tamburrino, M. B., Liberzon, I., Chan, P., Cohen, G. H., et al. (2016). Onset of alcohol use disorders and comorbid psychiatric disorders in a military cohort: Are there critical periods for prevention of alcohol use disorders? *Prevention Science, 17*(3), 347–356.

Fisher, C. A., Hoffman, K. J., Austin-Lane, J., & Kao, T. (2000). The relationship between heavy alcohol use and work productivity loss in active duty military personnel: A secondary analysis of the 1995 Department of Defense worldwide survey. *Military Medicine, 165*, 355–361.

Foa, E. B., Yusko, D. A., McLean, C. P., Suvak, M. K., Bux, D. A., Oslin, D., et al. (2013). Concurrent naltrexone and prolonged exposure therapy for patients with comorbid alcohol dependence and PTSD: A randomized clinical trial. *JAMA, 310*(5), 488–495.

Ford, J. D., Russo, E. M., & Mallon, S. D. (2007). Integrating treatment of posttraumatic stress disorder and substance use disorder. *Journal of Counseling and Development, 85,* 475–490.

Fuehrlein, B. S., Mota, N., Arias, A. J., Trevisan, L. A., Kachadourian, L. K., Krystal, J. H., et al. (2016). The burden of alcohol use disorders in U.S. military veterans: Results from the National Health and Resilience in Veterans Study. *Addiction, 111*(10), 1786–1794.

Fulton, J. J., Calhoun, P. S., Wagner, H. R., Schry, A. R., Hair, L. P., Feeling, N., et al. (2015). The prevalence of posttraumatic stress disorder in Operation Enduring Freedom/Operation Iraqi Freedom (OEF/OIF) veterans: A meta-analysis. *Journal of Anxiety Disorders, 31,* 98–107.

Gallaway, M. S., Fink, D. S., Sampson, L., Cohen, G. H., Tamburrino, M., Liberzon, I., et al. (2019). Prevalence and covariates of problematic gambling among a U.S. military cohort. *Addictive Behaviors, 95,* 166–171.

Gibbs, D. A., & Rae Olmsted, K. L. (2011). Preliminary examination of the confidential alcohol treatment and education program. *Military Psychology, 23*(1), 97–111.

Gooding, P., & Tarrier, N. (2009). A systematic review and meta-analysis of cognitive-behavioural interventions to reduce problem gambling: Hedging our bets? *Behaviour Research and Therapy, 47*(7), 592–607.

Grattan, L. E., Mengistu, B. S., Bullock, S. H., Santo, T. J., & Jackson, D. D. (2019). Restricting retail hours of alcohol sales within an army community. *Military Medicine, 184*(9–10), e400–e405.

Gunby, P. (1991). Service in strict Islamic nation removes alcohol, other drugs from major problem list. *JAMA, 265*(5), 560–562.

Harris, T., Kintzle, S., Wenzel, S., & Castro, C. A. (2017). Expanding the understanding of risk behavior associated with homelessness among veterans. *Military Medicine, 182*(9–10), e1900–e1907.

Harwood, H. J., Zhang, Y., Dall, T. M., Olaiya, S. T., & Fagan, N. K. (2009). Economic implications of reduced binge drinking among the military health system's TRICARE Prime plan beneficiaries. *Military Medicine, 174,* 728–736.

Hawkins, E. J., Grossbard, J., Benbow, J., Nacev, V., & Kivlahan, D. R. (2012). Evidence-based screening, diagnosis, and treatment of substance use disorders among veterans and military service personnel. *Military Medicine, 177*(Suppl. 8), 29–38.

Hoyt, T. (2013). Limits to confidentiality in U.S. Army treatment settings. *Military Psychology, 25,* 46–56.

Hoyt, T., Barry, D. M., Kwon, S. J., Capron, C., De Guzman, N., Gilligan, J., & Edwards-Stewart, A. (2018). Preliminary evaluation of treatment outcomes at a military intensive outpatient program. *Psychological Services, 15,* 510–519.

Hurt, L. (2015). Post-deployment screening and referral for risky alcohol use and subsequent alcohol-related and injury diagnoses, active component, U.S. Armed Forces, 2008–2014. *Medical Surveillance Monthly Report, 22*(7), 7–13.

Institute of Medicine. (2013). *Substance use disorders in the U.S. Armed Forces.* Washington, DC: The National Academies Press.

Jacobsen, L. K., Southwick, S. M., & Kosten, T. R. (2001). Substance use disorders in patients with posttraumatic stress disorder: A review of the literature. *American Journal of Psychiatry, 158,* 1184–1190.

Jones, F. D. (1995). Disorders of frustration and loneliness. In R. Zajtchuk & R. F. Bellamy (Eds.), *Textbook of military medicine: War psychiatry* (pp. 63–84). Washington, DC: Office of the Surgeon General, U.S. Department of the Army.

Joseph, B. S. (1974). Lessons on heroin abuse from treating users in Vietnam. *Hospital and Community Psychiatry, 25,* 742–744.

Kaner E. F., Dickinson H. O., Beyer F. R., Campbell F., Schlesinger C., Heather N., et al. (2007). Effectiveness of brief alcohol interventions in primary care populations. *Cochrane Database of Systematic Reviews,* Issue 2, Article CD004148.

Karlsson, A., & Håkansson, A. (2018). Gambling disorder, increased mortality, suicidality, and associated comorbidity: A longitudinal nationwide register study. *Journal of Behavioral Addictions, 7*(4), 1091–1099.

Kelsall, H. L., Wijesinghe, M. S. D., Creamer, M. C., McKenzie, D. P., Forbes, A. B., Page, M. J., & Sim, M. R. (2015). Alcohol use and substance use disorders in Gulf War, Afghanistan, and Iraq War veterans compared with nondeployed military personnel. *Epidemiologic Reviews, 37*(1), 38–54.

Kennedy, C. H., Cook, J. H., Poole, D. R., Brunson, C. L., & Jones, D. E. (2005). Review of the first year of an overseas military gambling treatment program. *Military Medicine, 170,* 683–687.

Kenney, S. R., Bailey, G. L., Anderson, B. J., & Stein, M. D. (2017). Heroin refusal self-efficacy and preference for medication-assisted treatment after inpatient detoxification. *Addictive Behaviors, 73,* 124–128.

Kessler, R. C., Hwang, I., Labrie, R., Petukhova, M., Sampson, N. A., Winters, K. C., et al. (2008). DSM-IV pathological gambling in the National Comorbidity Survey Replication. *Psychological Medicine, 38*(9), 1351–1360.

Klein, A. A., & Seppala, M. D. (2019). Medication-assisted treatment for opioid use disorder within a 12-Step based treatment center: Feasibility and initial results. *Journal of Substance Abuse Treatment, 104,* 51–63.

Klesges, R. C., Talcott, W., Ebbert, J. O., Murphy, J. G., McDevitt-Murphy, M. E., Thomas, F., et al. (2013). Effect of the Alcohol Misconduct Prevention Program (AMPP) in Air Force technical training. *Military Medicine, 178*(4), 445–451.

Korte, K. J., Bountress, K. E., Tomko, R. L., Killeen, T., Maria, M. S., & Back, S. E. (2017). Integrated treatment of PTSD and substance use disorders: The mediating role of PTSD improvement in the reduction of depression. *Journal of Clinical Medicine, 6*(1), 9.

Larson, M. J., Mohr, B. A., Adams, R. S., Wooten, N. R., & Williams, T. V. (2014). Missed opportunity for alcohol problem prevention among army active duty service members postdeployment. *American Journal of Public Health, 104*(8), 1402–1412.

Larson, M. J., Mohr, B. A., Jeffery, D. D., Adams, R. S., & Williams, T. V. (2016). Predictors of positive illicit drug tests after OEF/OIF deployment among Army enlisted service members. *Military Medicine, 181*(4), 334–342.

Lenz, J., Brown, J., Flagg, S., Oh, R., Batts, K., Ditzler, T., & Johnson, J. (2013). Cristalius: A case in designer drugs. *Military Medicine, 178*(7), e893–e895.

Lewy, J. (2014). The Army disease: Drug addiction and the Civil War. *War in History, 21*(1), 102–119.

Li, T., Waters, T. M., Kaplan, E. K., Kaplan, C. M., Nyarko, K. A., Derefinko, K. J., et al. (2017). Economic analyses of an alcohol misconduct prevention program in a military setting. *Military Medicine, 182*(1–2), e1562–e1567.

Lin, J., Zhu, K., Soliván-Ortiz, A. M., Larsen, S. L., Schneid, T. R., Shriver, C. D., & Lee, S. (2018). Smokeless tobacco use and related factors: A study in the U.S. military population. *American Journal of Health Behavior, 42*(4), 102–117.

Loeffler, G., Hurst, D., Penn, A., & Yung, K. (2012). Spice, bath salts, and the U.S. military: The emergence of synthetic cannabinoid receptor agonists and cathinones in the U.S. Armed Forces. *Military Medicine, 177*(9), 1041–1048.

Lorains, F. K., Cowlishaw, S., & Thomas, S. A. (2011). Prevalence of comorbid disorders in problem and pathological gambling: Systematic review and meta-analysis of population surveys. *Addiction, 106*(3), 490–498.

Mateczun, J. (1995). U.S. Naval combat psychiatry. In R. Zajtchuk & R. F. Bellamy (Eds.), *Textbook of military medicine, war psychiatry: Warfare, weaponry and the casualty* (pp. 211–242). Washington, DC: Office of the Surgeon General, U.S. Department of the Army.

McCarty, D., Braude, L., Lyman, D. R., Dougherty, R. H., Daniels, A. S., Ghose, S. S., & Delphin-Rittmon, M. E. (2014). Substance abuse intensive outpatient programs: Assessing the evidence. *Psychiatric Services, 65*(6), 718–726.

McCauley, J. L., Killeen, T., Gros, D. F., Brady, K. T., & Back, S. E. (2012). Post-traumatic stress disorder and co-occurring substance use disorders: Advances in assessment and treatment. *Clinical Psychology: Science and Practice, 19*(3), 283–304.

McDevitt-Murphy, M. E., Luciano, M. T., Tripp, J. C., & Eddinger, J. E. (2017). Drinking motives and PTSD-related alcohol expectancies among combat veterans. *Addictive Behaviors, 64,* 217–222.

Meadows, S. O., Engel, C. C., Collins, R. L., Beckman, R. L., Cefalu, M., Hawes-Dawson, J., et al. (2018). *2015 Department of Defense Health Related Behaviors Survey (HRBS)*. Santa Monica: RAND Corporation.

Mee-Lee, D. (2013). *The ASAM criteria: Treatment criteria for addictive, substance-related, and co-occurring conditions* (3rd ed.). Rockville, MD: American Society of Addiction Medicine.

Miller, S. M., Pedersen, E. R., & Marshall, G. N. (2017). Combat experience and problem drinking in veterans: Exploring the roles of PTSD, coping motives, and perceived stigma. *Addictive Behaviors, 66,* 90–95.

Miller, W. R., & Rollnick, S. (2002). *Motivational interviewing: Preparing people to change* (2nd ed.). New York: Guilford Press.

Mooney, S. R., Horton, P. A., Trakowski Jr., J. H., Lenard, J. H., Barron, M. R., Nave, P. V., et al. (2014). Military inpatient residential treatment of substance abuse disorders: The Eisenhower Army Medical Center experience. *Military Medicine, 179*(6), 674–678.

Najavits, L. M., Lande, R. G., Gragnani, C., Isenstein, D., & Schmitz, M. (2016). Seeking safety pilot outcome study at Walter Reed National Military Medical Center. *Military Medicine, 181*(8), 740–746.

Nayoski, N., & Hodgins, D. (2016). The efficacy of individual community reinforcement and family training (CRAFT) for concerned significant others of problem gamblers. *Journal of Gambling Issues, 33,* 189–212.

Oesterle, T. S., Thusius, N. J., Rummans, T. A., & Gold, M. S. (2019). Medication-assisted treatment for opioid-use disorder. *Mayo Clinic Proceedings, 94*(10), 2072–2086.

Oliva, E. M., Christopher, M. L., Wells, D., Bounthavong, M., Harvey, M., Himstreet, J., et al. (2017). Opioid overdose education and naloxone distribution: Development of the Veterans Health Administration's national program. *Journal of the American Pharmacists Association, 57*(2), S168–S179.

Ong, A. L., & Joseph, A. R. (2008). Referrals for alcohol use problems in an overseas military environment: Description of the client population and reasons for referral. *Military Medicine, 173*(9), 871–877.

Pack, A. J. (1983). *Nelson's blood: The story of naval rum.* Annapolis, MD: Naval Institute Press.

Pallesen, S., Mitsem, M., Kvale, G., Johnsen, B. H., & Molde, H. (2005). Outcome of psychological treatments of pathological gambling: A review and meta-analysis. *Addiction, 100*(10), 1412–1422.

Pemberton, M. R., Williams, J., Herman-Stahl, M., Calvin, S. L., Bradshaw, M. R., Bray, R. M., et al. (2011). Evaluation of two web-based alcohol interventions in the U.S. military. *Journal of Studies on Alcohol and Drugs, 72*(3), 480–489.

Petry, N. M. (2005). Gamblers anonymous and cognitive-behavioral therapies for pathological gamblers. *Journal of Gambling Studies, 21*(1), 27–33.

Petry, N. M., Stinson, F. S., & Grant B. F. (2005). Comorbidity of DSM-IV pathological gambling and other psychiatric disorders: Results from the National Epidemiologic Survey on Alcohol and Related Conditions. *Journal of Clinical Psychiatry, 66*(5), 564–574.

Priest, K. C., Gorfinkel, L., Klimas, J., Jones, A. A., Fairbairn, N., & McCarty, D. (2019). Comparing Canadian and United States opioid agonist therapy policies. *International Journal of Drug Policy, 74, 257–265.*

Prugh, G. S. (1975). *Law at war: Vietnam 1964–1973.* Arlington, VA: U.S. Department of the Army.

Quilter, C. J. (1993). *U.S. Marines in the Persian Gulf, 1990–1991: With the I Marine Expeditionary Force in Desert Shield and Desert Storm.* Arlington, VA: History and Museums Division, Headquarters U.S. Marine Corps.

Rash, C. J., Weinstock, J., & Van Patten, R. (2016). A review of gambling disorder and substance use disorders. *Substance Abuse and Rehabilitation, 7,* 3–13.

Rielage, J. K., Hoyt, T., & Renshaw, K. (2010). Internalizing and externalizing personality styles and psychopathology in OEF/OIF veterans. *Journal of Traumatic Stress, 23,* 350–357.

Robins, L. N., Helzer, J. E., & Davis, D. H. (1975). Narcotic use in Southeast Asia and afterward: An interview study of 898 Vietnam returnees. *Archives of General Psychiatry, 32*(8), 955–961.

Ronzitti, S., Loree, A. M., Potenza, M. N., Decker, S. E., Wilson, S. M., Abel, E. A., et al. (2019). Gender differences in suicide and self-directed violence risk among veterans with post-traumatic stress and substance use disorders. *Women's Health Issues, 29,* S94–S102.

Rosenberg, J. M., Bilka, B. M., Wilson, S. M., & Spevak, C. (2018). Opioid therapy for chronic pain: Overview of the 2017 US Department of Veterans Affairs and US Department of Defense Clinical Practice Guideline. *Pain Medicine, 19*(5), 928–941.

Ruzek, J. I. (2003). Concurrent posttraumatic stress disorder and substance use disorder among veterans: Evidence and treatment issues. In P. Ouimette & P. J. Brown (Eds.), *Trauma and substance abuse* (pp. 191–207). Washington, DC: American Psychological Association.

Santiago, P. N., Wilk, J. E., Milliken, C. S., Castro, C. A., Engel, C. C., & Hoge, C. W. (2010). Screening for alcohol misuse and alcohol-related behaviors among combat veterans. *Psychiatric Services, 61*(6), 575–581.

Saunders, J. B., Aasland, O. G., Babor, T. F., De la Fuente, J. R., & Grant, M. (1993). Development of the alcohol use disorders identification test (AUDIT): WHO collaborative project on early detection of persons with harmful alcohol consumption-II. *Addiction, 88*(6), 791–804.

Schmid, B., Tubman, D. S., Loomis, D. J., Grandela, J. E., Vernale, M. A., Messler, E. C., et al. (2017). Substance use disorders in the United States military: Current approaches and future directions. In S. Bowles & P. T. Bartone (Eds.), *Handbook of military psychology* (pp. 115–136). New York: Springer.

Schranz, A. J., Barrett, J., Hurt, C. B., Malvestutto, C., & Miller, W. C. (2018). Challenges facing a rural opioid epidemic: Treatment and prevention of HIV and hepatitis C. *Current HIV/AIDS Reports, 15*(3), 245–254.

Seal, K. H., Cohen, G., Waldrop, A., Cohen, B. E., Maguen, S., & Ren, L. (2011). Substance use disorders in Iraq and Afghanistan veterans in VA healthcare, 2001–2010: Implications for screening, diagnosis and treatment. *Drug and Alcohol Dependence, 116*(1–3), 93–101.

Sexual Assault Prevention and Response Office. (2019). *Department of Defense annual report on sexual assault in the military: Fiscal year 2018.* Arlington, VA: Office of the Under Secretary of Defense for Personnel and Readiness.

Sirratt, D., Ozanian, A., & Traenkner, B. (2012). Epidemiology and prevention of substance use disorders in the military. *Military Medicine, 177*(Suppl. 8), 21–28.

Skipper, L. D., Forsten, R. D., Kim, E. H., Wilk, J. D., & Hoge, C. W. (2014). Relationship of combat experiences and alcohol misuse among U.S. Special Operations soldiers. *Military Medicine, 179*(3), 301–308.

Sobocinski, A. (2004). A few notes on grog. *Navy Medicine, 95,* 9–10.

Sparrow, K., Kwan, J., Howard, L., Fear, N., & MacManus, D. (2017). Systematic review of mental health disorders and intimate partner violence victimisation among military populations. *Social Psychiatry and Psychiatric Epidemiology, 52*(9), 1059–1080.

Steenbergh, T. A., Whelan, J. P., Meyers, A. W., Klesges, R. C., & DeBon, M. (2008). Gambling and health risk-taking behavior in a military sample. *Military Medicine, 173*(5), 452–459.

Stein, M. B., Campbell-Sills, L., Gelernter, J., He, F., Heeringa, S. G., Nock, M. K., et al. (2017). Alcohol misuse and co-occurring mental disorders among new soldiers in the U.S. Army. *Alcoholism, Clinical and Experimental Research, 41*(1), 139–148.

Storer, R. M. (2003). A simple cost-benefit analysis of brief interventions on substance abuse at Naval Medical Center Portsmouth. *Military Medicine, 168,* 765–768.

Taj, N., Devera-Sales, A., & Vinson, D. C. (1998). Screening for problem drinking: Does a single question work? *Journal of Family Practice, 46*(4), 328–335.

Tiron, R. (2007, December 11). *Pentagon slots funding troops' vacation trips*. The Hill. Retrieved from *https://thehill.com/homenews/news/13865-pentagon-slots-funding-troops-vacation-trips.*

Tucker, J., Smolenski, D. J., & Kennedy, C. H. (2020). *Department of Defense Suicide Event Report: 2018 annual report*. Falls Church, VA: Defense Health Agency.

U.S. Africa Command. (2019). *Force health protection requirements and medical guidance for entry into the U.S. Africa Command theater*. Stuttgart, Germany: Author.

U.S. Army Medical Command. (2006). *Mental Health Advisory Team (MHAT) IV Operation Iraqi Freedom 05–07: Final report*. Fort Sam Houston, San Antonio, TX: Author.

U.S. Army Medical Command. (2008). *Mental Health Advisory Team (MHAT) V Operation Iraqi Freedom 06–08: Iraq Operation Enduring Freedom 8: Afghanistan*. Fort Sam Houston, San Antonio, TX: Author.

U.S. Army Medical Command. (2019). *Substance Use Disorder Clinical Care (SUDCC) operations manual for outpatient care*. Fort Sam Houston, San Antonio, TX: Author.

U.S. Central Command. (2020). *MOD fifteen to USCENTCOM individual protection and individual-unit deployment policy*. MacDill Air Force Base, Tampa, FL: Author.

U.S. Coast Guard. (2007). *Personnel security and suitability program* (Commandant Instruction M5520.12C). Washington, DC: U.S. Department of Homeland Security.

U.S. Coast Guard. (2012). *Coast Guard aviation medicine manual* (Commandant Instruction M6410.3A). Washington, DC: U.S. Department of Homeland Security.

U.S. Coast Guard. (2018a). *Coast Guard substance abuse prevention and treatment manual* (Commandant Instruction M6320.5). Washington, DC: U.S. Department of Homeland Security.

U.S. Coast Guard. (2018b). *Military drug and alcohol policy* (Commandant Instruction M1000.10A). Washington, DC: U.S. Department of Homeland Security.

U.S. Coast Guard. (2018c). *Military separations* (Commandant Instruction M1000.4). Washington, DC: U.S. Department of Homeland Security.

U.S. Government Accountability Office. (2017). *DoD and the Coast Guard need to screen for gambling disorder addiction and update guidance*. Washington, DC: Author.

U.S. Indo-Pacific Command. (2020). *USINDOPACOM FY 2021 force health protection guidance for USINDOPACOM AOR*. Camp H. M. Smith, HI: Author.

van Dam, D., Vedel, E., Ehring, T., & Emmelkamp, P. M. (2012). Psychological treatments for concurrent posttraumatic stress disorder and substance use disorder: A systematic review. *Clinical Psychology Review, 32*(3), 202–214.

Walker, D., Neighbors, C., Walton, T., Pierce, A., Mbilinyi, L., Kaysen, D., et al. (2014). Spicing up the military: Use and effects of synthetic cannabis in substance abusing army personnel. *Addictive Behaviors, 39*(7), 1139–1144.

Walker, D. D., Walton, T. O., Neighbors, C., Kaysen, D., Mbilinyi, L., Darnell,

J., et al. (2017). Randomized trial of motivational interviewing plus feedback for soldiers with untreated alcohol abuse. *Journal of Consulting and Clinical Psychology, 85*(2), 99–110.

Washington, G. (1776). *General orders, 26 February 1776.* National Historical Publications and Records Commission. Retrieved from *https://founders. archives.gov/documents/Washington/03–03–02–0269.*

Weathers, F. W., Litz, B. T., Keane, T. M., Palmieri, P. A., Marx, B. P., & Schnurr, P. P. (2013). The PTSD Checklist for DSM-5 (PCL-5)—Standard [Measurement instrument]. Retrieved from *www.ptsd.va.gov/professional/assessment/ documents/PCL5_Standard_form.PDF.*

Weaver, M. F., Hopper, J. A., & Gunderson, E. W. (2015). Designer drugs 2015: Assessment and management. *Addiction Science & Clinical Practice, 10*(1), 8.

Weis, D. R., & Manos, G. H. (2007). Prevalence and epidemiology of pathological gambling at Naval Medical Center Portsmouth psychiatry clinic. *Military Medicine, 172*(7), 782–786.

Welte, J. W., Barnes, G. M., Tidwell, M. C. O., Hoffman, J. H., & Wieczorek, W. F. (2015). Gambling and problem gambling in the United States: Changes between 1999 and 2013. *Journal of Gambling Studies, 31*(3), 695–715.

Wigham, S., Bauer, A., Robalino, S., Ferguson, J., Burke, A., & Newbury-Birch, D. (2017). A systematic review of the effectiveness of alcohol brief interventions for the UK military personnel moving back to civilian life. *BMJ Military Health, 163*(4), 242–250.

Wilk, J. E., Bliese, P. D., Kim, P. Y., Thomas, J. L., McGurk, D., & Hoge, C. W. (2010). Relationship of combat experiences to alcohol misuse among U.S. soldiers returning from Iraq war. *Drug and Alcohol Dependence, 108*, 115–121.

Witkiewitz, K., & Estrada, A. X. (2011). Substance abuse and mental health treatment in the military: Lessons learned and a way forward. *Military Psychology, 23*(1), 112–123.

Woodruff, S. I., Hurtado, S. L., & Simon-Arndt, C. M. (2018). U.S. Marines' perceptions of environmental factors associated with alcohol binge drinking. *Military Medicine, 183*(7–8), e240–e245.

Wortmann, J. H., Jordan, A. H., Weathers, F. W., Resick, P. A., Dondanville, K. A., Hall-Clark, B., et al. (2016). Psychometric analysis of the PTSD Checklist-5 (PCL-5) among treatment-seeking military service members. *Psychological Assessment, 28*(11), 1392–1403.

Yakovenko, I., Quigley, L., Hemmelgarn, B. R., Hodgins, D. C., & Ronksley, P. (2015). The efficacy of motivational interviewing for disordered gambling: Systematic review and meta-analysis. *Addictive Behaviors, 43*, 72–82.

Zinberg, N. E. (1972). Heroin use in Vietnam and the United States: A contrast and a critique. *Archives of General Psychiatry, 26*(5), 486–488.

APPENDIX 7.1. SUBSTANCE USE DISORDER INTAKE EVALUATION

NAME: John Doe
SSN: 000-00-1111
RANK/RATE/SERVICE: PO3/USN
DOB: 01 January 1998
DATE OF EVALUATION: 08 May 2022

Introduction: The patient is a 22-year-old single Caucasian male, E-4/AD/ USN, with approximately 4 years of continuous active-duty service. He was referred for treatment following a screening on 29 Apr 20 during which problematic alcohol use was identified. He has been stationed at White Beach Naval Facility for 7 months of a 24-month tour. He was seen on this date for an evaluation to begin treatment. He was advised of the limits of his confidentiality and rights, and consented to participate.

Chief Complaint: "I have a drinking problem."

History of Present Illness (HPI): The incident leading to the present evaluation occurred on 25 Apr 20 when the service member was involved in an alcohol-related incident (ARI) for being UA [unauthorized absence; the Navy's version of AWOL] to unit physical training. Regarding this event, he reported consuming approximately 16 drinks on the previous night and slept through the scheduled training.

The PO3 reported that his first introduction to alcohol was at age 16, and he began regular drinking when he was 19 years old. During the first year of his regular drinking, he consumed eight drinks per occasion two times per week. He stated that he felt the effects of his alcohol use after five drinks, and eight drinks were required before he was intoxicated. He estimated that during the past 12 months he had consumed alcohol three times per week. He normally consumed 10 drinks per occasion. He reported that he felt the effects of alcohol after 10 drinks, and 15 drinks were required before he was intoxicated. He endorsed a history of monthly blackouts during the last 7 months and denied withdrawal symptoms. He acknowledged a family history of alcoholism (paternal uncle and grandfather). The PO3 reported that his last consumption of alcohol was on 02 May 20, when he consumed approximately six drinks. The patient and records indicated no previous ARIs. The patient denied any previous alcohol treatment/education.

The PO3 reported a prior history of illicit substance use (marijuana), for which he indicates he has a drug waiver when enlisting in the Navy. Regarding the use of tobacco products, he reported that he smokes a pack of cigarettes per day and does not desire to quit at this time. He denied use of oral tobacco or vaping.

Diagnostic Criteria: The patient's substance misuse file and psychosocial assessment revealed the following information about DSM-5 criteria for an alcohol use disorder:

   a. The patient endorsed a marked tolerance or markedly diminished effect with continued use of the same amount. The patient noted that initially it took 8 drinks for him to become intoxicated and it now takes 15.
   b. The patient endorsed alcohol use in larger amounts or over a longer period than intended. The patient reported that he is often late to work due to drinking the night before but that he has been unable to limit his intake.
   c. The patient endorsed persistent desire or unsuccessful efforts to cut down or control substance use. The patient reported that he has tried to stop drinking independently on at least four occasions but has been unsuccessful.
   d. The patient endorsed continued alcohol use despite knowledge of having a persistent or recurrent psychological or physical problem that is caused or exacerbated by the use of the substance. The patient noted that he has experienced repetitive alcohol-related blackouts for the past 7 months.

Some symptoms of the disturbance have persisted for at least 1 month or have occurred repeatedly within the past 12-month period.

Results of Brief Screening Instruments: The PO3 was administered the Alcohol Use Disorders Identification Test (AUDIT) questionnaire on 29 Apr 20 with a raw score of 22 on his AUDIT and 3 out of 4 on the CAGE test. A value of 8 or greater on the AUDIT indicates a possible alcohol use disorder.

He was administered the PTSD Checklist for DSM-5 (PCL-5). There was no indication of PTSD symptoms. He received a raw score of 0 on the South Oaks Gambling Screen (SOGS), which is not indicative of problem gambling. The patient was administered a nutrition screening. There were no nutritional problems noted.

Mental Health History: The patient denied the following: suicidal ideation, gestures, or attempts. The patient denied self-mutilation. The patient denied previous hospitalizations for psychiatric treatment. The patient denied having difficulty concentrating, dysphoria, and anxiety. The patient also denied disturbances in sleep and in appetite. In the past year, he acknowledged some work-related difficulties and increased conflict or arguments with significant others. The patient denied anger control problems.

Past Developmental/Social History: The PO3 reported being the eldest of three siblings. He denied a history of emotional, physical, and sexual abuse. He graduated from high school on time and reported having several friends and typically maintained good relations with his peers. He reported that he is single and has no children. He noted no religious affiliation. The patient reported that he enjoys rock climbing. He denied financial problems. His upbringing included middle-class European American cultural/ethnic influences.

Psychological and Social Stressors: The PO3 denied significant psychosocial stressors. He rated his current ability to cope with stressors as fair. The following characteristic was chosen as being self-descriptive: "active." The patient endorsed "upbeat" as a descriptor of his mood. He was arrested for underage possession of alcohol and DUI (prior to his entering the service) for which he did community service.

Medical History: The PO3 acknowledged a family history of alcohol problems but denied a family history of illicit substance use. He denied a significant medical history and rated his general level of health as good. Currently, he is not under the care of a physician or taking any medication. He denied experiencing any current pain (0/10) or having a condition that frequently results in pain. He denied use of nutritional supplements.

The patient meets ASAM criteria for <u>admission to</u> IOP. The following dimensional criteria apply: AU: Please confirm underline under "admission to" is correct.

Dimension 1: Withdrawal Risk
Severity of condition was rated: High   Moderate   Minimal   *None*
Current withdrawal problems: Yes   *No*
Stated goal(s) in this dimension:
Progress toward goal: Worse   No Change   Improved   Resolved   *N/A*
See recommendations below: Patient reported his last drink was 02 May 20.

Dimension 2: Biomedical Conditions and Complications
Severity of condition was rated: High   Moderate   Minimal   *None*
Current medical conditions: Yes   *No*
Stated goal(s) in this dimension:
Progress toward goal: Worse   No Change   Improved   Resolved   *N/A*
See recommendations below.

*Dimension 3: Emotional/Behavioral/Cognitive Conditions
and Complications*

Severity of condition was rated: High   Moderate   Minimal   *None*
Based on: Stress Mgt.   Anger Mgt.   Unresolved Grief   Suicide   History
   PD   Dx
Other Specify:
Stated goal(s) in this dimension:
Progress toward goal: Worse   No Change   Improved   Resolved   *N/A*
See recommendations below.

Dimension 4: Resistance to Change

Severity of condition was rated: High   *Moderate*   Minimal   None
Based on: *Screening Evaluation*   Completion of Goals   Attendance
Group Behavior Other Specify:
Stated goal(s) in this dimension: To educate the patient on the effects of
   alcohol and the disease of alcoholism.
Progress toward goal: Worse   *No Change*   Improved   Resolved   N/A
See recommendations below:

Dimension 5: Relapse/Continued Use/Continued Problem Potential

Severity of condition was rated: *High*   Moderate   Minimal   None
Based on: BAC Group Interaction   *Urge to Use*   Prior Relapse   Other
   Specify:
Stated goal(s) in this dimension: To identify and apply coping skills for
   relapse triggers and high-risk situations.
Progress toward goal: Worse   *No Change*   Improved   Resolved   N/A
See recommendations below:

Dimension 6: Recovery Environment

Severity of condition was rated: High   *Moderate*   Minimal   None
Based on: *Barracks Environment*   AA Involvement   Spouse Support
Other Specify:
Stated goal(s) in this dimension: To identify a support network, drink
   refusal skills, and alternatives to drinking.
Progress toward goal: Worse   *No Change*   Improved   Resolved   N/A
See recommendations below:

Dimension 7: Operational

Severity of condition was rated: High   Moderate   *Minimal*   None
Based on: Command Support
Stated goal(s) in this dimension:
Progress toward goal: Worse   *No Change*   Improved   Resolved
See recommendations below.

Mental Status Examination (MSE): The patient arrived for the present evaluation appropriately groomed and properly dressed in the uniform of the day. Rapport was easily established and maintained. The patient did not appear defensive or anxious. The patient did not demonstrate psychomotor abnormalities. Attention and concentration were adequate during the present evaluation. Observation of the patient did not reveal evidence of memory, thought, or speech difficulties. Affect was broad and mood congruent. The patient denied hallucinations and delusions. The patient denied current suicidal or homicidal ideation, plan, or intent.

Diagnostic Impression: Alcohol Use Disorder, Moderate (ICD-10: F10.20)

Stage of Change: Contemplation

Recommendations:

1. Attend IOP classes Monday through Friday 0730–1130.
2. Attend at least two AA meetings per week.
3. Attend individual and group counseling sessions as scheduled.
4. Write in your journal daily.
5. Follow your treatment plan.
6. Abstain from alcohol.
7. Abstain from all establishments whose primary purpose is to sell alcohol.
8. The patient understands that he may page the Duty Counselor at 555-1000 if he is at risk of relapse.
9. Patient was assessed not to have any learning needs or barriers. The patient was educated about the diagnosis and rationale for treatment, and the patient expressed understanding.

J. A. Smith   D. E. Jones, PhD, ABPP
GSM2, USN   CAPT, MSC, USN
Navy Drug & Alcohol Counselor   *Clinical Psychologist*

APPENDIX 7.2.
PSYCHOLOGICAL EVALUATION

NAME: A. B. Jones
SSN: 123-45-6789
RANK/RATE/SERVICE: LCPL/USMC
DOB: 01 January 1998
DATE OF EVALUATION: 24 February 2020

Identifying Data: The service member is a 22-year-old married male with 1 year, 5 months of continuous active-duty service. He was encouraged to self-refer for gambling problems by an individual in his chain of command who is also a gambler in treatment.

History: The history of the present problem was taken from the service member and was considered reliable. He noted that he started gambling approximately 3 years ago and immediately developed a problem. He reported that at first he was betting on dogs, horses, and slot machines, but when transferring overseas, he began gambling solely on slot machines. He reported that in the past 9 months he has gambled $14,000, some of which was family savings, and that he is $3,800 in debt. The service member reported a preoccupation with gambling, chasing his losses, gambling more than he intended to, felt that he was unable to stop, lied to his wife about his gambling, and that this weekend she notified him that she wanted to file for marital separation after discovering financial loans that she was unaware of. The service member reported that after his wife told him about her desire to separate, he started drinking. He reported that he drank three to four beers and eight mixed drinks. He noted that he became suicidal and attempted to hang himself in his bathroom with a belt. He reported that his roommate heard the shower bar crash in the bathroom, forced his way in, and stopped him from trying again. Despite the suicide attempt this weekend, the service member denied symptoms of a mood, anxiety, psychotic, eating, and/or somatization disorder.

Psychological History: The service member noted that he sought help for his gambling in October 2019 and was prescribed sertraline to address the problem. He noted that he took the sertraline for a week and did not return to treatment. He denied a history of suicidal ideation or suicide attempts prior to this weekend.

Medical History: The service member denied a significant medical or surgical history. He denied current pain (0/10). He denied a history of head injuries and seizures.

Substance History: The service member denied a history of substance misuse and illegal drug use. He noted that he drinks three to four caffeinated sodas per day and smokes a pack of cigarettes daily.

Family Mental Health/Substance Abuse History: The service member denied a family history of mental health problems, pathological gambling, or substance abuse.

Personal History: The service member is the oldest of two siblings raised in an intact Arizona home. He denied a childhood history of emotional, physical, and sexual abuse. He noted some discipline/behavioral problems in grade school, but he graduated on time with a C average. The service member noted that he has been married for 1 year, 8 months, and he and his wife have one child. The service member reported serious marital conflict related to the lies that he has been telling about finances and gambling. He noted that if he cannot successfully get treatment for his gambling problem, he will lose his wife and child.

Psychological Testing: The service member was administered the South Oaks Gambling Screen. He scored a 15, which is considered indicative of a significant gambling problem. He was also administered the Beck Depression Inventory–II, on which he received a 6. This was not considered indicative of a clinical depression.

Mental Status Examination: Mental status examination at the time of the evaluation revealed an appropriately groomed male dressed in the uniform of the day. He was alert and oriented to person, place, time, and situation. He was cooperative, and eye contact was direct. There were no atypical behaviors or psychomotor disturbances noted. Speech was normal in range, rate, and intensity, though he often paused when answering questions or answered minimally when embarrassed. Cognitive functioning, judgment, insight, and impulse control appeared intact in the clinical interview. Thought processes appeared clear and goal-directed. Auditory and visual hallucinations were denied. His affect was restricted and congruent with his nervous mood. He adamantly denied current suicidal/homicidal ideation, plan, and intent.

Diagnostic Impression: Gambling Disorder, Moderate (ICD-10: F63.0)

Plan:

1. It is recommended that the service member attend the Gambling Treatment Program at the Substance Abuse Rehabilitation Program for cognitive-behavioral treatment related to his gambling disorder. His first group therapy appointment is at 1730 on 25 Feb 20.

2. The service member was referred to a financial counselor. He was accepted for a walk-in appointment as soon as he leaves SARP today.
3. The service member was provided with referral information for the community reinforcement and family training (CRAFT) program at the Family Clinic on base to discuss with his spouse.
4. The service member was instructed not to drink until this crisis stage has passed. He noted that he understood this rationale and would not have a problem abstaining from alcohol indefinitely.
5. The service member was encouraged to attend the weekly Gambler's Anonymous meeting (Thursdays at 1800).
6. The service member understands that he may call for an earlier appointment at any time (555-1234) or phone the after-hours counselor at 555-0000 if at risk for relapse.
7. The service member adamantly denied suicidal ideation, plans, rehearsal, or intent. He was able to articulate a thorough plan for safety.
8. These findings were discussed with the service member, who agreed with the results of the evaluation and the current plan.
9. Clinic POC is SSGT Smith or Dr. Watson at 555-1234.

C. H. Watson   J. A. Smith
CDR/MSC/USN   SSGT/USMC
Head, Substance Abuse   *Substance Abuse Counselor*
Rehabilitation Program

CHAPTER 8

Military Sexual Assault

Carrie L. Lucas, Ashley C. Schuyler, Sara Kintzle,
Kelly M. Wails, Hannah I. Nordwall, and Carl Andrew Castro

Military sexual assault (MSA) causes a range of adverse health, mental health, and professional problems and has garnered increased focus for the military in recent years (Forkus et al., 2021; Lofgreen, Carroll, Dugan, & Karnik, 2017; Suris & Lind, 2008; Turchik & Wilson, 2010). This chapter will review the historical background, rates, health and mental health variables, and military reporting rules. Four clinical cases will be presented in order to highlight military culture, reporting, confidentiality, resources, and treatment considerations.

A sexual assault in the military context is considered different than a sexual assault in general, given that elements specific to the military culture can compound the distress of MSA, complicate the process of disclosing or reporting the experience, and challenge the healing process. Service members who experience MSA, especially when they do not report the assault, often must continue living and working alongside their perpetrator, thereby prolonging states of fear and distress well after the initial incident. Feelings of betrayal, by the perpetrator and the broader military institution, may underlie MSA experiences and exacerbate psychological distress. Aspects of military culture, including a value on performance and a sense of team allegiance, can contribute to fears about disclosure or experiencing retaliation (including social and professional; Castro, Kintzle, Schuyler, Lucas, & Warner, 2015). Leadership and unit behavior that condones sexual prejudice, harassment, or discriminatory language are associated with increased incidence of both sexual assault and harassment (Castro et al., 2015; Sadler, Mengeling, Booth, O'Shea, & Torner, 2017). In addition, the inherent conflict between MSA and important military values (e.g., strength, self-sufficiency, loyalty) creates a dissonance that may inhibit opportunities for social support and contribute to a detrimental impact on well-being (Bell & Reardon, 2011; Castro et al., 2015).

HISTORICAL BACKGROUND

Serious attention to MSA began to emerge during the late 1980s and early 1990s, when the issue was forced to the forefront following the 1991 Tailhook incident. This was a Navy combat fighter pilot convention where an astonishing 83 women and 7 men reported experiencing MSA (Shields, 1998). Initial research sought to examine the extent of sexual assault within the military and early data primarily focused on small samples of female active-duty service members or veterans seeking care through the Department of Veterans Affairs (VA). Wolfe and colleagues (1998) examined data from 160 female service members who had recently returned from the Persian Gulf War and found that 7% reported MSA during the deployment. However, studies at VA medical centers found higher rates, ranging from 15 to 30% among female veterans (Coyle, Wolan, & Van Horn, 1996; Murdoch & Nichol, 1995). Because these samples were limited to individual VA medical centers, Hankin et al. (1999) sought to examine the prevalence of MSA in a large, national sample of female veterans. In a sample seeking VA outpatient primary care, the authors found that 23% of the 3,632 female veterans reported MSA. Furthermore, the discrepancies between rates of active-duty women reporting MSA while serving (7%) versus the reported rates (15–30%) once they were no longer serving indicated there might be significant problems that were going unaddressed.

RATES OF MSA

Despite systematic and comprehensive efforts over nearly two decades to address sexual assault in the military, the occurrence of MSA continues to be a significant concern. Recent data from the Department of Defense (DoD) indicate that during 2019 roughly 13,000 female (6%) and 7,500 male (0.7%) active-duty members experienced MSA (ranging from unwanted sexual contact to rape; DoD, 2020b). Similarly, a recent meta-analysis of studies that required a clear definition of MSA for inclusion found a mean prevalence of 24% among women and 2% among men across 43 studies (Wilson, 2018). Across veteran clinical and community samples, reports of MSA ranged from 3 to 54% among females and 0.2 to 9% among males (Kang, Dalager, Mahan, & Ishii, 2005; Sadler, Booth, Nelson, & Doebbeling, 2000; Schuyler et al., 2017; Street, Stafford, Mahan, & Hendricks, 2008; Stahlman et al., 2015). Risk of MSA is higher among enlisted service members, service members with premilitary trauma histories, and those service members identifying as sexual minorities (lesbian, gay, bisexual, or transgender [LGBT]; Castro et al., 2015; Lofgreen et al., 2017; Lucas, Goldbach, Mamey, Kintzle, & Castro, 2018; Schuyler et al., 2020; Suris & Lind, 2008; Turchik & Wilson, 2010). Compared to non-LGBT service members, LGBT service members are estimated to have double the risk of experiencing MSA (Schuyler et al., 2020).

HEALTH CONCERNS ASSOCIATED WITH MSA

A substantial body of research has investigated the relationships between MSA experiences and subsequent health outcomes, the bulk of which has been conducted among female veterans. In terms of physical health, MSA has been linked with poorer health status (Booth et al., 2012; Sadler et al., 2000) and a higher risk of chronic health problems (e.g., obesity, diabetes; Frayne et al., 1999; Sadler, Booth, Mengeling, & Doebbeling, 2004). Furthermore, MSA has been found to predict various health risk behaviors (Forkus et al., 2021), including tobacco use (Frayne et al., 1999; Schuyler et al., 2017) and sexual risk-taking behaviors (Turchik et al., 2012). Among a sample of over 2,500 veterans, women and men who experienced MSA were 2–4 times more likely to report current physical health symptoms and health risk-taking behaviors compared to those who did not experience MSA (Schuyler et al., 2017). One possible explanation for the link between MSA and physical health is a prolonged internal stress response and associated maladaptive coping behaviors (e.g., substance use), which may create increased vulnerability to subsequent health concerns (Lofgreen et al., 2017).

In terms of mental health, research among female service members has found that MSA is associated with increased anxiety, posttraumatic stress disorder (PTSD), psychological distress, and suicidality, as well as greater use of mental health care services (Rosellini et al., 2017; Stahlman et al., 2015). Unfortunately, many individuals who experience sexual assault do not seek services or report the assault. Among a sample of female veterans who experienced MSA, fewer than one-quarter indicated that they sought immediate support after the experience (Kintzle et al., 2015), and among a mixed sample of female and male civilians, only 32% reported it to police (Morgan & Kena, 2018).

Mental health outcomes associated with MSA among female and male veteran samples are similar to those observed among female active-duty service members, and include PTSD, (Kang et al., 2005; Schuyler et al., 2017; Kimerling et al., 2010), depression (Hankin et al., 1999; Kearns et al., 2016; Schuyler et al., 2017), sexual dysfunction, sexual dissatisfaction (McCall-Hosenfeld, Liebschutz, Spiro, & Seaver, 2009; Turchik et al., 2012), suicidality (Bryan, Bryan, & Clemans, 2015), other trauma-related outcomes such as dissociation, interpersonal difficulties, and emotional dysregulation (Bell & Reardon, 2011), and, among female veterans specifically, eating disorders (Forman-Hoffman, Mengeling, Booth, Torner, & Sadler, 2012). Although some outcomes have been more commonly associated with MSA among women (e.g., depression; Kearns et al., 2016) or men (e.g., suicidality; Bryan et al., 2015), there is evidence of a substantial mental health risk regardless of sex or gender. For instance, among a large sample of Gulf War veterans, women and men with MSA histories had approximately 5 and 6 times the odds, respectively, of reporting PTSD compared to veterans without MSA (Kang et al., 2005). Among another sample of veterans, women and men who experienced MSA were 3–6 times more likely to report clinical levels of PTSD or depression than those without MSA (Schuyler et al., 2017). In the context of other military stressors or traumas, a study of female veterans found that combat exposure and general harassment were significantly associated with PTSD, while MSA, combat exposure, and general harassment were significantly associated with depression (Kearns et al., 2016).

The relationship between MSA and substance use behaviors is less clear (Forkus et al., 2021). For instance, while some studies have found MSA to confer a greater risk of alcohol problems among female veterans (e.g., Frayne et al., 1999; Hankin et al., 1999), others have not (e.g., Booth et al., 2012; Creech & Borsari, 2014; Schuyler et al., 2017). One study involving a large, longitudinal sample of current and former military personnel found MSA to predict alcohol relapse among female veterans who were former problem drinkers, as well as smoking relapse among males who were former smokers (Seelig et al., 2017). It may be that MSA contributes to prolonged distress that, if left unresolved, facilitates extended use of emotion-focused coping behaviors such as alcohol use.

REPORTING MSA

The reporting of sexual assault within the military has faced a number of obstacles. Prior to the current reporting system, MSA could only be reported if the individual named the perpetrator and went on record as filing a complaint (House Armed Services Committee, 1994). Anonymous reporting was prohibited by DoD and Service policies. There were two main ideas that drove these restrictions: (1) It was the duty of service members to report all crimes and aid in the investigations, and this could not be achieved if MSAs were reported anonymously, and (2) those accused had the right to confront their accuser, and this was only possible by knowing who made the accusation. The consequence was that few official reports were made and it was suspected that this represented substantial underreporting. Without filing formal charges, service members were unable to access important resources, such as a victim advocate and focused medical and mental health care. Moreover, without reporting the assault, veterans did not have the necessary documentation in their military records to receive health care and support from the VA, as there was no evidence the sexual assault occurred while the individual was serving in the military.

Pressure by members of Congress resulted in a series of task forces that led to changes to DoD policies, most notably the Care for Victims of Sexual Assault Task Force formed in 2004 and the Joint Task Force for Sexual Assault Prevention and Response formed in 2006. As a result of these efforts, the Sexual Assault Prevention and Response Office (SAPRO)[1] was formed, which currently serves as DoD's single point of authority for sexual assault policy. One of the defining results of this work was the creation of the improved reporting processes used in the military today, namely restricted and unrestricted reporting (described in more detail below). Other policy improvements include more stringent guidelines for commanders to address concerns about the leadership response to disclosures, problematic in-house investigations, and retaliation (Castro et al., 2015; DoD Instruction 6495.02 in DoD, 2020b). Additionally, any veteran may now receive care from the VA for health care problems related to MSA, regardless of whether it can be demonstrated to be service connected (Department of Veterans Affairs, 2020). Importantly, all reporters of MSA are entitled to a Special Victims Counsel (SVC) provided by the military, a lawyer who is specifically trained in handling these cases, thereby ensuring that the rights of the individual who was assaulted are protected (Directive-Type Memorandum [DTM] 14–003; DoD, 2017). Perhaps in what is the most far-reaching decision involving MSA, the U.S. Supreme Court unanimously ruled in *U.S. v. Briggs* (2020) that a previous 5-year statute of limitations on rape cases that occurred between 1986–2006 did not apply in military rape cases. In 2006, Congress had amended the Uniformed Code of Military Justice (UCMJ) that removed any time limits on all military rape charges. Combined, these actions have effectively removed any statutes of limitations involving military rape.

CURRENT REPORTING OPTIONS

With regard to reporting, individuals who have been sexually assaulted in the military have three options: not report, file a restricted report, or file an unrestricted report.[2] While the goal and hope are that sexual assaults will

---

[1] For clinicians seeing service members who report or are being treated for sexual assault trauma, it is recommended that they be familiar with the SAPRO website (*www.sapr. mil*). This site contains the military sexual assault annual reports, up-to-date military sexual-assault-related policies, and a number of other useful resources.

[2] MSA perpetrated by a spouse or intimate partner does not fall under the SAPR Program and is managed by the Family Advocacy Program (DoD Instruction 6495.01; DoD, 2020b), which handles all cases involving domestic violence. Services listed in Table 8.1 are available to the spouse or intimate partner with the addition of a domestic abuse victim advocate, which replaces active-duty SAPR programming (DoD DTM 64001.01; DoD, 2016).

be reported, many individuals (see above) do not report the assault. This is depicted by the following case.

Case 8.1. *The Soldier Who Opted Not to Report a Rape*

The specialist (SPC) was raped during a party in a fellow soldier's barracks room. Everyone at the party had been drinking, and the SPC was intoxicated at the time. She was embarrassed and blamed herself for the rape. She began to experience significant self-doubt and distrust of others, withdrew from her friends, avoided her fellow soldiers from the party, became increasingly isolated and her work performance suffered. She did not want to report the rape, but she felt she needed mental health support. Fortunately, she saw a flyer for the inTransition Program in the women's bathroom, and after phoning its number, she was connected to confidential care at the local Vet Center.

While most sexual assault resources are necessarily provided once a service member reveals an assault to a military health care provider and/or the SAPR POC, local Vet Centers and the inTransition Program (*https://health.mil/Military-Health-Topics/Centers-of-Excellence/Psychological-Health-Center-of-Excellence/inTransition*) are exceptions. The inTransition program, a confidential program that assists service members and veterans in finding mental health care, provides assistance for active-duty personnel who have experienced sexual assault in finding confidential mental health care at a local Vet Center. Alternately, service members may contact their local Vet Center directly and receive care without a TRICARE referral and at no cost for mental health concerns arising from a sexual assault. Contacting either of these resources does not trigger a report.

Restricted Report

A service member can elect to initiate a restricted report (1) by disclosing to a health care provider, who will notify the Sexual Assault Response Coordinator (SARC), or (2) by independently contacting the SAPR Program (DoD Instruction 6495.02; DoD, 2020b). If a service member reports MSA to a health care professional, health care providers are required to notify SAPR to verify individuals are made aware of the reporting options. Upon notification, the SARC explains the service member's rights, resources, and reporting options. It is notable that service members may decline all SAPR services (6495.02; DoD, 2020b). A service member who initiates mental health care (regardless of the reporting option selected) will be afforded protected communication by *Psychotherapist-Patient Privilege* (Military Rule of Evidence [MRE] 513; Uniform Code of Military Justice [UCMJ], 2012a). Mental health providers are only able to discuss details of the assault or care provided with other entities when a release of information is signed by the individual prior to disclosure. The primary limitations include

concern for harm to self, harm to others, harm to mission, or a need for inpatient care; if any of these exist, then leadership must be notified (DoD Instruction 6490.08; DoD, 2011). However, the concerns can be discussed without disclosing the assault. Support varies due to the reporting option selected and is further explained below (see also Table 8.1).

Initiating a restricted report allows a service member access to a SAPR Victim Advocate (SAPR VA) who provides supportive services 24/7 as requested. Support services can include being present during a Sexual Assault Forensic Examination (SAFE), medical appointments, legal appointments, and any time further support is requested by the service member (DoD Instruction 6495.02; DoD, 2020b). Communication with the SAPR VA is protected communication through *Victim Advocate-Victim Privilege* (MRE 514; UCMJ, 2012b). There are some rare exceptions when communication can be shared by the SAPR VA with others. These exceptions include: if the victim is deceased, if there is concern for fraud or a crime, or if there are high-risk safety concerns for military personnel (e.g., suicidal/homicidal intent).

A service member may also request legal aid and counsel through the SVC. The SVC is a specially trained military lawyer who prosecutes crimes on behalf of the military. SVCs provide legal support to service members and "collaborate effectively with SARCs (and SAPR VAs) to facilitate a victim's welfare, security and recovery from sexual assault" (DTM 14–003; DoD, 2017, p. 7).

For restricted reports, information with non-personal identifiable information (PII) is provided to the installation commander for "public safety and command responsibility" (DoD Instruction 6495.02; DoD, 2020b). This information is used to verify that leadership is tracking trends on the installation, but it does not afford leadership an opportunity to support those who have experienced MSA, as specific individuals are not known.

A restricted report also allows for anonymous reporting of perpetrator information to the DoD, in what is known as the CATCH (Catch a Serial Offender) Program (*www.sapr.mil/catch*; DTM; Sexual Assault Prevention and Response Office [SAPR], 2019), to assist in identifying serial offenders. The information entered into the CATCH Program is analyzed at a headquarters level to assist in identifying a "match" between two or more submissions. If a match is identified, the CATCH Program notifies the local SAPR Program to offer the individual who made an unrestricted report the opportunity to convert it to an unrestricted report, which then allows for a criminal investigation (DTM; SAPR, 2019).

To demonstrate some of the variables involved in an unrestricted report, we offer the following case.

Case 8.2. *The Sailor Who Eventually Filed a Restricted Report*

The sailor, a Master-at-Arms Chief Petty Officer (MAC or simply "Chief"), presented to the on-base mental health clinic with anxiety symptoms. She had been raped 6 months before by a fellow service member, but did not disclose this to the provider. Consequently, her provider began a course of cognitive-behavioral therapy (CBT) to reduce her anxiety and anticipated a short-term treatment period given her superior past performance and no prior history of mental health concerns. However, little progress was made in the course of treatment, and after six sessions, the provider, who by now had established a good relationship with the MAC, initiated a conversation about the lack of progress. The MAC disclosed that her anxiety symptoms began following the rape. She noted that the perpetrator had since PCS'd (permanent change of station, i.e., transferred). Additionally, she disclosed that her consumption of alcohol had increased dramatically over the past 4 months. Given this new information and further evaluation, her diagnosis was changed to PTSD, the treatment plan was altered to include cognitive processing therapy, and the provider started to closely monitor her alcohol use, which declined rapidly once she began receiving appropriate treatment.

In addition to the clinical diagnostic and treatment changes, the MAC was offered SAPR services. She declined a SAPR VA, but elected to file a restricted report and agreed to participate in the CATCH Program.

Her leadership was not contacted during her mental health treatment as her initial presentation did not require it, the restricted report negated command notification, and the MAC did not present a danger to self, others, or the mission. With appropriate treatment, a concerted increase in her healthy coping strategies, and participation in an off-base support group once she had completed formal treatment, her anxiety symptoms were brought under control and she remained fit for duty.

The pattern demonstrated by this sailor, in which she had difficulty disclosing her trauma and had increased her use of alcohol to cope, is not uncommon. The positive outcome in this case is that she independently sought treatment, optimizing her chances of maintaining her mental health and her career. The rapport she developed with her provider eventually facilitated disclosure, a restricted report, and effective treatment (for more on evidence-based treatments for trauma, see Chapter 4, this volume).

Unrestricted Report

A service member may elect to initiate an unrestricted report (1) by contacting the chain of command or the military criminal investigative organization, (2) by independently contacting the SAPR Program, or (3) by contacting the health care personnel who notifies the SARC. It is notable that a service member may elect to change a restricted report to an unrestricted report at any time (DoD Instruction 6495.02; DoD 2020b). It is critical for service members to understand that a restricted report will be automatically converted to an unrestricted report if anyone in the individual's chain

TABLE 8.1. Comparison of Restricted and Unrestricted Reporting

Restricted report	Unrestricted report
Can switch to unrestricted report	Cannot revert to restricted report

Sexual Assault Prevention and Response (SAPR)	
• SARC coordinates care • Protection from retaliation and reprisal • Personal Identifiable Information stays in SAPR Office (command not informed of name/no charges are filed) • May participate in CATCH Program	• SARC coordinates care • Protection from retaliation and reprisal • SARC may be present during interviews • SARC may be present during legal proceedings • May participate in CATCH Program
Sexual Assault Prevention and Response Victim Advocate (SAPR-VA)	
• Service member may decline • Attends to needs and provides supportive services	• Service member may decline • Attends to needs and provides supportive services • May be present during interviews • May be present during legal proceedings
Special Victims' Counsel (SVC)	
• Service member may decline • Can request services (i.e., legal aid/ counsel)	• Service member may decline • Can request services (i.e., legal aid/counsel) • May be present during interviews • Support during any legal proceedings
Mental Health (Therapist)	
• Service member may decline • Assessment, support, and evidence-based treatment	• Service member may decline • Assessment, support, and evidence-based treatment
Chaplain	
• Service member may decline • Non-denominational/denominational confidential counseling	• Service member may decline • Non-denominational/denominational confidential counseling
Medical Care	
• Service member may decline • Emergency care • SAFE Kit tracked and retained for 5 years	• Service member may decline • Emergency care • SAFE Kit processing
	Commanders (Leadership)
	• Service member may not decline notification • Command notification
	Law Enforcement (i.e., Special Investigations, Military Police, and Others)
	• Incident investigation initiated • Service member may decline to participate in investigation • Service member can utilize restraining orders/military protective orders
	Other Services
	• Expedited transfer available

Note. CATCH = Catch a Serial Offender (*www.sapr.mil/catch*; DTM; DoD, 2019); SAFE = Sexual Assault Forensic Examination (DoD Instruction 6495.02; DoD, 2020b); SARC = Sexual Assault Response Coordinator (DoD Instruction 6495.02; DoD, 2020b). The authors acknowledge that the findings from the 2021 Independent Review Commission on Sexual Assault in the Military will provide updates to the above (Department of Defense, 2022).

of command becomes aware of the assault, even if the service member does not want the report to become unrestricted (DoD Instruction 6495.02; DoD, 2020b). The services listed above for restricted reporting are made available during an unrestricted case along with the addition of command notification and availability of support within the duty section; incident investigation through special investigations, military police, and others; as well as expedited transfer to assist the service member in moving to a location away from the perpetrator if he or she desires this (see also Table 8.1).

Unrestricted reports require command training that highlights "official need to know" to protect the confidentiality of individuals (DoD Instruction 6495.02; DoD, 2020b, p. 45). An unrestricted report allows the command to better support individuals who experience MSA and to manage dynamics within the command, should the alleged perpetrator belong to the same command. Additionally, the service member may have the SVC present during legal proceedings or investigations to "provide victims with a comprehensive understanding of their rights and information required to be provided during the investigation and court-martial process" (DTM 14–003; DoD, 2017, p. 7). Let's examine a case in which the service member opted to file an unrestricted report.

Case 8.3. The Airman Who Filed an Unrestricted Report

A senior airman (SrA) presented to her command's Sexual Assault Response Coordinator (SARC) and made an unrestricted report of a rape that occurred a week prior. She also sought treatment at the on-base behavioral health clinic at the recommendation of her SAPR VA. The SrA had a supportive command, and she was comfortable with their involvement in her case and in receiving information from the SAPR VA and SVC. She also voluntarily kept them apprised of her mental health appointments, though she understood that this was not necessary or expected. While she had optimal command support and was actively utilizing all available resources, she experienced increased distress, which was believed by her therapist to be complicated by a history of childhood trauma necessitating previous mental health treatment. Consequently, she received a referral to an intensive outpatient program (IOP) specializing in sexual assault trauma. She made good progress in the IOP and returned to the on-base clinic, where she continued to improve and receive support during the trial. Unfortunately, the trial exacerbated her symptoms, and after the perpetrator was found not guilty, her mental health declined further. After 6 months of no clinical improvement despite evidence-based trauma treatment, she was referred for a Medical Evaluation Board (MEB; see Chapter 2, this volume).

Unfortunately, the treatment of sexual trauma can be complex, and both individual history (i.e., childhood trauma) and external variables (e.g., seeing the perpetrator go unpunished, having to relive an assault during a trial) can significantly impact mental health.

MALE SEXUAL ASSAULT

The previous cases focused on female service members, but it is critical to identify the needs and reporting behaviors of male service members. A recent study by the RAND Corporation found male victims are more likely to focus on legal needs, rather than mental health needs due to concerns over stigma causing reduced reporting (Matthews, Farris, Tankard, & Dunbar, 2018). Men also struggle more with sexual identity or a loss of masculinity, as well as fears of being perceived as gay. Due to these varying concerns, military bases and providers need to post the availability of free and anonymous resources. Examples include the (1) Safe Helpline (*https:// safehelpline.org*), a 24/7, free, anonymous, and confidential hotline for service members needing support following a sexual assault, providing one-on-one support, peer support, and information about resources; and (2) Safe HelpRoom (*https://safehelpline.org/safe-helproom*), a 24/7 chat service where individuals who have experienced MSA can log on anytime to talk to other individuals who have experienced MSA (Safe HelpRoom also offers a 2-hour block of time each week that is reserved for males only). Let's examine a case involving a male service member.

Case 8.4. The Male Soldier Who Was Raped

The soldier, an Army Sergeant (SGT), called the military's Safe Helpline following a violent rape by another male. He began to participate in the weekly Safe HelpRoom chat service for male service members dealing with MSA. Through this resource, he decided to contact his local SARC and file an unrestricted report. During course of this process, he also decided to transfer to a new duty station, an option that was presented to him by his command. Following his transfer, he sought care at the on-base mental health clinic. He declined SAPR VA services and noted that he just wanted to focus on mental health treatment. Upon evaluation, he was diagnosed with PTSD. Additionally, he began to experience significant problems at work, despite a concerted effort to perform well, significant efforts to employ healthy coping strategies, and motivation to continue his military career.

He began a trial of prolonged exposure (PE) treatment, but only completed two sessions due to an increase in symptoms. Consequently, his provider referred him to a residential trauma-focused treatment program that specializes in military populations. His command was supportive of his need to be absent for medical care, and he successfully completed the 30-day program. Following his discharge from the residential program, he returned to outpatient care and resumed his military duties. He completed a full course of PE and was able to return to previous levels of work performance. Although his symptoms were under control and he was doing well at work, he requested a monthly appointment for monitoring and support until he felt comfortable with treatment termination.

The military has a number of programs that provide services and care for individuals who experience MSA. In the case of this service member, he was able to use anonymous services that led him to feel confident in utilizing the SARC and filing an unrestricted report, which in turn made an expedited transfer available.

CONCLUSION

Over the past 40 years, the literature on MSA has expanded our awareness of (1) obstacles to addressing reports effectively, (2) rates of MSA within the military, and (3) adverse health outcomes for individuals who experienced MSA. The establishment of the Sexual Assault Prevention and Response (SAPR) Office in 2005 helped facilitate a system for individuals who experience MSA to initiate a report and seek services. SAPR provides an option for anonymity, checks and balances that remove undue command influence, and advocacy for the individuals who experienced MSA through SAPR-VAs (Victim Advocates) and the SVC. As shown in Table 8.1, there are multiple avenues to report MSA and seek on-base treatment. There are also aforementioned services beyond the installation, such as inTransition, Safe Helpline, and Safe HelpRoom that provide individuals who have experienced MSA with support. Finally, the clinical case samples highlight the various ways in which an individual who experienced MSA can move through treatment and support services, and emphasize the varying levels of confidentiality and how every patient's experience is ultimately impacted by how much is disclosed, when it is disclosed, and to whom it is disclosed.

REFERENCES

Bell, M. E., & Reardon, A. (2011). Experiences of sexual harassment and sexual assault in the military among OEF/OIF veterans: Implications for health care providers. *Social Work in Health Care, 50*(1), 34–50.

Booth, B. M., Davis, T. D., Cheney, A. M., Mengeling, M. A., Torner, J. C., & Sadler, A. G. (2012). Physical health status of female veterans: Contributions of sex partnership and in-military rape. *Psychosomatic Medicine, 74*(9), 916–924.

Bryan, C. J., Bryan, A. O., & Clemans, T. A. (2015). The association of military and premilitary sexual trauma with risk for suicide ideation, plans, and attempts. *Psychiatry Research, 227*(2–3), 246–252.

Castro, C. A., Kintzle, S., Schuyler, A. C., Lucas, C. L., & Warner, C. H. (2015). Sexual assault in the military. *Current Psychiatry Reports, 17*(7), 54.

Coyle, B. S., Wolan, D. L., & Van Horn, A. S. (1996). The prevalence of physical and sexual abuse in women veterans seeking care at a Veterans Affairs Medical Center. *Military Medicine, 161*(10), 588–593.

Creech, S. K., & Borsari, B. (2014). Alcohol use, military sexual trauma, expectancies, and coping skills in women veterans presenting to primary care. *Addictive Behaviors, 39*(2), 379–385.

Department of Defense. (2011). *Command notification requirements to dispel stigma in providing mental health care to service members* (Department of Defense Instruction 6490.08). Retrieved from *https://jpp.whs.mil/public/docs/03_Topic-Areas/03-Victim_Privacy/20150116/41_DoDI6490_08_CmdNotificationReq_DispelStigma_20110817.pdf*.

Department of Defense. (2016). *Family Advocacy Program FAP: Clinical Case Staff Meeting (CCSM) and Incident Determination Committee (IDC)* (Department of Defense Manual 6400.01, Vol. 3). Retrieved from *www.esd. whs.mil/Portals/54/Documents/DD/issuances/dodm/640001m_vol3.pdf*.

Department of Defense. (2017). *DoD implementation of Special Victim Capability (SVC) prosecution and legal support* (DTM 14–003). Retrieved from *www. secnav.navy.mil/sapro/Documents/DTM14003_SVC%20LEGAL.pdf*.

Department of Defense. (2019). *Investigation of adult sexual assault in the Department of Defense* (Department of Defense Instruction 5505.18). Retrieved from www.esd.*whs.mil/Portals/54/Documents/DD/issuances/dodi/550518p.pdf*.

Department of Defense. (2020a). *Annual report of sexual assault in the military, fiscal year 2019*. Retrieved from *www.sapr.mil/sites/default/files/1_ Department_of_Defense_Fiscal_Year_2019_Annual_Report_on_Sexual_Assault_in_the_Military.pdf*.

Department of Defense. (2020b). *Sexual Assault Prevention and Response (SAPR) Program procedures* (Department of Defense Instruction 6495.02). Retrieved from *www.esd.whs.mil/Portals/54/Documents/DD/issuances/dodi/649502p.pdf?ver=2020–09–11–115130–333*.

Department of Defense. (2022). *Spotlight: Independent Review Commission on Sexual Assault in the Military*. Retrieved from *www.defense.gov/Spotlights/Independent-Review-Commission-on-Sexual-Asssault-in-the-Military*.

Department of Veterans Affairs. (2020). Disability compensation for conditions related to military sexual trauma (MST). Retrieved from *www.benefits. va.gov/BENEFITS/factsheets/serviceconnected/MST.pdf*.

Forkus, S. R., Weiss, N. H., Goncharenko, S., Mammay, J., Church, M., & Contractor, A. A. (2021). Military sexual trauma and risky behaviors: A systematic review. *Trauma, Violence, & Abuse, 22*(4), 976–993.

Forman-Hoffman, V. L., Mengeling, M., Booth, B. M., Torner, J., & Sadler, A. G., (2012). Eating disorders, post-traumatic stress, and sexual trauma in women veterans, *Military Medicine, 177*(10), 1161–1168.

Frayne, S. M., Skinner, K. M., Sullivan, L. M., Tripp, T. J., Hankin, C. S., Kressin, N. R., et al. (1999). Medical profile of women Veterans Administration outpatients who report a history of sexual assault occurring while in the military. *Journal of Women's Health & Gender-Based Medicine, 8*(6), 835–845.

Hankin, C. S., Skinner, K. M., Sullivan, L. M., Miller, D. R., Frayne, S., & Tripp, T. J. (1999). Prevalence of depressive and alcohol abuse symptoms among women VA outpatients who report experiencing sexual assault while in the military. *Journal of Traumatic Stress, 12*(4), 601–612.

House Armed Services Committee. (1994). *Sexual harassment of military women and improving the military complaint system.* 103rd Congress, Second Session.

Kang, H., Dalager, N., Mahan, C., & Ishii, E. (2005). The role of sexual assault on the risk of PTSD among Gulf War veterans. *Annals of Epidemiology, 15,* 191–195.

Kearns, J. C., Gorman, K. R., Bovin, M. J., Green, J. D., Rosen, R. C., Keane, T. M., et al. (2016). The effect of military sexual assault, combat exposure, postbattle experiences, and general harassment on the development of PTSD and MDD in female OEF/OIF veterans. *Translational Issues in Psychological Science, 2*(4), 418–428.

Kimerling, R., Street, A. E., Pavao, J., Smith, M. W., Cronkite, R. C., Holmes, T. H., et al. (2010). Military-related sexual trauma among Veterans Health Administration patients returning from Afghanistan and Iraq. *American Journal of Public Health, 100,* 1409–1412.

Kintzle, S., Schuyler, A. C., Ray-Letourneau, D., Ozuna, S. M., Munch, S., Xintarianos, E., et al. (2015). Sexual trauma in the military: Exploring PTSD and mental health care utilization in female veterans. *Psychological Services, 12,* 394–401.

Lofgreen, A. M., Carroll, K. K., Dugan, S. A., & Karnik, N. S. (2017). An overview of sexual trauma in the U.S. military. *Focus, 15*(4), 411–419.

Lucas, C. L., Goldbach, J. T., Mamey, M. R., Kintzle, S., & Castro, C. A. (2018). Military sexual assault as a mediator of the association between posttraumatic stress disorder and depression among lesbian, gay, and bisexual veterans. *Journal of Traumatic Stress, 31*(4), 613–619.

Matthews, M., Farris, C., Tankard, M., and Dunbar, M. S. (2018). *Needs of male sexual assault victims in the U.S. Armed Forces.* Santa Monica, CA: RAND Corporation. Retrieved from *www.rand.org/pubs/research_reports/RR2167. html.*

McCall-Hosenfeld, J. S., Liebschutz, J. M., Spiro III, A., & Seaver, M. R. (2009). Sexual assault in the military and its impact on sexual satisfaction in women veterans: A proposed model. *Journal of Women's Health, 18*(6), 901–909.

Morgan, R. E., & Kena G. (2018). *Criminal victimization, 2016: Revised.* Washington, DC: U.S. Department of Justice. Retrieved from *www.bjs.gov/content/pub/pdf/cv16.pdf.*

Murdoch, M., & Nichol, K. (1995). Women veterans' experiences with domestic violence and with sexual harassment while in the military. *Archives of Family Medicine, 4,* 411–418.

Rosellini, A. J., Street, A. E., Ursano, R. J., Chiu, W. T., Heeringa, S. G., Monahan, J., et al. (2017). Sexual assault victimization and mental health treatment, suicide attempts, and career outcomes among women in the U.S. Army. *American Journal of Public Health, 107*(5), 732–739.

Sadler, A. G., Booth, B. M., Mengeling, M. A., & Doebbeling, B. N. (2004). Life span and repeated violence against women during military service: Effects on health status and outpatient utilization. *Journal of Women's Health, 13*(7), 799–811.

Sadler, A. G., Booth, B. M., Nielson, D., & Doebbeling, B. N. (2000). Health-related consequences of physical and sexual violence: Women in the military. *Obstetrics and Gynecology, 96,* 473–480.

Sadler, A. G., Mengeling, M. A., Booth, B. M., O'Shea, A. M., & Torner, J. C. (2017). The relationship between U.S. military officer leadership behaviors and risk of sexual assault of Reserve, National Guard, and active component servicewomen in nondeployed locations. *American Journal of Public Health, 107*(1), 147–155.

Schuyler, A. C., Kintzle, S., Lucas, C. L., Moore, H., & Castro, C. A. (2017). Military sexual assault (MSA) among veterans in Southern California: Associations with physical health, psychological health, and risk behaviors. *Traumatology, 23*(3), 223–234.

Schuyler, A. C., Klemmer, C., Mamey, M. R., Schrager, S. M., Goldbach, J. T., Holloway, I. W., et al. (2020). Experiences of sexual harassment, stalking, and sexual assault during military service among LGBT and non-LGBT service members. *Journal of Traumatic Stress, 33*(3), 257–266.

Seelig, A. D., Rivera, A. C., Powell, T. M., Williams, E. C., Peterson, A. V., Littman, A. J., et al. (2017). Patterns of smoking and unhealthy alcohol use following sexual trauma among US service members. *Journal of Traumatic Stress, 30*(5), 502–511.

Sexual Assault Prevention and Response Office. (2019). *Procedures to implement the "Catch a Serial Offender" program* (DTM). Retrieved from *www.sapr.mil/sites/default/files/public/docs/victim-assistance/%21%20CATCH%20Program%20Procedures_FINAL%20SIGNED%2010%20June%202019.pdf.*

Shields, P. M. (1998). The mother of all hooks: The story of the U.S. Navy's Tailhook scandal [Book review]. *Armed Forces and Society, 24*(4), 606–608.

Stahlman, S., Javanbakht, M., Cochran, S., Hamilton, A. B., Shoptaw, S., & Gorbach, P. M. (2015). Mental health and substance use factors associated with unwanted sexual contact among US active duty service women. *Journal of Traumatic Stress, 28*(3), 167–173.

Street, A. E., Stafford, J., Mahan, C. M., & Hendricks, A. (2008). Sexual harassment and assault experienced by Reservists during military service: Prevalence and health correlates. *Journal of Rehabilitation Research and Development, 45*(3), 409–419.

Suris, A., & Lind, L. (2008). Military sexual trauma: A review of prevalence and associated health consequences in veterans. *Trauma, Violence, & Abuse, 9*(4), 250–269.

Turchik, J. A., Pavao, J., Nazarian, D., Iqbal, S., McLean, C., & Kimerling, R. (2012). Sexually transmitted infections and sexual dysfunctions among newly returned veterans with and without military sexual trauma. *International Journal of Sexual Health, 24*(1), 45–59.

Turchik, J. A., & Wilson, S. M. (2010). Sexual assault in the U.S. military: A review of the literature and recommendations for the future. *Aggression and Violent Behavior, 15*(4), 267–277.

Uniform Code of Military Justice Manual. (2012a). *Psychotherapist-patient privilege* (Military Rule of Evidence [MRE] 513). Retrieved from *www.sapr. mil/public/docs/ucmj/UCMJ_MRE513_Psychotherapist-Patient_Privilege_2012.pdf.*

Uniform Code of Military Justice Manual. (2012b). Military Rule of Evidence (MRE) 514, *Victim advocate-victim privilege* (MRE 514). Retrieved from *www.sapr.mil/public/docs/ucmj/UCMJ_MRE514_Advocate-Victim_Privilege_2012.pdf.*

Wilson, L. C. (2018). The prevalence of military sexual trauma: A meta-analysis. *Trauma, Violence, & Abuse, 19*(5), 584–597.

Wolfe, J., Sharkansky, E. J., Read, J. P., Dawson, R., & Ouimette, P. C. (1998). Sexual harassment and assault as predictors of PTSD symptomatology among U.S. female Persian Gulf war military personnel. *Journal of Interpersonal Violence, 13*(1), 40–57.

CHAPTER 9

Suicide Prevention
and the Military Psychologist

Aaron D. Werbel, Mathew B. Rariden,
Patricia J. Razuri, and Stephanie M. Long

When discussed in a military context, suicide prevention usually centers around epidemiology, risk and protective factors, associated factors, Service prevention programs and screening, or the initial assessment or identification of individuals at risk for suicide. The suicide prevention chapters in the previous two editions of this book also focused on these topics (Jones, Kennedy, & Hourani, 2006; Jones, Hourani, Rariden, Hammond, & Werbel, 2012). While briefly summarizing these important areas, this chapter addresses the elements missing from the previous editions as a guide to the behavioral health provider with regard to treatment intervention, interactions with a service member's command administrative responsibilities during and after treatment, and both clinical and administrative investigative expectations in the event of a death by suicide. In addition, with the increase in embedded psychologists, we also address the unique role a command psychologist plays in suicide prevention as it differs from that of a specialty medical clinic provider.

HISTORICAL CONTEXT

The military has been collecting and reporting on deaths by suicide since the middle of the 19th century (Smith, Doidge, Hanoa, & Frueh, 2019); however, military suicide prevention in modern times received heightened attention following the death of Chief of Naval Operations Admiral

Jeremy Boorda in 1996. This resulted in significant examination of prevention policies and programs across the Services (Shaffer, 1997), and the U.S. Air Force pioneered an interdisciplinary designed program in collaboration with the Centers for Disease Control and Prevention (CDC) with a community-wide approach (Knox, Litts, Talcott, Feig, & Caine, 2003; Litts, Moe, Roadman, Janke, & Miller, 1999). By end of the decade, the U.S. Army, U.S. Navy, and U.S. Marine Corps also engaged military and civilian experts with renewed attention on suicide prevention programs in keeping with the distinct organizational cultures and missions of their Service, and the Department of Defense (DoD) formally established the Suicide Prevention and Risk Reduction Committee (SPARRC) (Army Chief of Public Affairs, 2000; Jones et al., 2001). The SPARRC established a Suicide Rate Standardization Work Group in 2005; a Suicide Nomenclature Standardization Work Group in 2006; and a standardized suicide data collection form and database work group in 2007. The SPARRC also expanded the annual suicide prevention conference, from approximately 50 attendees in 2002 to approximately 850 attendees by 2010 to include international attendees from foreign military organizations (DoD, 2010).

As suicide rates increased during Operation Enduring Freedom (OEF) and Operation Iraqi Freedom (OIF), the Army collaborated with the National Institute of Mental Health (2009) to better understand risk and related factors for soldier suicides. The original Study to Assess Risk and Resilience in Servicemembers (STARRS) ran from 2009 to 2015 and consisted of eight separate studies (U.S. Department of Army, 2020). It was renewed from 2015 to 2020 as the Army STARRS-LS (Longitudinal Study) to follow the original 72,000 soldier participants, and will continue its work until 2024 to better understand risk and related factors for soldier suicides (Naifeh et al., 2019). In August 2010, the DoD Task Force on the Prevention of Suicide by Members of the Armed Forces released a report that noted "extraordinary effort," more than any other employer in the nation, to prevent suicides (DoD, 2010). Noting a lack of centralized strategic planning, the report called for a DoD-level office under the Secretary of Defense to coordinate strategy and programs and the appointment of Service headquarters and Installation Directors of Psychological Health (IDPH) to coordinate the many installation resources that support suicide prevention efforts. This led directly to the creation of the DoD Suicide Prevention Office in November 2011 (DoD, 2013), numerous policy and strategy documents (Defense Suicide Prevention Office [DSPO], 2012; DSPO, 2015; Office of the Under Secretary of Defense for Personnel and Readiness [OUSDP&R], 2017), Service-level Directors of Psychological Health who collaborate with the Defense Health Agency on the Behavioral Health Clinical Community (OUSDP&R, 2011), and Service-specific policies regarding the appointment of IDPH at all installations (U.S. Army Medical Command [MEDCOM], 2017). While these Service-level and installation positions are not specifically suicide prevention program officers, they do facilitate the coordination of behavioral health support that contributes significantly to suicide prevention success. With regard to surveillance, the Services implemented a standardized DoD Suicide Event Report (DODSER) on January 1, 2008, to collect and analyze data from deaths by suicide (Hilton et al., 2009; DoD, 2009).

EPIDEMIOLOGY

A brief review of the latest in epidemiological investigations provides the military psychologist value for identification of individuals at risk and can inform relative effectiveness of prevention and intervention strategies. In the United States, the latest face-to-face household survey results of 67,791 adults by the Substance Abuse and Mental Health Services Administration (2019) estimated that in 2018, 10.7 million adults ages 18 or older thought seriously about trying to kill themselves (4.3% of adults), 3.3 million made suicide plans (1.3%), and 1.4 million made a nonfatal suicide attempt (0.6%). Young adults (18–25) reported higher rates of suicide-related thoughts and planning than in 2008 to 2016 and similar to 2017, sustaining a decade-long trend of increasing suicide-related risk. Suicide attempts by young adults in 2018 were higher than 2008–2014 and similar to the rates from 2015 to 2017. The survey specifically excluded active-duty military members, making it a convenient comparison sample to military epidemiology studies. The latest CDC reports place suicide as the 10th leading cause of death for all ages, but the 2nd leading cause of death for 15- to 34-year-olds (accidental injury is first) and 4th for 35- to 54-year-olds (CDC, 2020). The suicide rate increased 35% from 1999 to 2018, from 10.5 to 14.2 per 100,000. The rate of increase accelerated in the latest decade, approximately 0.8% each year from 1999 to 2006 and 2.1% each year from 2006 through 2018 (Hedegaard, Curtin, & Warner, 2020). In addition to the direct impact in loss of lives, research suggests that an average of 135 additional individuals are impacted by each death (Cerel et al., 2018). As a result, these individuals are often at increased risk for their own suicide-related behaviors.

Military suicide epidemiology is tracked and analyzed with the DOD-SER, and previously with the DONSIR (Navy), ASER (Army), and SESS (Air Force) (DoD, 2009). Between 1991 and 2000, the annual suicide rates fluctuated between 10 and 15 per 100,000. Suicide rates increased significantly from 2000 to 2010 (Reger, 2015). According to the latest DODSER report (Tucker, Smolenski, & Kennedy, 2020), the pace of increase began to slow in the next decade; however, the 2018 suicide rate for active-duty service members was statistically significantly greater than the average for 2015–2017. The 2018 suicide rates for the active and reserve components did not differ from the U.S. adult population suicide mortality rates for CY17 when adjusted for age and gender composition of the military population. The National Guard, however, had a higher suicide rate than expected from the U.S. adult population data. The latest DODSER report analyzed 278 active-duty service member deaths and 1,375 suicide attempts from CY 2018 and reported the following trends:

- Six deaths and 101 suicide attempts were associated with one or more previous DODSER-reported suicide attempts since 2010, with the median number of days from the last attempt to the death being 41 and to the most recent attempt being 61.
- The most common service member to die by suicide was a non-Hispanic, white male aged 17–29, which accounted for 38.9% of submitted forms. Female service members accounted for 6.9% of suicide DODSER forms and 30.6% of suicide-attempt DODSER forms.
- Firearm use was the most common (60.4%) method, resulting in death with almost all (92.3%) privately owned rather than service weapons.
- Drug and/or alcohol overdose was the most frequently reported method for attempts (59.7%), followed by trauma from a fall or sharp/blunt object (16.7%) and hanging/asphyxiation (13.2%).
- Forty-five percent of those who died by suicide had at least one current or past behavioral health diagnosis in their medical record compared to just over 60% for attempts.
- 52.9% of those who died by suicide had contact with the Military Health System (MHS) in the 90 days prior to death, 48.2% of which were general medical appointments, while 30.2% were in behavioral health. Attempt survivors had more contact with MHS, with 62.4% being seen in the 90 days prior to the event (50.3% for general medicine and 49.5% in behavioral health).
- The most common associated stressors for military members who died by suicide were related to relationship (39.2%), legal/administrative (32.4%), and work (18.7%); for suicide attempts, the top stressors were relationship (38.5%), work (31.5%), and legal/administrative (29.5%).

COMMAND SUICIDE PREVENTION PROGRAMS

The stereotypical command suicide prevention "program" as identified by most service members is a 1- to 2-hour annual training best known as an effective insomnia remedy. Unfortunately, when the command-level program is a "check in the box" annual training delivered by a junior member of the command selected without regard to public speaking skills to meet the annual requirement, it is the worst-case example of a suicide prevention program. Annual training, even when most effective, is only one part of a required robust command-level suicide prevention program. Each Service has specific requirements for its comprehensive suicide prevention programs, all inspectable by the offices of the Service Inspector General (IG) (U.S. Air Force Suicide Prevention Program, 2020; U.S. Army Suicide Prevention Program, 2020; U.S. Marine Corps Suicide Prevention Program, 2020; U.S. Navy Suicide Prevention Program, 2020). These requirements vary between Services, but typically include the following core elements:

1. Involvement of Service and command leadership
2. Appointment of a suicide prevention program officer or coordinator
3. Ensuring a climate supportive of treatment intervention
4. Annual gatekeeper-style training (face-to-face or online; peer-to-peer or led by subject matter expert)
5. Intervention skill guidance distilled into an easy to recall acronym (e.g., Army/Air Force: ACE (Ask, Care, Escort): Navy: ACT (Ask, Care, Treat); Marine Corps: RACE (Recognize, Ask, Care, Escort)
6. Reporting (DODSER) and investigative actions (psychological autopsies, Service-level "deep dives")

Command-level suicide prevention programs are most effective when everyone in the unit identifies the program as a commander's priority. This is best accomplished by selecting a nonmedical, nonchaplain senior enlisted leader or officer as coordinator of the program; this avoids the common perception that suicide prevention is the purview of a medical or religious ministry program. Suicide prevention must be the priority of every member of a unit. A common failing of command-level programs is the exclusion of all related resources that address associated stressors and risk factors. A suicide prevention coordinator should include programs related to financial health, relationship building, sexual assault/harassment response and prevention, resilience building, spouse and dependent resilience, and the like in the overall rubric of a robust suicide prevention program. Suicide prevention programs are often considered "soft skills" by commands and thus Service IG inspections are hindered by incomplete training completion records. Commands are often meticulous at maintaining records of weapons qualifications, searchable by both individual and unit to show percent of command readiness at any given time. In contrast, a request for suicide prevention training records is often met with a stack of attendance sheets, rather than a searchable database without an ability to determine full compliance by a unit. The recent increase in embedded or organic behavioral health assets in operational units (see Chapter 10, this volume) has great potential to further improve command-level suicide prevention programs.

EMBEDDED COMMAND BEHAVIORAL HEALTH

Throughout the rest of this chapter, we will return to a specific case study to illustrate how the practices discussed apply directly to preventing and treating suicide-related risk and behaviors in the military.

Case 9.1a. The Soldier with Thoughts of Suicide

The corporal is a 22-year-old, mixed-race, single, never-married male with no children. After high school, John began to struggle with motivation and decided to remain at home with his parents while working part-time. At the age of 20, he felt that his peers from high school were excelling in life while he was stagnating, which drove him to the local recruiting office to enlist in the Army. His parents were strongly against his enlistment and made their dissatisfaction known. Boot camp led to high hopes for a better future. At his advanced individual training, John noticed that his positive mood and sense of hope began to decline. This downturn in his mood was captured by a routine screening assessment that led to an in-person safety assessment by a mental health provider at the local medical treatment facility (MTF). The SPC denied both past and present safety concerns and expressed a strong motivation to complete his training and report to his first operational command. He was cleared by mental health and returned to complete his training. After reporting to his first command, John began losing hope that his mood would improve with time, and he reported suicidal thoughts of hanging himself in a secluded corner of the unit. He joked about suicide to a peer, who reported the comment to their supervisor. The supervisor brought him to the unit medic, who assessed him for safety. The medic's persistence led the corporal to admit the full extent of his current thoughts of wanting to die. His command decided to send a situational report to higher leadership, prompting the decision to medically evacuate the corporal with the embedded psychologist and then to the nearest MTF.

Suicide prevention, at the command level, is a responsibility that should never rest solely on the shoulders of a single person, but most commands appoint a single suicide prevention coordinator (SPC) tasked with carrying out the annual training plan. Some SPCs are very dedicated and a good fit for the role, while others were assigned the SPC role as a dreaded collateral duty. At best, the SPC has sufficient clout, expertise, and motivation to make a meaningful impact, while at worst, the SPC conducts a single annual brief to "check the box." An embedded command psychologist (or chaplain) should not be appointed as the SPC but is in a unique position, to facilitate the establishment and sustainment of a command culture where all members are empowered to prevent suicide. The maturing expertise of embedded military psychology has demonstrated three critical lines of effort: (1) program development and management, (2) acquisition of nonconventional intervention and engagement skills, and (3) leadership of formal and informal teams.

Program Development and Management

The most effective, responsive, and robust suicide prevention programs, in any military environment, have at their core a system for engagement and management of service members by a diverse array of peers, leaders, force multipliers, and helping professionals spread throughout the organization. Such programs work best when leadership has a clear vision, established goals, invested personnel, and readily available options to reliably connect the right service member with the right path forward. However, personnel turnover, role confusion, diffusion of responsibility, administrative and bureaucratic inefficiencies, and the necessary focus on the command's mission—all serve to undermine programmatic efforts to prevent suicide.

The first task for a new command or embedded psychologist is to fully understand all the personnel and their roles in the command and under what systems of logic they operate. This process takes at least 90 days, involves a systematic assessment of the command, and requires a deep-seated curiosity about the new environment. It is easy to assume every current practice is done for a reason, or alternatively, that current practice is flawed and stands to benefit from a complete overhaul; the truth often lies somewhere in the middle as programs always mature and change with time. Taking the time for an initial assessment period with an open mind can go a long way toward identification of the path forward. During this stage, the embedded provider should review DoD-level suicide prevention policy and regional/local suicide prevention instructions, while ensuring the SPC does the same. Converse with as many members of the command as possible and consult with peers in similar operational communities. When serving as a command consultant, an important recommendation to the commanding officer made at the end of this stage is whether existing command instructions are sufficient, need updating, or need to be written for the first time.

Following a robust assessment of the organization, the next step is to help the SPC assemble the respective stakeholders within the command(s) (e.g., commanding officer, executive officer, senior enlisted leader, medical officers, mental health officers, chaplains, legal officers, etc.) to discuss best practices to date, areas for attention/improvement, and any specific tasks for the group. If indicated, this meeting is a prime opportunity for any discussion regarding standard operating procedures and their codification within command specific instructions. With or without an effective instruction or programmatic document, which can be established over time, the outcome of the meeting with stakeholders should produce a plan to prevent suicides—at the smallest unit level.

Imagine the following scenario as it follows two possible paths. Path 1: A junior service member, new at the command, makes the following statement to a peer, "Maybe I should just kill myself." The peer immediately engages the service member on this statement, develops a concern for the service member's safety, reports the concern to a supervisor who locates and accompanies the junior service member to the command's Medical Department, where risk is assessed, and the decision to transport the member to the local Emergency Department is made. Path 2: The individual makes the comment to the peer, who tells the supervisor, who does nothing with this information, believing that it was an innocent comment made during a transient moment of exasperation.

Typically, supervisors have the best intentions, but without a reliable, command-driven notification system of people in place for the supervisor to follow in what can be accurately described as an ambiguous moment in time, which path is followed is also determined by chance. In Path 1, the supervisor was well trained, clearly understood the order of operations given the information on hand, and maintained faith that the correct action was carried out for the Service member, the work-center, the command, and the Service. Successful suicide prevention programs, explicitly and implicitly embraced by a command, engender trust, faith, and confidence during crucial points in time where effective decision making must occur. From the point of identification of a safety concern to the point of resolution, maintaining a sense of continuous momentum is key. The hallmark of a successful suicide prevention program is the systematic empowerment to ask, care, and treat at all levels—every member of the command is a potential first responder and every member knows it.

Acquisition of Nonconventional Skills

Embedded behavioral health providers have a relatively straightforward role when a service member is identified as mentally ill—disposition management and treatment by mental health and medical staff. However, the command psychologist must participate in a unique way when the service member or work-center in question is free of identifiable pathology, but struggling nonetheless. Often a service member is struggling to connect the task of the day (e.g., cleaning, studying, working long grueling hours) with the desire of the future (e.g., attending college, beginning a future career, starting or reintegrating with a family). Maybe a leader with a strong record of performance recently experienced a professional setback and is feeling lost. What can be done when a unit's morale is low, but no toxic leadership practices or specific contributing factors have been identified? If ignored, these situations, usually driven by operational and combat stress, will have significant negative effects on individual and group coping abilities.

In operational communities, where stress is omnipresent and individual autonomy is low, stress injuries can multiply and lead to suicide-related thoughts without effective prevention efforts; feeling stuck with no hope for improvement can lead to a festering sense of entrapment (Shelef, Levi-Belz, Fruchter, Santo, & Dahan, 2016). The suicide prevention mission within a unit demands nonconventional skills. The command psychologist, SPC, and their team should learn new skills to address these problems and find the time to teach these skills in small and large venues, and then regularly assess skill acquisition across the command. Such skills range from organizational consulting to personal coaching. Each time an individual service member or unit-level concern is brought to their attention, the command team will need to determine if the issue rests within the clinical, organizational, or resilience realm, and engage with skills that are suitable to the task. Having a powerful presence for a command suicide prevention team is, by its very nature, aspirational. A command presence, tangibly felt by the members of the command, requires continuous time and attention in order to remain effective, and the most effective way to move in this aspirational direction is to lead teams made up of force multipliers.

Leadership of Formal and Informal Teams

In the operational environment, neither the command psychologist nor the SPC is likely to have direct authority over other members of a command suicide prevention team or stakeholders. Nonetheless, both, if properly empowered by instruction, with explicit support from the commanding officer, can harness the right confluence of knowledge, skills, and abilities to lead an effective team spread across the enterprise. Once the team is assembled, the embedded provider can help empower the SPC to provide clear direction and supervision throughout the year. Providing direction and guidance to a loose association of force multipliers spread throughout a large organization is a challenge that requires a working knowledge of group dynamics, management strategies, and policy implementation.

The command psychologist and SPC cannot, nor should they attempt to, advance the suicide prevention mission all on their own. Both will have other primary duties that constantly demand their time and attention; maintaining effective suicide prevention programs necessitates the involvement of dedicated, well-directed team members and stakeholders.

SCREENING AND ASSESSMENT

Screening

The new VA (Veterans Affairs)/DoD Clinical Practice Guidelines (CPG) for Management of Patients at Risk for Suicide (2019), as formulated by the Assessment and Management of Suicide Risk Work Group, recommend universal screening for suicide. Universal screening means asking every patient, every visit, if he or she has current or recent suicide-related thoughts at all primary-care and specialty clinic appointments. While less than half of military suicide decedents have a history of behavioral health care, more than half have received other health care within the 90 days prior to their deaths (Tucker, Smolenski, & Kennedy, 2020). Though universal screening will not accurately identify every at-risk individual, it does have enough predictive value to identify some who may otherwise not disclose their suicide-related thoughts and no evidence for causing harm (VA/DoD, 2019). There is some evidence for using the Patient Health Questionnaire 9 (PHQ-9) for universal screening, particularly Question 9: "Over the past two weeks, how often have you been bothered by thoughts that you would be better off dead or of hurting yourself in some way?" While further research on this topic is necessary, military clinics (including within operational units) would benefit from including universal screening for suicide risk for all patients in their standard protocols.

Assessment

Providers should conduct a comprehensive suicide risk assessment in a caring empathic manner critical to gathering sufficient and accurate information. The elements of a suicide risk assessment must include at a minimum: current suicidal ideation, prior suicide attempts, current psychiatric diagnoses, psychiatric hospitalization history, current psychiatric symptoms, recent biopsychosocial stressors, and availability of firearms (VA/DoD, 2019). Evidence referenced below is cited in more detail in the CPG report. Suicide risk evaluations should include questions about self-directed violence, specifically regarding current suicidal ideation and a history of prior suicide attempts. These two data points have strong evidence for predicting future suicide risk. There is some evidence for including assessment of preparatory behavior, past or present suicidal intent, and nonsuicidal self-directed violence, also described as self-injurious behavior or self-harm. Several psychiatric diagnoses, including mood disorders, anxiety disorders, substance use disorders, eating disorders, and psychotic disorders, have strong evidence for suicide risk. There exists some evidence for personality disorders being associated with suicide risk, but the evidence is not as strong as for the other psychiatric diagnoses listed. Additionally, there exists strong evidence for history of psychiatric hospitalizations as a risk factor. Multiple psychiatric symptoms have strong evidence for inclusion in a comprehensive suicide risk assessment: agitation, anger, anxiety/panic, depressed mood, hopelessness, impulsivity, insomnia, intoxication, problem-solving difficulties, and rumination. There is some evidence for including assessment of decreased psychosocial functioning and hallucinations as psychiatric symptoms in the risk assessment.

Assessment of various recent biopsychosocial stressors should also be included in a comprehensive suicide risk evaluation. These stressors are often retrospectively identified in suicide data analyses and case reviews as having existed prior to a decedent's suicide: relationship loss (i.e., breakup, divorce, death), job loss, risk of job loss/homelessness, legal/disciplinary problems, social isolation, and traumatic exposure (Tucker et al., 2020). Exposure to trauma may include bullying, emotional abuse, interpersonal violence, sexual assault, physical assault, and suicide of known acquaintance, coworker, friend, or family member. There is some evidence for inclusion of the following stressors: financial problems, transition of care, barriers to accessing care, physical health problems (specifically, history of moderate to severe traumatic brain injury and cancer diagnosis), and sexual orientation or gender identity minority status (specifically, lesbian, gay, bisexual orientation or transgender identity). The strongest evidence for availability of lethal means in a suicide risk assessment focuses on availability of firearms. There is some evidence for asking about other lethal means (i.e., large amounts of medication), but firearms are the most lethal method of suicide and have received the most attention (Shenassa, Catlin, & Buka, 2003). Many suicide prevention efforts focus on lethal means safety as a public health approach to suicide prevention. Clinicians must develop comfort with asking about access to firearms (personal and military), as well as asking how a service member's personal weapons and ammunition are stored. This information will be incorporated into stabilization planning discussed in the next section.

Finally, a comprehensive suicide risk assessment should identify protective factors, particularly reasons for living. There are not many protective factors with strong empirical support, but the reasons for living are a vital part of the suicide risk assessment and also factor into stabilization planning.

An Important Note on Risk Stratification

Much of the work in suicide prevention over the past 50 years focused on clarifying and using risk and protective factors to identify those at increased risk of suicide-related behavior, inform the assessment of suicide risk, and guide treatment goals (e.g., increase modifiable protective factors while reducing modifiable risk factors). There are numerous listings of risk and protective factors often stratified as permanent and nonmodifiable (e.g., personal demographics, history of suicide attempt); predisposing and potentially modifiable (e.g., mental illness, low self-esteem); acute (e.g., anxiety, rage, ideations); precipitating or triggering (e.g. legal problems, shame); or contributory (e.g., access to weapons, grief) (Western Michigan University, 2020). VA/DoD CPG (2019) recommends "an assessment of risk factors as part of a comprehensive evaluation of suicide risk, including but not limited to: current suicidal ideation, prior suicide attempt(s), current psychiatric conditions (e.g., mood disorders, substance use disorders) or symptoms (e.g., hopelessness, insomnia, and agitation), prior psychiatric hospitalization, recent bio-psychosocial stressors, and the availability of firearms." While acknowledging that there are many more risk factors relevant for a comprehensive assessment, the factors listed above were highlighted as having the strongest evidence for their use and, as such, should never be excluded from consideration.

Quite possibly the most important note about risk and protective factors is that a comprehensive assessment of suicide risk should never be based on an additive or subtractive model of identified factors. There is no magic number of risk factors that leads to an accurate assessment of high or acute risk and no magic number of protective factors that grants immunity from suicide-related behaviors. The combination of risk and protective factors is idiopathic and, while an essential part of a comprehensive risk assessment, is thus not sufficient in and of itself in determining risk or treatment recommendations.

Stratification of risk levels is another important consideration for providers that uses risk and protective factors to help guide intervention and disposition. Notably, the CPG (VA/DoD, 2019) reports that "while it is an expected standard of care, there is insufficient evidence to recommend for or against the use of risk stratification to determine the level of suicide risk." This may be a shocking statement for many psychologists who base their clinical decisions on risk stratification. While the CPG reports insufficient evidence for risk stratification, it does acknowledge that risk stratification is an accepted standard of care practice that should continue to be used by providers to inform risk mitigation strategies and treatment decisions within the context of a comprehensive risk assessment. The CPG proposes use of the VA model of therapeutic risk stratification (Rocky Mountain MIRECC, 2020).

TREATMENT INTERVENTION

Case 9.1b. The Soldier Who Was Admitted to the Hospital

The corporal reported suicide-related thoughts since the age of 12, beginning after cyberbullying at school and his parents' marital problems. Between the ages of 15 and 19, he attempted suicide four times: (1) overdosing on over-the-counter (OTC) pills, (2) crashing his car into a wall, (3) drinking alcohol and taking OTC pills, and (4) increasing the amount of alcohol and OTC pills he used. With each incident, the corporal reported an expectation of death. He reported a history of symptoms consistent with major depressive disorder, recurrent and severe, and inpatient treatment was indicated. As a result, he was escorted to the nearby MTF Emergency Department, where he was evaluated for inpatient hospitalization. The provider finished the evaluation, paged and consulted with on-call psychiatry at the MTF, and liaised with the unit chain of command who would assume responsibility for their soldier following his discharge from the MTF; the corporal was evaluated by on-call psychiatry, who convinced him that inpatient treatment would help keep him safe and begin the process of establishing a treatment program tailored to his specific needs.

Stabilization or Safety Planning

One intervention that is not typically considered a specific therapeutic approach, but can be effectively utilized within psychotherapy, is stabilization planning, more commonly referred to as *safety planning*. It is a collaborative process between the provider and the patient, designed to help prepare the patient for potential future suicidal crises. Although there is limited research currently available for stabilization planning interventions, this process has replaced the former practice of safety or no-suicide contracts. No-suicide contracts originated in the late 1960s, but despite common adoption, often with the most at-risk patients, they lacked a standard definition and theoretical conceptualization (Rudd, Mandrusiak & Joiner, 2006). Rudd and colleagues (2006) found that most studies of no-suicide contracts focused on frequency of use rather than effectiveness, and those that did address effectiveness suffered from significant methodological problems. Drew (2001) actually found that patients with no-suicide contracts were, in fact, more likely to engage in subsequent self-harm. Stabilization planning reflects a collective shift in the conceptual framework of suicide prevention (Jobes & Chalker, 2019). It is considered a best practice by clinicians and should be conducted with every patient at risk for suicide (VA/DoD, 2019).

Several approaches to stabilization planning exist, with the most widely recognized including: Stanley and Brown's Safety Plan Intervention (SPI) (Stanley et al., 2018) used throughout the VA and throughout much of the DoD; the Crisis Response Plan (CRP) developed by Rudd, Joiner, and Rajad, but more recently researched and advocated for by Bryan (Bryan et al., 2018); and the Crisis Stabilization Plan within the Collaborative Assessment and Management of Suicidality (CAMS) framework created by Jobes (2012). These all have the following elements in common: identification of warning signs and/or triggers, specific coping strategies, resources, and reasons for living. Although stabilization planning is not commonly considered to be a stand-alone psychotherapy approach, it can be considered an excellent application of problem-solving therapy, discussed later in this chapter. The SPI and CRP both also specifically address lethal means

234MILITARY PSYCHOLOGY

safety, which is critical for suicide prevention. Numerous studies have demonstrated the importance of means restriction for safety (Bryan et al., 2019; Butterworth, Daruwala, & Anestis, 2018; Jin, Khazem, & Anestis, 2016), and the CPG recommends reducing access to lethal means to decrease suicide rates. The DoD also offers guidance for providers on the voluntary temporary safekeeping of weapons by the command when suicide risk is identified (Wright, 2014). One particularly comprehensive review with recommendations for both providers and commanders was presented by Hoyt and Duffy (2015), in which the authors strive to balance the need to ensure safety from suicide risk with the rights of service members (see Table 9.1).

Psychotherapy Treatment Approaches

The evidence-based literature in treatment for suicide risk is still maturing, and according to the 2019 CPG, only two therapy approaches have sufficient evidence to recommend them for intervention with suicidal patients: cognitive-behavioral therapy (CBT) for suicide prevention and problem-solving therapy (PST). Furthermore, these two therapies only have a recommendation for treating patients with multiple previous suicide attempts. The recommendation in preventing suicide attempts for at-risk individuals is neutral. Additionally, the research basis regarding interventions for suicidality in patients with comorbid conditions (i.e., borderline personality disorder, substance use disorders) is largely insufficient. For example, dialectical behavior therapy (DBT), initially specifically developed for treating borderline personality disorder overall, of which suicidality is one of nine diagnostic criteria, is reported as having insufficient evidence for treating suicidality in patients with borderline personality disorder. Needless to say, there is further work to be completed in establishing a robust research basis of adequate breadth and depth in the field of suicide intervention.

The majority of current evidence-informed psychotherapy approaches to treating suicidal patients, in light of the paucity of research, fall within the category of CBT. In general, CBT endeavors to assist patients in changing their maladaptive behaviors, beliefs, emotional responses, and interpersonal interactions in order to improve their condition. CBT also is frequently utilized as a short-term therapy approach, typically concluded within 12 sessions. CBT for suicide prevention focuses on changing the same elements, but specifically with regard to suicide. The goals of CBT for suicide prevention are to identify antecedents, beliefs, emotions, and behaviors related to suicidality; challenge maladaptive beliefs and behaviors; develop alternative effective beliefs and behaviors; and practice utilizing the alternative beliefs and behaviors (VA/DoD, 2019; Stanley et al., 2009). CBT for suicide prevention also includes relapse prevention strategies toward the end of treatment, designed to help the patient identify warning signs that a

TABLE 9.1. Summary of Recommendations for Providers and Commanders

Providers should . . .	Commanders should . . .
• Assess access to both military-issued and privately owned firearms as a core component of risk assessment and safety planning. • Collaborate with patient, command, and family members to temporarily remove firearms from the home when a patient is at risk for suicide. • Engage all involved parties, including family members and commanders at all levels, in the process of means restriction counseling when recommending firearms restriction. • Be aware of state-specific laws regarding the temporary transfer of firearms between individuals. • Be aware of the potential impact of firearms restriction on unit readiness and deployability, taking care to use the least restrictive means to ensure safety. • Forge relationships with local Veteran Service Organizations (VSO) as a potential mechanism for voluntary, short-term transfer of firearms to a trusted peer. • Engage unit command teams through outreach activities, to include baseline training in the process of means restriction counseling.	• Provide space in unit arms rooms for potential short-term voluntary storage of privately owned weapons. • Require registration of all privately owned firearms stored on military installations (to include on-base housing) with the provost marshal. • Emphasize weapons safety, such as firearms storage in commercial safes or cases rather than out in the open, in a nightstand, or under a bed/pillow in order to decrease impulsive use of firearms. This may also include emphasizing securely storing ammunition separately from firearms. • Exercise creativity to ensure that weapons-restricted soldiers can still be gainfully employed within the unit at the level of their rank and experience without calling undue attention to the soldier or exacerbating behavioral health stigma. • As a last resort only, restrict a soldier to the barracks or military installation in order to temporarily prevent access to privately owned weapons stored in a private residence.
Providers should not . . .	Commanders should not . . .
• Take possession of firearms or encourage soldiers to bring firearms into medical clinics. • Make blanket recommendations that soldiers "give away" their firearms. • Recommend or imply that a soldier is incapable of carrying a firearm. • Imply that a soldier is "mentally unsound" from a legal perspective, unless in a court-appointed role that specifically authorizes such determinations or recommendations.	• Enact blanket policies requiring disclosure of privately owned weapons not stored on a military installation. • Attempt to confiscate or order service members to turn over privately owned weapons. • Increase stigma by calling attention to a soldier who has been placed on weapons restriction.

Note. From Hoyt and Duffy (2015). In the public domain.

suicidal crisis may be developing and to preidentify coping strategies that can be utilized. PST is based on the premise that individuals experience difficulties when their problems overwhelm their resources, with suicidality being one example of a maladaptive coping response to overwhelming stressors. PST teaches individuals to identify the connection between their distress and problems, define their problems, and apply problem-solving techniques to them to resolve their distress. DBT, arguably a form of CBT, is based on the premise that certain individuals experience greater emotional dysregulation and that this dysregulation leads to suicidal thoughts and behaviors. DBT endeavors to teach individuals mindfulness, emotion regulation, distress tolerance, and interpersonal effectiveness skills, all of which may be effective in decreasing emotional dysregulation and improving coping skills for emotional dysregulation, thereby theoretically reducing further suicide attempts.

In addition to considering specific treatment approaches and modalities for suicidal patients, it is also important to consider other supplemental approaches. One such approach is Caring Contacts. The literature on Caring Contacts began in the 1970s, and there continues to be interest and support for this approach to the present day (Carter, Clover, Whyte, Dawson, & D'Este, 2005; Comtois et al., 2019; Motto & Bostrom, 2001). Caring Contacts involves communicating concern for the patient's well-being without any expectation of return contact. This communication was initially delivered via postcard but has continued to evolve with technological advances such that some Caring Contacts are now delivered via text message (although some continue to be delivered via postcard). While the research on Caring Contacts was insufficient for a CPG recommendation, it does appear to have small to moderate benefits for decreasing future suicide attempts and may also help individuals become more involved in treatment. On its own, Caring Contacts is not considered a treatment approach, but can be a valuable supplemental intervention. While it may present numerous challenges, a future best practice worth considering would be for military treatment clinics to collaborate with command personnel shops to develop protocols for implementing Caring Contacts with personnel following treatment for significant risk. Taking into account appropriate confidentiality requirements, there is a role for both medical and administrative personnel in Caring Contacts.

Pharmacological Approaches

Pharmacological approaches have largely focused on treating suicidality as associated with an underlying mental health disorder (i.e., major depressive disorder), rather than as an independent condition. According to the 2019 VA/DoD CPG, ketamine has shown some evidence as an adjunctive, short-term treatment for suicidality in major depressive disorder; there is also some evidence for the use of lithium as a stand-alone treatment for suicidality in bipolar disorder and in combination with another psychotropic for suicidality in unipolar or bipolar depression; clozapine, too, has the support of some evidence for treating suicidality in schizophrenia or schizoaffective disorder. There is no recommended pharmacological approach for suicidality overall, particularly when exhibited outside the context of one of the serious mental illnesses listed above.

ADMINISTRATIVE RESPONSIBILITIES

Case 9.1c. The Soldier Who Was Placed on a Profile

After a week on the inpatient unit, the corporal was discharged to his command with recommendations for outpatient treatment and placed on a profile. Because his duty assignment was in a specialty that required additional levels of personal reliability, his previous diagnosis of a depressive disorder meant that he was not only unfit for full duty but also unsuitable for continued service in his career specialty. John voiced a strong desire to get better during his outpatient treatment, with the goal of returning to full duty in a new career path. The embedded psychologist assured John that the guiding principle for a temporary profile was the belief that service members benefit from treatment and may return to duty.

Military psychologists often find themselves in multiple roles within a command, the most common being as a provider to their patients and a consultant to the command. While occasional fodder for ethical conflicts to be discussed with mentors, most often these two roles are well aligned with each other, and the military clinician must be aware of administrative implications for treating service members at risk for suicide.

The first consideration is the commanding officer's (CO) need-to-know. The CO's need-to-know is a recognized Health Insurance Portability and Accountability Act (HIPAA) exclusion and typically covered during the informed consent process, written formally into the treatment agreement signed when commencing outpatient care (HIPAA Privacy of Individually Identifiable Health Information, 2000; OUSDP&R, 2011). The CO has a clearly defined right to be informed of limited information about service members receiving behavioral health care to include: serious risk of harm to self, serious risk of harm to others, serious risk of harm to mission, special personnel (e.g., nuclear, aviation), inpatient medical care, acute conditions interfering with duty, substance use disorder treatment, command-directed mental health evaluations, and other special circumstances as determined by an O6 or higher-ranking officer (OUSDP&R, 2011). The military clinical psychologist must discern which patients' conditions may necessitate informing the CO and convey that information in a clear, succinct manner. In regard to suicidality, initial determination of serious risk of harm to self would be made during the initial and all subsequent suicide risk assessments, but the serious risk of harm to mission, special personnel, and acute conditions interfering with duty (related to treatment recommendations) are more dependent on the unique circumstances of the service member, occupation within the military, specific role within the command, and the command's mission (e.g., high-level security clearance or the Personnel Reliability Program [Office of the Under Secretary of

Defense for Acquisition, Technology, and Logistics (OUSDAT&L), 2015]).
For example, some service members have specific skill sets that are not
widely acquired throughout the military or work in small teams that are
highly interdependent. If a service member is being recommended for more
intensive treatment that conflicts with a command's mission or training
schedule, and the member has a specific unique skill set required for that
mission or training, it may be necessary to inform the CO of the risk to
the mission because of the potential conflict between the recommended
treatment and the command's needs. The clinician does not always have
access to this information and may need to proactively communicate with
the command to ensure a decision process about need-to-know is fully
informed. This process may feel like an intricate dance between asking
questions to obtain sufficient information to make these determinations
while not divulging information that could violate confidentiality, privacy,
and the tenants of this "need-to-know."

A second consideration is the member's occupation within the military.
Many military occupations have specific requirements directly or peripher-
ally related to mental health. Perhaps the most restrictive are within the
aviation community and nuclear field duty. Being part of an air crew has
stringent health requirements, and even OTC medication usage can temporarily affect someone's ability to fly. Suicidality, even when effectively
treated, can be cause for concern within these occupations. Additionally,
a common recommendation for service members at risk for suicide is to
restrict their access to weapons at their command. This recommendation
can interfere with the performance of duties, particularly for occupations
requiring weapons and ordnance-handling. If placement on a restricted
access to weapons list extends past 90 days, they may need to cross-rate
to an occupation that does not require the ability to handle weapons or
ordnance. Furthermore, many occupational specialties within the military
require a basic-level security clearance, with some requiring the highest levels of clearance. With a few exceptions, being diagnosed with and treated
for a mental health condition will at the very least require disclosure by
service members when they are renewing their security clearance. Counseling for adjustment related to serving in a combat zone, grief, marital/family
problems (with the exclusion of any domestic violence incident), and sexual
assault—all do not require disclosure during application or renewal of a
security clearance (Office of the Secretary of Defense, 2012). Furthermore,
COs are often encouraged to make their personnel aware that seeking mental health care, particularly early when problems are more easily treated,
is aligned with national security (OUSDP&R, 2011). If a service member
has a high-level security clearance, the clinician may have a lower threshold to contact that member's CO if the member is enrolled in a special
program like the Personnel Reliability Program or if the member's unique
circumstances may result in harm to the mission, but this communication

should be in line with guidance for commander's need-to-know covered above (USDAT&L, 2015).

A third consideration is the operational tempo (OPTEMPO) of the service member's command. Many evidence-based psychotherapies require consistent attendance and engagement in treatment. Service members with high OPTEMPO and frequent field or underway activities may not be able to attend treatment consistently, which reduces the effectiveness of care. This situation requires a conversation with the member's CO to discuss treatment recommendations that necessitate keeping the service member on the installation. These recommendations may result in a profile or limited-duty period, discussed in greater detail in the next section.

Temporary Duty Limitations

In military settings, clinicians may recommend an array of duty limitations and administrative measures to help manage and monitor risk in outpatient and operational environments. Service members should not deploy if they are identified as at risk for suicide (Woodson, 2013; OUSDP&R, 2010). One of the most common means to communicate short-term modifications or limitations in deployment and duties is for the clinician to provide the service member with a temporary profile (in the Army, Air Force) or limited duty (LIMDU; in the Navy, Marine Corps), often ranging between 30 and 180 days in accordance with the branch of Service, diagnosis, and prognosis. Rationale for duty limitations may include stabilization on a new medication, reestablishing a consistent sleep pattern, participating in ongoing treatment, or referral for necessary specialty services that would otherwise be hindered by the individual's routine schedule or scope of work. Recommendations for specific limitations may relate to restricting access to weapons (including removal of a firing bolt or pin), prohibiting use of alcohol, ordering a move into the barracks, limiting contact with individuals having a negative impact on the service member's functioning, and facilitating the service member's attendance at scheduled appointments (Hassinger, 2003; Hill, Johnson, & Barton, 2006; Payne, Hill, & Johnson, 2008).

Particularly in deployed settings, where weapons and ammunition may be readily accessible, mental health resources limited, and medical evacuation not immediately available or operationally viable, clinicians can help delineate appropriate guidelines for more persistent monitoring as a part of a *unit watch*. Documented examples range from direct observation from first formation until lights out for lower-risk service members (e.g., military-specific suicidal ideation, self-injurious behavior while intoxicated the night prior, or step-down from inpatient hospitalization) to a 24-hour watch, where the service member is observed at all times when deemed to be of low to moderate risk (Payne et al., 2008). In such instances, the recommending clinician is encouraged to provide both verbal consultation and written instructions to the identified escort and command, document-ing a description of the service member's safety concerns, warning signs of and actions to take in case of deterioration or decompensation, any restric-tions to be placed on the service member, and contact information for the provider (Hassinger, 2003; Payne et al., 2008). It is important to remember that duty limitations and related measures are not a form of treatment, but rather useful tools to be used in conjunction with empirically based inter-ventions. Continual monitoring of a service member's status is also criti-cal to determine whether limitations should be terminated as symptoms resolve, duty restrictions extended to accommodate additional treatment, or if the service member should be considered for separation through medi-cal or administrative channels when concerns do not adequately resolve for continued service despite treatment efforts.

Medical Separation/Fitness for Duty

In the military, diagnostic decisions, estimates of risk, and intervention options are closely tied to fitness-for-duty considerations (see also Chap-ter 2, this volume). Although the concept of fitness implies a dichotomous decision (fit vs. unfit), in practice, there are gradations that permit some flexibility in personnel decisions. For example, after a course of treatment, a service member whose suicidal ideation has fully resolved or who engaged in significant self-harm or risky behavior without intent to die may ulti-mately return to the unit as fit for full duty. The immediate responsibility for diagnostic decisions about a military member's psychiatric fitness for duty rests with the local clinician and is often driven by the acuity or chronicity of the presenting problem. When it is determined that a service member's condition cannot be adequately stabilized within an appropriate period of time (generally 6–12 months depending on Service policy) or the individual has been diagnosed with a severe mental illness with limited probability of returning to full-duty status, the clinician may refer the service member to a Medical Evaluation Board (MEB). However, the ultimate determination for medical retirement and any disability rests with the Physical Evaluation Board (PEB) located in Washington, D.C. (OUSDP&R, 2014b).

Administrative Separation/Suitability for Service

Another concept pertinent to risk management and military dispositions is suitability for continued military service as it relates to personality traits, coping skills, and interpersonal abilities of service members to perform their duties in a safe and effective manner. Members deemed unsuitable for further service on the basis of an adjustment or personality disorder may be recommended for administrative separation from the Armed Ser-vices pursuant to service-specific regulations and governing authorities

(OUSDP&R, 2014a). A personality disorder diagnosis in and of itself, however, does not mean that a person is unsuitable for the military. Rather, a recommendation for separation is typically made only if the member's personality disorder results in problematic behaviors that have been documented as directly interfering with performance of duty. Particularly when a service member presents with co-occurring conditions, such as a personality disorder and medical, substance use, or other psychiatric condition(s), it should be noted that any administrative or medical separation procedure can become lengthy and complex. Especially in such instances, service members with elevated suicide-related risk warrant ongoing monitoring and should remain informed of their administrative status to decrease potential for escalating distress and suicide-related ideation or behavior as they await final disposition of their case.

POSTVENTION

Case 9.1d. The Soldier Who Died by Suicide

The corporal engaged in weekly CBT and met with his medical officer for medication management. Rumors of heavy alcohol consumption began to circulate. The chain of command reported these concerns to the embedded psychologist, and when confronted, the corporal admitted to drinking alcohol but denied excessive intake. He was hospitalized a second time for 2 weeks when he was found in the barracks heavily intoxicated and inconsolable. Upon discharge, the command safety plan was updated to include twice daily check-ins with superiors. He was scheduled to meet with the embedded psychologist once per week and had an intake interview with the intensive outpatient treatment program at the MTF. Medications were prescribed in 1-week supplies to prevent the safety risk of hoarding, and he was referred to outpatient psychiatry to take over management of his medications from the medical officer. Despite these efforts, the corporal continued to decompensate and was hospitalized under similar circumstances two additional times. He was scheduled for residential alcohol treatment (not considered an emergent admission program), but 2 weeks after his fourth inpatient stay, he consumed a toxic amount of alcohol and OTC medications resulting in his death.

Clinical Investigation Requirements

Specific clinical actions taken in the wake of a service member's suicide attempt or death by suicide can vary across and within military branches. In such instances, clinicians may accordingly be called on to perform a number of different requirements and roles in suicide surveillance, quality control measures, and investigatory proceedings. As directed by the DoD, clinicians must, at minimum, submit standardized reporting on any suicide attempts in the Department of Defense Suicide Event Report (DODSER) system, and support the command unit with the submission for deaths within 30 and 60 days, respectively (OUSDP&R, 2017). For instances in which a service member dies by suicide while in the care of a clinician, a treatment facility will first determine if the death meets the Joint Commission criteria to be considered a *sentinel event* (Comprehensive Accreditation Manual for Behavioral Health Care, 2020). If the death by suicide occurred within 72 hours of discharge from an inpatient psychiatric admission or the Emergency Department, the command will conduct a comprehensive systematic analysis and provide a corrective action plan.

Whether or not considered a sentinel event, all treatment facilities determine additional incidents that are considered patient safety events which require a standard quality of care review in which leadership evaluates whether clinical procedures and guidelines met appropriate standards of care (Defense Health Agency, 2019). The first step of conducting a standard of care review following a suicide is determining all significantly involved providers (SIP) based on health record documentation. While this is often stressful for providers who are suddenly coping with the tragic loss of a patient and naturally experiencing self-doubt, it is important to note it is not a punitive investigatory process but one with a goal in accord with the principles of high reliability to ensure a continuous learning environment that ensures process improvement. A peer professional will be assigned to review documented care in the case.

Administrative Investigation Requirements

In addition to clinically specific requirements, each Service directs several actions be taken by leadership following the death of a service member by suicide. Immediately following the death of a service member, individuals are tasked to (1) notify the service member's next of kin and (2) serve as casualty assistance officers that advise and assist the next of kin. As part of command investigations, appointed individuals are also charged with identifying circumstances surrounding the death and determining whether any misconduct was involved. This is often referred to as a *line of duty* (LOD) investigation. Military psychologists are often asked to prepare a formal mental health assessment in memorandum format for suicides and attempted suicides as part of the LOD. Clinicians should remain cognizant of these proceedings, and the potential for such individuals to seek out support as they perform their often challenging duties and professional consultation as part of their investigatory procedures. The Postvention Toolkit for a Military Suicide Loss provides a detailed timeline for investigation processes, as well as postvention practices, following a suicide (DSPO, 2020).

Unit Postvention Support

As found in younger civilian populations, recent empirical analysis suggests increased risk for suicide attempts among military units with a history of the same in the preceding year, particularly in units of smaller size (i.e., ≤ 40 soldiers; Ursano et al., 2017). These and related findings suggest increased risk for mental health concerns and need of heightened suicide awareness and prevention methods following suicide attempts and deaths—particularly when considering the type, closeness, and length of relationship (Pitman, Osborn, King, & Erlangsen, 2014). Available research highlights the degree to which an active (vs. passive) postvention program can effectively support prevention efforts by decreasing the risk of suicide among impacted survivors (Aguirre & Slater, 2010; Campbell, Cataldie, McIntosh, & Millet, 2004). Although there is no single, standardized postvention model across the Services, the DoD has begun adopting the three-phase process promoted by the Tragedy Assistance Program for Survivors (TAPS): stabilization, grief work, and posttraumatic growth (DSPO, 2020). Specific clinical elements of a postvention model may also include increasing awareness, providing training, promoting self-care, and identifying those at increased risk (Ramchand et al., 2015). Delivery of care can range from individual to group sessions and often emphasizes the degree to which individuals experience and process grief differently. Alongside chaplains, military providers may be asked to facilitate and attend memorials and remembrance events. Particularly when embedded in a unit, command elements may similarly seek out clinical guidance and best practices on how to effectively communicate and relate to family members of the deceased service member. Throughout the support process, clinicians should be mindful of the range of reactions one might encounter, such as potential for fellow service members to harbor resentment toward actions of the deceased, or for family members toward the unit or military service in general. The Army requires that a command or senior behavioral health provider lead the Suicide Response Team in support of the unit following a suicide at the discretion of the commander (Department of the Army, 2015).

Provider Postvention Support

Providers practicing in both embedded elements and traditional clinical settings alike should anticipate the potential for increased workload and clinical demands following suicide attempts and deaths. With the increased likelihood of dual roles and responsibilities amongst clinicians practicing in military settings, providers may also find themselves grieving the loss of service members they personally knew as either colleague or patient. It is not uncommon for clinicians to question their competency and clinical practices following the death of a service member who was in their care. During such times, clinician self-care is vital to help combat compassion fatigue and distress (Ramchand et al., 2015). Increased consultation and collaboration with other providers can prove critical in maintaining ethical and appropriate standards of care. Some military facilities recently expanded the role of the Army directed Suicide Response Teams to support not only local units but fellow providers in the MTF in the event of a death by suicide. The Fort Belvoir Community Hospital team offers pre- and postvention educational programing, and voluntary group and individual support to providers who experience a patient death by suicide (Fort Belvoir Suicide Response Team, 2020).

CONCLUSION

After years of proactive, groundbreaking attention and programs, service member deaths by suicide remain tragic events of increasing frequency. As described in this chapter, this parallels the trend of increasing suicide-related ideations, attempts, and deaths by similar-age civilian peers across the country. It would be reductive to presume this increase resulted from a lack of improvement in suicide risk assessment, treatment, prevention programs, and postvention support implemented over the last 10 years: How devastatingly high would the suicide rate be without the programs described in this chapter? Yet, our efforts remain insufficient. Rather than focus on epidemiology, risk and protective factors, and historical efforts, this chapter is a guide for the military behavioral health provider to implement evidence-based assessment strategies and treatment interventions for working with service members at risk for suicide; and to improve consultation and liaison with commands to include administrative responsibilities both during and after treatment. In addition, as the embedding of psychologists within operational units continues to increase, such providers have a unique role to play in preventing suicide from within the warfighter's midst. This chapter is but one guide for the skills and tools necessary for these providers to employ to win this war against suicide.

REFERENCES

Aguirre, R. T. P., & Slater, H. (2010). Suicide postvention as suicide prevention: Improvement and expansion in the United States. *Death Studies, 34,* 529–540.
Army Chief of Public Affairs. (2000, Spring). Hot topics: Suicide prevention. *Soldiers,* pp. 1–15.
Bryan, C. J., Bryan, A. O., Anestis, M. D., Khazem, L. R., Harris, J. A., May, A. M., et al. (2019). Firearm availability and storage practices among military personnel who have thought about suicide. *JAMA Network Open, 2*(8), e199160.

Bryan, C. J., May, A. M., Rozek, D. C., Williams, S. R., Clemans, T. A., Mintz, J., et al. (2018). Use of crisis management interventions among suicidal patients: Results of a randomized controlled trial. *Depression and Anxiety, 35*(7), 619–628.

Butterworth, S. E., Daruwala, S. E., & Anestis, M. D. (2018). Firearm storage and shooting experience: Factors relevant to the practical capability for suicide. *Journal of Psychiatric Research, 102,* 52–56.

Campbell, F. R., Cataldie, L., McIntosh, J., & Millet, K. (2004). An active postvention program. *Crisis, 25,* 30–32.

Carter, G. L., Clover, K., Whyte, I. M., Dawson, A. H., & D'Este, C. (2005). Postcards from the Edge project: Randomized controlled trial of an intervention using postcards to reduce repetition of hospital treated deliberate self-poisoning. *BMJ, 331*(7520), 805.

Centers for Disease Control and Prevention, National Center for Injury Prevention and Control. (2020). *WISQARS leading causes of death reports, 1981–2018.* Retrieved from *webappa.cdc.gov/sasweb/ncipc/leadcause.html.*

Cerel, J., Brown, M. M., Maple, M., Singleton, M., van de Venne, J., Moore, M., et al. (2018). How many people are exposed to suicide? Not six. *Suicide and Life-Threatening Behavior, 9*(2), 529–534.

Comtois, K. A., Kerbrat A. H., DeCou C. R., Atkins D. C., Majeres J. J., Baker J. C., et al. (2019). Effect of augmenting standard care for military personnel with brief caring text messages for suicide prevention. *JAMA Psychiatry, 76*(5), 474.

Defense Health Agency (2019, August 29). *Clinical quality management in the Military Health System* (DHA-PM 6025.13). Falls Church, VA: Author.

Defense Suicide Prevention Office. (2012). *Defense Suicide Prevention Office strategic plan 2012–2016* (Booklet No. 1002). Washington, DC: Office of the Secretary of Defense.

Defense Suicide Prevention Office. (2015). *Department of Defense strategy for suicide prevention.* Retrieved from www.dspo.mil/Portals/113/Documents/TAB%20B%20-%20DSSP_FINAL%20USD%20PR%20SIGNED.PDF.

Defense Suicide Prevention Office. (2020). *Postvention Toolkit for a Military Suicide Loss.* Retrieved from *www.dspo.mil/Portals/113/Documents/PostventionToolkit.pdf?ver=MKd_y1Ab8NuHB-fsO34WuA%3d%3d.*

Department of the Army. (2015, April 14; revised 2019, March 11). *Army health promotion* (AR 600–63). Retrieved from *https://armypubs.army.mil/epubs/DR_pubs/DR_a/pdf/web/ARN15595_R600_63_admin_FINAL.pdf.*

Department of the Army. (2020). *STARRS studies.* Retrieved from *https://starrs-ls.org/#/page/army-starrs-studies.*

Department of Defense. (2009). *Department of Defense Suicide Event Report (DODSER): Calendar year 2008 annual report.* Washington, DC: National Center for Telehealth and Technology, Defense Center of Excellence for Psychological Health & Traumatic Brain Injury.

Department of Defense. (2010). *The challenge and the promise: Strengthening the force, preventing suicide and saving lives: Final report of the Department of Defense Task Force on the prevention of suicide by members of the Armed Forces.* Retrieved from *www.health.mil/dhb/downloads/Suicide%20Prevention%20Task%20Force%20final%20report%208-23-10.pdf.*

Department of Defense. (2013). *Department of Defense, Defense Suicide Prevention Office, annual report—FY 2012.* Arlington, VA: Defense Suicide Prevention Office. Retrieved from *www.dspo.mil/Portals/113/Documents/DSPO-2012-Annual-Report-MARCH-2013-FINAL.pdf.*

Department of Veterans Affairs and Department of Defense. (2019). *VA/DoD clinical practice guideline for the assessment and management of patients at risk for suicide* (Version 2.0). Retrieved from *www.healthquality.va.gov/guidelines/MH/srb/VADoDSuicideRiskFullCPGFinal5088212019.pdf.*

Drew, B. L. (2001). Self-harm behavior and no-suicide contracting in psychiatric inpatient settings. *Archives of Psychiatric Nursing, 15*(3), 99–106.

Fort Belvoir Suicide Response Team. (2020). *Fort Belvoir Community Hospital.* Unpublished manual.

Hassinger, A. D. (2003). Mentoring and monitoring: The use of unit watch in the 4th Infantry Division. *Military Medicine, 168*(3), 234–238. Retrieved from *https://academic.oup.com/milmed/article/168/3/234/4820101.*

Hedegaard, H., Curtin, S.C., & Warner, M. (2020). *Increase in suicide mortality in the United States, 1999–2018* (NCHS Data Brief No. 362). Hyattsville, MD: National Center for Health Statistics.

Hill, J. V., Johnson, R. C., & Barton, R. A. (2006). Suicidal and homicidal soldiers in deployed environments. *Military Medicine, 171*(3), 228–232.

Hilton, S., Stander, V., Werbel, A., & Chavez, B.R. (2009). *Department of the Navy Suicide Incident Report (DONSIR): Summary of Findings, 1999–2007.*

HIPAA Privacy of Individually Identifiable Health Information, 45 C.F.R. §164.512(k)(1) (2000).

Hoyt, T., & Duffy, V. (2015). Implementing firearms restriction for preventing U.S. Army suicide. *Military Psychology, 27*(6), 384–390.

Jin, H. M., Khazem, L. R., & Anestis, M. D. (2016). Recent advances in means safety as a suicide prevention strategy. *Current Psychiatry Report, 18*(10), 96.

Jobes D. A. (2012). The Collaborative Assessment and Management of Suicidality (CAMS): An evolving evidence-based clinical approach to suicidal risk. *Suicide & Life-Threatening Behavior, 42*(6), 640–653.

Jobes, D. A., & Chalker, S. A. (2019). One size does not fit all: A comprehensive clinical approach to reducing suicidal ideation, attempts, and deaths. *International Journal of Environmental Research and Public Health, 16*(19), 3606.

Joint Commission. (2020). *Comprehensive accreditation manual for behavioral health care.* Update 2. Retrieved from *www.jointcommission.org/-/media/tjc/documents/resources/patient-safety-topics/sentinel-event/20200101_6_cambhc_21_se.pdf.*

Jones, D. E., Kennedy, K. R., Hawkes, C., Hourani, L. L., Long, M. A., & Robbins, N. L. (2001). Suicide prevention in the Navy and Marine Corps: Applying the public health model. *Navy Medicine, 92*(6), 31–36.

Jones, D. E., Kennedy, K. R., & Hourani, L. L. (2006). *Suicide prevention in the military.* In C. H. Kennedy & E. A. Zillmer (Eds.), *Military psychology: Clinical and operational applications* (pp. 130–162). New York: The Guilford Press.

Jones, D. E., Hourani, L. L., Rariden, M. B., Hammond, P. J., & Werbel, A. D. (2012). *Suicide prevention in the military.* In C. H. Kennedy & E. A. Zillmer

(Eds.), *Military psychology: Clinical and operational applications* (pp. 211–250). New York: The Guilford Press.

Knox, K. L., Litts, D. A., Talcott, G. W., Feig, J. C., & Caine, E. D. (2003). Risk of suicide and related adverse outcomes after exposure to a suicide prevention programme in the U.S. Air Force: Cohort study. *British Medical Journal, 327,* 1376–1378.

Litts, D. A., Moe, K., Roadman, C. H., Janke, R., & Miller, J. (1999, November 26). Suicide prevention among active duty Air Force personnel: United States, 1990–1999. *Morbidity and Mortality Weekly Report, 48*(46), 1053–1057.

Motto, J. A., & Bostrom, A. G. (2001). A randomized controlled trial of postcrisis suicide prevention. *Psychiatric Services, 52*(6), 828–833.

Naifeh, J. A., Mash, H. B., Stein, M. B., Fullerton, C. S., Kessler, R. C., & Ursano, R. J. (2019). The Army Study to Assess Risk and Resilience in Servicemembers (Army STARRS): Progress toward understanding suicide among soldiers. *Molecular Psychiatry, 24,* 34–48.

National Institute of Mental Health. (2009). *Evidence-based prevention is goal of largest ever study of suicide in the military.* Retrieved from *www.nimh.nih. gov/archive/news/2009/evidence-based-prevention-is-goal-of-largest-ever-study-of-suicide-in-the-military.shtml.*

Office of the Secretary of Defense. (2012, September 4). *Department of Defense guidance on Question 21, Standard Form 86, Questionnaire for National Security Positions* [Department of Defense Memorandum]. Washington, DC: U.S. Department of Defense.

Office of the Under Secretary of Defense for Acquisition, Technology, and Logistics. (2015, January 13). *Nuclear weapons personnel reliability program* (Department of Defense Manual 5210.42). Washington, DC: U.S. Department of Defense. Retrieved from *www.esd.whs.mil/Portals/54/Documents/DD/issuances/dodm/521042m.pdf?ver=2018–11–19–100837–003.*

Office of the Under Secretary of Defense for Personnel and Readiness. (2010, February 5). *Deployment-limiting medical conditions for service members and DoD civilian employees* (Department of Defense Instruction 6490.07). Washington, DC: U.S. Department of Defense. Retrieved from *www.esd.whs.mil/Portals/54/Documents/DD/issuances/dodi/649007p.pdf.*

Office of the Under Secretary of Defense for Personnel and Readiness. (2011, August 17). *Command notification requirements to dispel stigma in providing mental health care to service members* (Department of Defense Instruction 6490.08). Washington, DC: U.S. Department of Defense. Retrieved from *www.esd.whs.mil/Portals/54/Documents/DD/issuances/dodi/649008p.pdf.*

Office of the Under Secretary of Defense for Personnel and Readiness. (2014a January 27; Change 5, 2020, June 12). *Enlisted administrative separations* (Department of Defense Instruction 1332.14). Washington, DC: U.S. Department of Defense. Retrieved from *www.esd.whs.mil/Portals/54/Documents/DD/issuances/dodi/133214p.pdf?ver=2019–03–14–132901–200.*

Office of the Under Secretary of Defense for Personnel and Readiness. (2014b, August 5). *Disability Evaluation System (DES)* (Department of Defense Instruction 1332.18). Washington, DC: U.S. Department of Defense. Retrieved from *https://warriorcare.dodlive.mil/files/2016/03/DoDI_1332.18.pdf.*

Office of the Under Secretary of Defense for Personnel and Readiness. (2017,

November 6; Change 2, 2020, September 11). *Defense Suicide Prevention Program* (Department of Defense Instruction 6490.16). Washington, DC: U.S. Department of Defense. Retrieved from *www.esd.whs.mil/Portals/54/Documents/DD/issuances/dodi/649016p.pdf?ver=2020–09–11–122632–850.*

Payne, S. E., Hill, J. V., & Johnson, D. E. (2008). The use of unit watch or command interest profile in the management of suicide and homicide risk: Rationale and guidelines for the military mental health professional. *Military Medicine, 173*(1), 25–35.

Pitman, A., Osborn, D., King, M., & Erlangsen, A. (2014). Effects of suicide bereavement on mental health and suicide risk. *The Lancet Psychiatry, 1*(1), 86–94.

Ramchand, R., Ayer, L., Fisher, G., Osilla K. C., Barness-Proby, D., & Wertheimer, S. (2015). *Suicide postvention in the Department of Defense: Evidence, policies and procedures, and perspectives of loss survivors.* Santa Monica, CA: RAND Corporation.

Reger, M. A., Smolenski, D. J., Skopp, N. A., Metzger-Abamukang, M. J., Kang, H. K., Bullman, T. A., et al. (2015). Risk of suicide among U.S. military service members following Operation Enduring Freedom or Operation Iraqi Freedom deployment and separation from the U.S. military. *JAMA Psychiatry, 72*(6), 561–569

Rocky Mountain MIRECC. (2020). *Therapeutic risk management—risk stratification table.* Retrieved from *www.mirecc.va.gov/visn19/trm.*

Rudd, M. D., Mandrusiak, M., & Joiner, T. E., Jr. (2006). The case against no-suicide contracts: The commitment to treatment statement as a practice alternative. *Journal of Clinical Psychology, 62*(2), 243–251.

Shaffer, D. (1997). *Suicide and suicide prevention in the military forces: Report of a consultation.* New York: Columbia University.

Shelef, L., Levi-Belz, Y., Fruchter, E., Santo, Y., & Dahan, E. (2016). No way out: Entrapment as a moderator of suicide ideation among military personnel. *Journal of Clinical Psychology, 72*(10), 1049–1063.

Shenassa, E. D., Catlin, S. N., & Buka, S. L. (2003). Lethality of firearms relative to other suicide methods: A population based study. *Journal of Epidemiology and Community Health, 57*(2), 120–124.

Smith, J. A., Doidge, M., Hanoa, R., & Frueh, B. C. (2019). A historical examination of military records of U.S. Army suicide, 1819 to 2017. *JAMA Network Open, 2*(12), e1917448.

Stanley, B., Brown, G. K., Brenner, L. A., Galfalvy, H. C., Currier, G. W., Knox, K. L., et al. (2018). Comparison of the Safety Planning Intervention with follow-up vs. usual care of suicidal patients treated in the Emergency Department. *JAMA Psychiatry, 75*(9), 894–900.

Stanley, B., Brown, G., Brent, D. A., Wells, K., Poling, K., Curry, J., et al. (2009). Cognitive-behavioral therapy for suicide prevention (CBT-SP): Treatment model, feasibility, and acceptability. *Journal of the American Academy of Child and Adolescent Psychiatry, 48*(10), 1005–1013.

Substance Abuse and Mental Health Services Administration. (2019). *Key substance use and mental health indicators in the United States: Results from the 2018 National Survey on Drug Use and Health* (HHS Publication No. PEP19–5068, NSDUH Series H-54). Rockville, MD: Center for Behavioral

Health Statistics and Quality, Substance Abuse and Mental Health Services Administration. Retrieved from *www.samhsa.gov/data*.

Tucker, J., Smolenski, D., & Kennedy, C. (2020). *Department of Defense suicide event report: Calendar year 2018 annual report*. Silver Spring, MD: Psychological Health Center of Excellence, Defense Health Agency.

U.S. Air Force Suicide Prevention Program. (2020). Retrieved from *www.resilience.af.mil/Suicide-Prevention-Program*.

U.S. Army Medical Command. (2017). *Behavioral health service line Department of Behavioral Health* (MEDCOM Policy Memo 17–029). Fort Sam Houston, San Antonio, TX: Author.

U.S. Army Suicide Prevention Program. (2020). Retrieved from *www.armyg1.army.mil/hr/suicide*.

U.S. Marine Corps Suicide Prevention Program. (2020). Retrieved from *www.usmc-mccs.org/services/support/suicide-prevention*.

U.S. Navy Suicide Prevention Program. (2020). Retrieved from *www.public.navy.mil/bupers-npc/support/21st_Century_Sailor/suicide_prevention/Pages/default.aspx*.

Ursano, R. J., Kessler, R. C., Naifeh, J. A., Herberman Mash, H., Fullerton, C. S., Bliese, P. D., et al. (2017). Risk of suicide attempt among soldiers in Army units with a history of suicide attempts. *JAMA Psychiatry, 74*(9), 924–931.

Western Michigan University. (2020). *Suicide prevention program: Risk factors*. Kalamazoo, MI: Author. Retrieved from *www.wmich.edu/suicideprevention/basics/risk*.

Woodson, J. (2013, October 7). *Clinical practice guidance for deployment-limiting mental disorders and psychotropic medications* [Department of Defense Memorandum]. Arlington, VA: U.S. Department of Defense. Retrieved from *https://health.mil/Reference-Center/Policies/2013/10/07/Deployment-Limiting-Mental-Disorders-and-Psychotrophic-Medications*.

Wright, J. (2014, August 28). *Guidance for commanders and health professionals in the Department of Defense on reducing access to lethal means through the voluntary storage of privately-owned firearms* (Department of Defense Memorandum). Arlington, VA: U.S. Department of Defense. Retrieved from *www.dspo.mil/Portals/113/Documents/Guidance-for-Commanders-and-HP-in-DoD-on-Reducing-Access-to-Lethal-Means.pdf*.

CHAPTER 10

Embedded and Expeditionary Mental Health Practice in the Military

Robert D. Lippy, Stephanie N. Pagano,
Thomas J. Patterson, and Alan D. Ogle

One of the most unique aspects of military psychology is the setting in which psychological services are provided—both physically and culturally. When we speak of embedded or expeditionary mental health, we are largely discussing these physical and cultural differences between traditional, civilian psychological practice and military psychology. Each service has its own unique terminology and ways of executing these concepts.[1]

Throughout this chapter, we will discuss a brief history of the concepts of embedded and expeditionary mental health, describe the common roles that embedded and expeditionary psychologists fill, and identify common tasks for embedded and expeditionary mental health work.[2] We will conclude with some unique challenges, suggestions for self-care, and a lessons-learned summary for the next generation of embedded and expeditionary psychologists.

---

[1]*Mental health versus behavioral health:* In the military, these words are often used interchangeably to refer to the scope of services provided by psychologists and other mental health professionals. The Army uses the term behavioral health (BH), and the Navy and Air Force tend to use the term mental health (MH). For consistency's sake, this chapter will use the general term *mental health* unless referring to a specific program.

[2]*Expeditionary mental health:* Mental health personnel who deploy away from their permanent duty station to support a combat or non-combat military operation. While many embedded psychologists deploy with their units, some may deploy assigned to other units, such as combat operational stress control (COSC) detachments. These personnel are traditionally in the military themselves, but civilians may also be employed in an expeditionary capacity in some, limited circumstances.

EMBEDDED AND EXPEDITIONARY
MENTAL HEALTH ACROSS THE SERVICES

The history of military psychology (see Chapter 1, this volume) demonstrates that the unique skills of psychologists as experts in human behavior are valuable to the military. One shift that has been notable is the integration of embedded models of practice across the military health system. Mental health providers have typically been centralized in hospital or clinic settings, where they provide diagnostic and therapy services to service members and sometimes to family members and retirees. The U.S. military also found beneficial effects from providing clinical services in a forward deployed environment (e.g., Moore & Reger, 2007). Early concepts of expeditionary mental health essentially meant moving a clinic from the garrison environment to a forward deployed environment and conducting the same mission—the provision of diagnostic and treatment services for those suffering from mental health disorders. Line commanders found this beneficial, and thus the embedded mental health (EMH) provider concept was born. One can think of an EMH provider as merging clinical and consultative support roles to help a line commander meet mission.[3]

In addition to providing clinical care to specific operational units, EMH providers, unlike traditional, clinically focused military treatment facility (MTF) providers, also conduct various nonclinical care activities in direct support of operational units (e.g., unit circulation/"walk-abouts," consultation to leaders, outreach education, performance enhancement, etc.) with the goal of improving unit readiness across the deployment cycle. The goal of embedding mental health personnel within operational units is to provide a more efficient path to care with providers who are better positioned to understand the culture and needs of the unit. To accomplish these goals, they must leverage both clinical and nonclinical skills. In addition to these skills, certain professional strengths and traits have been found important to serving effectively in an embedded position (see Table 10.1).

Each service takes a slightly different approach in implementing embedded and expeditionary mental health. EMH in the U.S. Navy and U.S. Marine Corps (recall that the Navy provides all medical care to the Marine Corps) maintains the core concept of assigning providers and technicians to line units. These personnel may have offices on a ship, in a building owned by the line commander, in a building owned by the MTF, or in

---

[3]*Embedded mental health*: Mental health personnel who are assigned to, or organic to, a line unit (as opposed to a hospital or clinic). Professional disciplines may include psychologists, psychiatrists, nurses, social workers, enlisted mental health technicians, and others. Embedded psychologists are charged with working closely with the unit's command structure, and may or may not deploy with the unit. Examples of EMH are Army brigade behavioral health officers, Navy aircraft carrier psychologists, and Air Force command psychologists.

TABLE 10.1. Traits of an Effective EMH Provider

- Confident/assertive
- Clinical competence
- Military culturally competence (deep understanding of unit mission, commander's priorities/philosophy, unit organization, individual job types/responsibilities
- Previous embedded experience or training
- Comfort working independently/autonomously
- Adaptable to changing demands, schedules
- Skilled in rapport building/emotional intelligence (with leaders and service members)
- Comfort with calculated risk taking, balanced against firm understanding of professional limits/boundaries
- Effective self-care

multiple locations. Regardless of where they work, their primary privileging is through the senior medical officer attached to the line unit they serve and not through an MTF. EMH in the Navy traces its roots to first embedding psychologists on aircraft carriers in the late 1990s (Johnson, Ralph, & Johnson, 2005), which showed a dramatic reduction of costly medical evacuations for mental health reasons during deployments. In 1999, the Marine Corps implemented the Operational Stress Control and Readiness (OSCAR) program within the 2nd Marine Division at Camp Lejeune, North Carolina, to establish a "new type of partnership between warfighters and mental health professionals . . . [enabling the] prevention, early identification, and effective [mental health] treatment . . . at the lowest level possible" (Nash, 2006, pp. 25–26). Following the successful deployment of OSCAR providers during Operation Iraqi Freedom (OIF) and Operation Enduring Freedom (OEF), the Marine Corps institutionalized the OSCAR program in all infantry divisions and regiments (Pierce, Broderick, Johnston, & Holloway, 2020). More recently, Marine logistics groups (MLGs) acquired mental health assets for the provision of organic mental health support to its units.

EMH across the Navy has expanded since the 1990s (Naval Center for Combat & Operational Stress Control [NCCOSC], 2020). In 2010, mental health providers were embedded within the explosive ordnance disposal (EOD) community and shortly thereafter to the Naval Coastal Riverine Force and Naval Construction Force. In 2012, mental health providers began routinely deploying with amphibious ready groups (ARGs; amphibious assault ships providing troop transport of Marines) as members of embarked fleet surgical teams (FSTs). A successful pilot starting in 2013 (e.g., decrease in unplanned losses for mental health reasons; increased retention of sailors) resulted in the expansion of the program in 2016 to include the permanent assignment of active-duty mental health providers in every submarine homeport. In 2018, Naval Surface Forces added 33 new EMH billets to provide increased mental health support directly at the waterfront in support of surface combatant ships. As of early 2020, approximately 29% of Navy mental health active-duty officer billets and 21% of enlisted BHT billets were embedded billets. This percentage is expected to increase as more Navy and Marine Corps operational commands gain EMH assets.

The U.S. Army's EMH model (EBH) has two core elements: the behavioral health officer (BHO; the part of the team that is directly embedded with the deployable unit) and the Embedded Behavioral Health Team (EBHT) (unique to the Army model). The BHO is a uniformed psychologist or social worker assigned to a brigade-sized line unit (approximately 3,500–4,500 soldiers). The BHO concept arose in an effort to ensure that deployable combat units in the Army had access to organic mental health support, similar to how these units have medical support from organic physicians. Mental health providers were assigned at the division level and eventually to the brigade level as demand increased for their services and brigades became the primary deployable unit in the Army. BHOs originally were assigned to the combat arms brigades (i.e., infantry, Stryker, and armor) but have recently expanded to other brigade-sized elements, including units of engineers, field artillery, signal, aviation, support, and military police, due to the positive response of line commanders to having an organic behavioral health asset in their formation. The Army EBHT is a civilian interdisciplinary team that consists of therapists and one prescriber who belong to the MTF, but are allocated to provide services for a specific brigade-sized element. The Army had success with the development of its first EBHT at Fort Carson, Colorado, when in 2009 they began working to make behavioral health care more accessible to the brigade combat teams. "The program improved access to care, improved continuity of care, enhanced BH provider communication with commanders, decreased inpatient hospitalizations, decreased referrals to the TRICARE network for behavioral healthcare and garnered high rates of commander and Soldier satisfaction" (Department of the Army, 2011, p. 1). The program has expanded and is now the norm across the Army. Typically, these clinics are located in an area of the installation where that unit is also located (the unit's "footprint") to reduce barriers to accessing care. Furthermore, the concept aligns each psychologist or social worker with a specific battalion (approximately 400–700 soldiers) within the brigade. Each provider's schedule has dedicated time for command outreach and prevention activities.

The Army BHO and EBHT work closely together to provide the full range of behavioral health support to their assigned unit. While both the BHO and EBHT serve the same population, only the BHO is truly embedded as a member of the unit and will have the opportunity to deploy with his or her assigned unit. However, the EBHT is expected to develop a high degree of cultural competence and strong relationships with the unit. The EBH model is a hybrid where MTF assets acknowledge the value in aligning with the line commanders' mission and supporting it by engaging in some nonclinical tasks (U.S. Army Medical Command, 2014).

Development of EMH in the U.S. Air Force occurred later than in the other services. Beginning in 2012, EMH supports were assigned to units that perform high-risk, high-impact operational missions. This included mental health and other specialists assigned to special operations units under the Preservation of Force and Family (POTFF) initiative. Also, in response to the growth of units able to execute combat missions from home station, Airman Resiliency Teams (ART) of mental, medical, and religious support providers were assigned to remotely piloted aircraft (RPA) and intelligence, surveillance, and reconnaissance (ISR) units that conduct real-time remote attack operations (i.e., execute air strikes from drone aircraft). The addition of ART was due to challenges and barriers to normal supports specific to these units (e.g., classified nature of work, 24/7 operations, perpetual combat engagement rather than time-limited by deployment cycle), the high rates of stress and human factors' challenges experienced in these units (see. e.g., Langley, 2012), as well as the high risk and high impact that human factors' errors can have in remote warfare. As a result of the positive impacts of POTFF, ART, and other pilot EMH programs, the Air Force is expanding embedded mental and medical teams to conventional forces units under the overall term integrated operational support (IOS), and is developing policies and training to support success (Office of the Secretary of the Air Force, 2020; USAF IOS Mental Health Practice Guide, 2020).

WHY EMH SERVICES?

In 2007, the Department of Defense (DoD) Task Force on Mental Health urged the military services to embed organic mental health professionals in line units due to service members' lack of familiarity with, or trust of, mental health supports. The goal was to have an "approachable resource for SMs and command, and provide a full range of preventative intervention services that build resilience, improve recovery and enhance the unit's mission" (DoD Task Force on Mental Health, 2007, p. 17). This finding represented a cultural shift toward providers who are not simply present, but are integrated within their units' culture. In 2009, the Army Mental Health Advisory Team (MHAT) found several barriers to mental health care, including the following: Often, soldiers did not know who their behavioral health asset was, they had difficulty accessing care and simultaneously maintaining confidentiality, and they were concerned about trust and rapport outside of the unit. These findings led to the recommendation that the number of BHOs per brigade be increased to two (Office of the Command Surgeon, U.S. Forces Afghanistan, and Office of the Surgeon General, United States Army Medical Command, 2009; Russell et al., 2014; U.S. Army Public Health Center, 2015).

COMMON ROLES AND ACTIVITIES OF EMH

EMH provides a range of mental health supportive services to unit members and leaders (NCCOSC, 2020). Indeed, the *raison d'être* for being embedded is to build unit knowledge and relationships that allow members and leaders rapid access to leverage mental health expertise in support of health and mission readiness. Although the allure of the embedded and expeditionary contexts often extends beyond the more traditional competencies of clinical assessment and intervention, these skill sets remain at the core of what psychologists must be able to provide in an embedded assignment or expeditionary environment. Additional competencies in a variety of consultation, prevention, and intervention skills, the ability to effectively supervise paraprofessionals, a firm grasp of the culture of the individual unit and their mission, alongside the solid ethical reasoning skills to navigate this complex system are often considered to be what sets the EMH provider apart from a traditional MTF provider.

Outreach/Unit Engagement Activities

One of the key elements of EMH is being seen, known, and trusted by unit members and leaders. This builds rapport and decreases the stigma for seeking mental health services. One of the best ways to gain this trust and familiarity is to get out of the clinic and into the unit spaces. This type of activity has many names, such as *walkabouts* or *unit circulation,* but the key component is to become integrated into the unit as much as possible. This activity can be as simple as walking about in work spaces and talking with service members. This time can also be an opportunity to share helpful psychological resources or tips, contact information for intervention options (such as where to locate the mental health clinic, Military Family Life Counselors [MFLC], Military OneSource, etc.), and give informal/desk side support to both service members and commanders. Consider the following example.

Case 10.1. The Typical Walkabout

The BHOs and behavioral health technician (BHT) went to the motor pool to conduct informal outreach (a so-called walkabout). Not long into their rounds, a company commander pulled the BHOs aside to consult on a soldier who was causing her some concern (he was having relationship problems and making vague statements about not wanting to go on). The company commander wanted to know her options for getting him help, both formally and informally. After educating the commander on the command-directed behavioral health evaluation process and talking through options, the commander said that she would talk with the soldier and get back to the BHOs with her decision. They confirmed that they had each other's cell phone numbers, and continued to move through the motor pool to talk with more soldiers. Meanwhile, the BHT encountered a specialist (SPC) working on his high mobility multipurpose wheeled vehicle (better known as a Humvee). The SPC noted not wanting to talk to any "shrinks" but asked for some tips on sleeping better. The BHT shared information about sleep hygiene and informed him of other resources if that didn't work. As they spoke, a small group grew around the BHT as the SPC wasn't the only soldier who could use some advice on better sleep. In a few minutes, another soldier mentioned difficulty with irritability; the BHT was also able to share some information about this.

Participating in unit activities such as physical training, range training, unit marches, and field exercises are effective ways to earn the respect of unit members and break down the stigma of mental health providers by being seen as "one of us." Engagement activities also help the provider gain insight into stressors faced by unit members as well as learn about the duties and responsibilities of the various occupational specialties in the unit, which is critical in helping the provider make informed fitness-for-duty determinations (see also Chapter 2, and Case 14.2, this volume). This deepened understanding of the duties and mission of the unit and its members, and also allowed EMH to provide care and other services that are contextually relevant and tailored to meet the needs of individual service members as well as the unit.

EMH personnel should participate in unit briefings, staff meetings, and officer calls. These provide information on important mission objectives, activities, and upcoming events, and allow opportunities to provide input when appropriate (e.g., relevant human factors or medical readiness concerns). Attendance at important unit social activities (e.g., unit gatherings, dining in/out, service birthday balls, Family Readiness Group (FRG) meetings, coffee socials, spouse socials) helps to build rapport and awareness of the EMH provider and services.

Prevention Activities

EMH providers leverage their skill set by conducting various resilience-building activities for the command. These activities include psychoeducation classes on common problems such as anger management, stress management, conflict resolution, self-care, peer/buddy aid, suicide aware-ness/prevention, and relationship problems. Some providers have been able to facilitate resilience programs, such as Operational Stress Control (e.g., Department of the Navy, 2016) and Master Resilience Training (e.g., Department of the Army, 2014). These psychoeducation classes can be con-ducted as requested, or as recurrent trainings, especially on deployment when the unit is free from garrison distractions. Some EMH personnel con-duct leadership seminars, emotional intelligence workshops, Psychological First Aid (PFA) skills trainings, book clubs, or even teach formal distance education college courses (e.g., introduction to psychology, abnormal psy-chology) during extended deployments. EMH providers extend their reach by teaching these resilience skills to other unit medical personnel, as well as chaplains and other religious ministries personnel. For a comprehensive discussion of prevention activities as it pertains to the prevention of serious military stress reactions, see Kennedy, 2020.

Disaster Mental Health

EMH personnel may be called on to provide unit-level crisis stabilization after a traumatic event (e.g., suicide, training accident; see also Chapter 11, this volume). For this reason, it is recommended that personnel have training in evidence-informed disaster mental health such as PFA (Brymer et al., 2006). In these situations, an EMH provider will advise unit-level leadership on additional support resources (e.g., chaplains, nonmedical counselors) that may be needed. The EMH provider can also liaison with these outside resources to coordinate the disaster response. Crisis interven-tions may include basic psychoeducation on topics such as common grief reactions, acute stress symptoms, and self-care. The provider is well posi-tioned with knowledge of the unit and any vulnerable service members, and can provide tailored interventions to these groups, such as smaller focus groups and consultation advice to unit leaders on how best to support indi-viduals (e.g., more frequent leader contact, peer support, or time off). The EMH provider is able to provide one-on-one individual counseling and is well positioned to provide follow-on care and support after other outside resources have left the unit.

Clinical Care

Similar to serving in a traditional mental health clinic in an MTF, most EMH providers spend some of their time providing clinical care for com-mon mental health diagnoses including adjustment disorders, depression, and anxiety. The amount of time spent in clinical work may vary depend-ing on the position the EMH provider holds, the local culture of the unit he or she serves, and the availability of other treatment resources in his or her location. For example, the Army requires BHOs to spend 50% of their time engaged in clinical activities (U.S. Army Medical Command, 2014). This clinical time includes providing direct patient care and may also include facilitation of ongoing care to unit members through consulting with civilian providers and serving as a liaison between the unit and the providers. Due to clinical needs and the availability of other treatment resources, some EMH providers may spend in excess of 40 hours per week engaged in patient care activities (e.g., shipboard providers while under way).

Clinical care while embedded is often limited in scope because of limited resources, including limited time and little support staffing (e.g., schedulers, medical support assistants, coders)—especially while expeditionary. It may also be limited by medical requirements such that higher risk (e.g., suicidal patients, family maltreatment) and/or the need for longer-term care can only be provided in the MTF. An essential skill EMH professionals must have, then, is to accurately triage a service member's presenting complaint and functional impairment to then provide the appropriate level of services to that individual (Ogle et al., 2019). It is critical to accurately determine if the need is for emergency or routine mental health treatment, as well as to assess for what may be handled in the embedded or expeditionary environment or what might be required to be handled elsewhere, such as a referral to a different treatment location or evacuation from an expeditionary location.

Clinical care in an embedded environment includes intake assessments, fitness-for-duty evaluations (see Chapter 2, this volume), and short-term problem-focused treatment. The treatment offered in the embedded setting may depend on whether it is being provided on deployment (expeditionary) or in garrison. For example, in a deployed setting, an EMH provider may have the time and flexibility in his or her schedule to provide traditional evidence-based psychotherapies such as prolonged exposure (PE), eye movement desensitization and reprocessing (EMDR), or cognitive processing therapy (CPT; for more on evidence-based treatment, see Chapter 4, this volume). For some providers, the opposite may be true on deployment, with higher demand and less access to full-scope mental health services requiring more focused, short-term interventions. The degree to which EMH providers are mobile and providing services across a geographically dispersed area also impacts the frequency with which they can conduct clinical care, and will need to be accounted for when deciding on what scope of clinical services they are able to provide.

Clinical Liaison/Care Coordination

In general, if a service member requires a higher level of care such as long-term outpatient therapy, intensive outpatient therapy, or inpatient treatment, he or she will need to be referred to the closest MTF for care. Under these circumstances, the EMH provider will place the referral to the MTF and provide a warm handoff. Although the MTF will take over the mental health care of these individuals, the EMH provider will continue to liaise with MTF providers if the service member continues to be assigned to the operational unit. This continued liaison is important to allow the EMH provider to consult with the service member's commanding officer (CO) as necessary.

Another example of an EMH provider making a referral includes the use of psychotropic medications. Referral to a primary-care provider or mental health prescriber may mean seeing an embedded physician assistant in the unit or seeing a hospital staff physician. Psychiatrists and prescribing psychologists deploying as part of forward operations (e.g., Navy fleet surgical teams, COSC detachments, etc.) may prescribe psychotropic medications commensurate with their scope of practice, although psychotropic medications in the formulary onboard a ship (or in another expeditionary environment) are limited. Complicating this issue is the fact that certain psychotropics may temporarily (e.g., within first 90 days of a new medication or with a dosage change) or permanently disqualify a service member from engaging in special duties (e.g., nuclear field duty) or deploying to certain geographic regions (e.g., Central Combatant Command Area of Responsibility or CENTCOM). Some expeditionary units may have organic medical assets such as physicians, physician assistants, or independent duty corpsman (Navy) whose scope of practice includes prescribing psychotropic medications.

Service members have access to numerous support resources other than EMH providers. These resources include other medical providers within their units, chaplains, and civilian nonmedical counseling (short-term, solution-focused counseling for common personal and family issues that do not warrant medical or behavioral health treatment) resources such as Military and Family Life Counselors (MFLCs) and counseling provided by Military OneSource (Trail et al., 2017). Part of the role of an EMH provider is to effectively call on these supportive resources to ensure access to levels of services that are appropriate to individual needs. Demand for clinical care often exceeds the capacity of one or two EMH providers, so these complementary programs and professionals play important roles in supporting line units. An EMH provider who has good working relationships with other support systems makes referrals and facilitates warm handoffs when appropriate. Similarly, if a service member decompensates to a level where one of these other resources cannot provide an appropriate level of support, if that individual has an established relationship with the EMH provider, the probability of an effective transfer of care increases significantly.

Consultation

Leader consultation is another activity core to the EMH mission to assist operational commanders in maintaining a ready and effective fighting force (Schendel & Kennedy, 2020). Topics of consultation range from recommendations regarding an individual to policy advice and/or organizational interventions that affect specific groups of service members or the whole unit. These types of consultations can be complex and multifaceted and require operational knowledge of the unique culture and mission of the unit, expertise in mental health treatment and processes in the military, and expertise as a consultant to organizations (see Tables 10.2 and 10.3 for recommendations on communicating with operational leaders). EMH providers are well suited to this role by virtue of their direct membership, or an ongoing and close working relationship, in the unit with which they are consulting. DoD guidance (DoD Instruction 6490.08) provides guidelines about what types of clinical information may be (or must be) released to unit officials, as well as who from the unit is authorized to receive this communication (usually those in command positions). The EMH provider must maintain appropriate patient protection and releases in support of service members and military mission requirements (see also Chapter 17, this volume).

Individual-Based Consultation

One of the most common consultation topics an embedded psychologist will address is providing recommendations to the unit related to an individual service member. An embedded provider may have primary knowledge of the individual in question from clinical work conducted directly with that service member. In other cases, the EMH provider may further consult with other treating providers, or conduct a review of medical record documentation, to inform his or her consultation with the unit. The majority of these consultations involve questions of risk and how the unit can implement risk mitigation strategies to protect the service member or others from potential harm (for a comprehensive discussion of suicide risk, see Chapter

---

TABLE 10.2. Best Practices for Communicating with Leadership

- Concise (Bottom line up front/BLUF)
- No psycho-babble; use clear language
- Communicate early and often on a service member's fitness for duty
- Provide actionable recommendations
- Timely communication of significant harm to self, others, or mission
- Remember military etiquette/proper protocol

TABLE 10.3. Best Practices for Gaining Command Buy-In

- Figure out what the unit's priorities are and find ways to help the commander do his or her job (leverage organizational skills to make an impact)
- Seek to enhance the unit's mission
- Develop a strategic partnership mentality
- Be present, be a team member (build social capital)
- Get out of your office (i.e., walkabouts)
- Participate in unit activities as much as possible
- Promote primary prevention/unit resilience
- Decrease mental health stigma by focusing on return to duty/preservation of the force
- Promote unit readiness through early identification

9, this volume). Common recommendations in these consultation sessions include restricting access to lethal means, limiting duty obligations, ensuring access to follow-up therapy services, providing increased support or supervision, or a combination of these and other creative strategies. The following case demonstrates an example of consultation with the command of an individual service member.

Case 10.2. *The Sailor with Marital Difficulties*

The Chief was concerned about one of his sailors who was having marital difficulties; he had uncharacteristically started to arrive late to work and his job performance had declined. He recommended to the sailor that he speak with the ship's psychologist. The sailor met with the psychologist, who then learned that his sleep had been deteriorating because the sailor was temporarily sleeping on an uncomfortable couch at a friend's house (when ships are in port, sailors do not live on their ship). This, in conjunction with the stress from the marital discord, were causing him significant problems. Following this session, the sailor provided written consent for the Chief and psychologist to talk. The psychologist recommended that the Chief give the sailor permission to sleep onboard the ship while he worked through his marital problems. The psychologist also connected the sailor to marital counseling at the Fleet and Family Service Center on base. The open communication between the psychologist and command, at the time the sailor's problems were initially noticed, allowed him to obtain appropriate resources, receive valuable support from his supervisor, and may have prevented an accident at work.

Issues such as the above are fairly typical and resources are generally easy to access. However, in expeditionary or deployed environments, the availability of other, formal psychological services and care (e.g., inpatient treatment) may be severely restricted. Especially in these cases, the use of unit resources is crucial to maintaining both individual health and readiness to complete the mission, and the provider often uses these resources to assist in meeting the clinical goals of a patient (e.g., reduce suicide risk) while limiting the impact to the overall mission. In some cases, the service member will necessarily be evacuated from theater.

In addition to suicide risk, EMH providers may also be called on to consult with unit officials regarding other clinical topics that fall within the limits of confidentiality. The majority of treatment information remains confidential unless excepted through HIPAA for military necessity (e.g., impact to mission) or as mandated by law or regulation. For example, service members who report domestic violence or illegal use of drugs must be reported to their leadership in order to engage in both risk mitigation and treatment services. These types of command consultation are often impromptu as they are triggered by specific circumstances or reports by the service member to a treating provider, but should be a part of the informed consent process with any new patient (see also Chapter 8, regarding confidentiality and sexual assault, and Chapter 17, regarding confidentiality in the military in general).

Group-Based Consultation

While many command consultations are triggered by specific events, in some cases EMH providers will engage in ongoing meetings to review specific or general topics related to mental health (e.g., Force Preservation Council, Human Factors Board, Command Resilience Team). Unit leaders may regularly hold meetings to discuss service members who require a higher level of command involvement, often referred to as *individuals of concern* or *at risk*. The designation of at risk may or may not be related to psychological well-being, but the presence of other at-risk indicators that rise to the level of command involvement (e.g., legal problems) warrants EMH providers' awareness to offer additional support or to provide information to treatment team members that may assist with a service member's care and risk mitigation. The level of disclosures available to the provider in these meetings may be reduced depending on who is in attendance, but at minimum these forums provide an opportunity to synchronize who the leadership is most concerned about with who the clinical staff is most concerned about.

As previously mentioned, one activity that makes EMH unique from MTF care is a focus on population health and primary prevention. Beyond care to individuals, EMH providers generally have the skill set to advise the CO on the psychological health of the entire unit. EMH providers conduct both informal and formal surveillance. Informally, they track trends in individual service members that may provide insight on a larger environmental problem (e.g., command climate). These data on trends, patterns, and clusters are invaluable to unit leadership, and psychologists are uniquely suited to gather, interpret, and present these data in terms that are useful to a nonmedical audience. For example, several patients from a small unit may reveal an underlying leadership problem in that unit. Other examples that may prove useful to unit commanders include the general morale and sentiment of the unit, patterns in relationships back home, and responses to work–rest cycles. Other formal surveillance can include pre- and post-deployment mental health screenings or meetings with service members for routine mental health checkups (e.g., Navy EMH providers in the Submarine Forces conduct routine "checkup, from the neck up"), or a unit needs assessment.

Psychological Testing

Psychological testing is an essential job requirement (e.g., aeromedical psychological evaluations, clearances for submarine duty, sniper school, security clearances, fitness for duty, etc.). However, there are challenges to purchasing, securely storing, and transporting materials, as well as relying on computerized testing software, in an austere environment or an area with information technology restrictions (e.g., shipboard). When providers are able to utilize testing, the batteries are often short with an emphasis on screening or answering a fairly narrow referral question, though some are necessarily rigorous. All embedded clinical psychologists should possess training in administration and interpretation of screening batteries, as well as comprehensive psychometric evaluations.

Performance Enhancement/Optimization

Performance optimization involves providing interventions and skills training drawn from sport psychology, industrial–organizational psychology, and organizational development areas to enhance the performance of unit members, teams, leaders, and the unit as a whole. Through use of these interventions, EMH providers are able to positively impact the effectiveness of unit members and the unit to better perform their operational missions. Examples include: mental skills training for pilots of high-performance aircraft (e.g., arousal control, visualization, performance self-talk), interventions to improve functioning and cohesion of a Special Operations team, leadership skills coaching, organizational development interventions, and human factors' consultation to mission planning. Performance optimization is distinct from EMH prevention and treatment in that the focus is on the enhancement of operational mission performance. These services are inherently nonclinical and therefore are not documented in a service member's medical record. It is notable that providers who undertake these functions must receive additional training and education, above and beyond that necessary to perform basic EMH functions. The following case provides an example of an intervention to enhance leadership skills.

Case 10.3. *Improving Team Effectiveness*

An Air Force Captain in an intelligence unit has been tasked with building a multispecialty team of analysts to provide rapid analyses and recommendations on potential targets for air strikes. The analysts' skill sets are very different (e.g., some review visual imagery; others analyze electronic signals/sounds; others conduct research), and each traditionally works individually or only with others within their specialty. The Captain requests the EMH psychologist's assistance to build an effective, interoperable team. The psychologist has all team members, team leaders, and the Captain educate the others on their background and specialty skills to promote mutual understanding and connectedness. They then complete self-assessment instruments on personality style, communication and work behavior preferences, followed by an interactive class on what the results may mean for working together as a team. Discussion includes understanding differences and ways to engage with others that may be most effective given members' personal styles. This is followed by group-based activities of team members working together to solve a problem or complete a complex task as a team, with debriefing and discussion on how personal and communication styles manifested in how the team worked together. The Captain and team leaders develop work-specific scenarios and exercises to practice together. The psychologist collaborates with team leaders and the Captain to provide debriefing and coaching to continue to enhance team interoperability, cohesion, and effectiveness. The team begins working together with improved communication and comfort to give and receive feedback with each other in order to collaboratively deliver the best team product.

Utilization of Behavioral Health Technicians/Specialists

Behavioral health technicians (BHTs) are enlisted service members and civilians who undergo extensive training and, in many cases, have considerable experience in MTF clinical care as well as operational and deployed environments (Psychological Health Center of Excellence [PHCoE], 2019). With appropriate supervision, training, and structure, BHTs extend an EMH provider's reach and greatly assist in accomplishing the broad mission and tasks of EMH. Beyond assisting providers with administrative tasks (e.g., scheduling, record keeping), BHTs support a wide range of clinical, consultation, and outreach services in support of the EMH mission, including, but not limited to, triage screenings, supporting intake evaluations, group psychoeducation, supplementing aspects of evidence-based psychotherapy, psychoeducational groups/presentations/training, outreach and prevention, care coordination, crisis intervention, and command consultation (PHCoE, 2019).

BHTs offer a unique perspective as enlisted personnel. They are able to use their peer status to help break down the mental health stigma in units by conducting frequent unit circulation. In addition, they are better able to obtain valuable unfiltered information (i.e., deckplate gouge) about the status of the unit that enlisted personnel may be reluctant to share with a mental health officer. Best practices for utilizing BHTs consists of using a paired-team model to incorporate BHTs into the workflow, ideally with at least one BHT for every EMH provider (PHCoE, 2019). When a BHT works side-by-side with the provider as they perform various tasks, optimal learning occurs through observation and role-modeling. Also, this model helps build the trust necessary for a provider to feel confident in the skills of the BHT.

Pre-deployment Services

EMH providers are often expected to deploy with their unit and, even if not deploying, will still have a key role in preparing the unit for deployment. They work closely with unit leadership and other members of the medical team to provide training, medical clearance, and education. Often, the EMH provider is also training for deployment with their unit. These training activities might include preparatory field exercises or shipboard underways. Trainings usually culminate with a validation exercise, where observers from other units watch the unit conduct mission essential tasks and rate their performance. In addition to being validated in key medical tasks (e.g., caring for simulated patients, facilitating medical evacuation), EMH providers have a real-world mission of providing clinical care and unit consultation during these events. The training serves to both bond the provider to his or her unit and to test that the provider is prepared for the type of work that he or she will be doing in an austere environment.

Medical prescreening and clearance are guided by policy for the theater of operations where the unit will be deploying as well as the unit commander's guidance (e.g., CENTCOM MOD15; United States Central Command Central [USCENTCOM], 2020), and an EMH provider plays an important role in this prescreening. Using these policies and their commander's intent as a guide, EMH providers will work with other medical personnel to provide mental health screening to service members who are scheduled to deploy. Each service member may have his or her medical record reviewed to ensure that the member's mental health history and needs are compatible with the deployed environment. In some cases, the EMH provider may recommend deploying a service member who is diagnosed with a disqualifying condition or who is taking a disqualifying medication if, in the provider's clinical judgment, he or she believes the individual is capable of deploying safely and successfully. In those cases, the EMH provider will work with the medical team to submit a waiver for adjudication by the senior medical officer of the theater of operations to determine if an exception to policy can be granted enabling that individual to deploy. Common considerations when determining deployability criteria include availability of mental health support (both psychotherapy and medication), host nation capabilities, the likely consequences of symptom return or exacerbation, possible medication side effects, the likely level of danger and stress in the operational environment, the specific duties performed by the service member, and the level of importance of the mission (i.e., training missions vs. combat missions may have different levels of acceptable risk in the eyes of the commander).

The deployment process itself can be stressful. Meetings, briefings, classes, extra paperwork, uncertainty, and last-minute changes are all very common experiences for both service members and providers. In an effort to bolster unit resilience, predeployment briefings or classes are often requested on various topics related to mental health. Educating deployers and their families about common stressors, effective coping, expectation management, and other topics is important to ensure the well-being of the force and family. Mobilizing other supportive resources such as the Family Readiness Group (FRG)/Key Spouses and other professional agencies such as Military OneSource, MFLCs, the Red Cross, and local community partners can be instrumental for both the home front and the deploying service member.

Despite meticulous prescreening and resilience training, it is not uncommon for mental health utilization to increase prior to deployment. Some individuals may request to remain behind and not deploy, while others may feign medical or mental illness in an effort to be disqualified from deployment. How these cases are handled varies greatly across services, units, and deployments. Regardless of the particular processes followed, EMH providers are encouraged to engage in thoughtful ethical decision making as they navigate potential conflicts between their two duties: to the unit and to the individual (see Chapter 17, this volume). In navigating these concerns, consultation with other professionals and mentors may be an important resource to access. It is important to remember that in many cases, EMH providers are not final decision makers but are instead advisors who recommend actions to commanders.

Even though nearly everyone in the unit may be deploying, ensuring that the service members who are not are taken care of is another responsibility of the EMH provider. These nondeployers are often called the *rear detachment* or *remain-behind element/unit*. This may mean coordinating with the local MTF, EBHT, or fellow EMH provider who is not deploying to ensure that those in the rear detachment have their needs met and are connected to care. Warm handoffs, case consultation, and frequent communication are necessary components to a smooth transition.

create and, as necessary, revise a self-care plan, focusing on physical, emotional, mental, spiritual, and social health.

Deployment self-care looks similar to what may happen at home, yet there are clear differences. Typical activities are available to some extent, such as exercising, reading, listening to music, watching movies, eating, and using video chat programs to interact with loved ones. However, many conveniences are missing on deployment. Food options may not be great, or may not adequately cater to dietary preferences. Work hours are long. The Internet can be slow (if available at all). Communication back home can be challenging based on time zone differences and connection issues that are common in austere environments. The lack of personal freedom and privacy are ever present. Features of home that we take for granted such as running water, hot water, electricity, and easily accessible restrooms may be luxuries on deployment. Deployments often feature environmental stressors, such as extreme temperatures, loud noise, cramped quarters, offensive smells, and severe weather. Walking is usually the primary mode of transportation, which can exacerbate the impacts of an unpleasant environment. Noncombat deployments or missions are often just as austere, or more so, and should not be discounted

Self-care in a deployed or expeditionary setting can be challenging for anyone, but may be even more challenging for female providers. Maintaining relationships and not feeling isolated are important, yet women are almost always in the minority. It's also not uncommon for women to report constantly feeling as if they are being observed or watched, like being in a glass bowl (Ritchie, 2001, p. 1036; Todd, 2008). Military regulations about fraternization and inappropriate relationships as officers and professionals may lead women to feel even more isolated as cross-gender interactions are at risk of being misperceived. Hence, women have to balance not isolating with constantly being aware of perceptions/misperceptions of the type of relationships they are maintaining with others. In addition, safety concerns and the requirements to have a battle buddy while traveling are emphasized for women, though this applies equally to men. Culturally, host nations may also view and treat women differently than is normative in the United States, which can add additional layers of consideration and complexity, including safety, to various activities. In summary, for women there is often the added stress and pressure of double standards, and constantly having to be aware of the risk of sexual assault and sexual harassment, which can take a toll on one's mental/emotional energy.

Even though deployment is often considered a stressful experience, albeit a rewarding one, there are some aspects of expeditionary work that may be simpler than life in garrison. Family and personal demands on your time are usually less intense while deployed. The near-singular focus on work obligations and the presence of support systems that provide food, cleaning, and laundry services help to mitigate stress.

While self-care is important for providers, it's also a skill set to teach to others. Research has found that self-care and health-promoting leadership are inversely related to issues like secondary traumatic stress (Penix, Kim, Wilk, & Adler, 2019). From a provider and leadership perspective, it's imperative to the team that EMH providers encourage other care providers (e.g., medical staff, chaplains) to engage in self-care. In an embedded position, the ability to impact and create change systemically sets the stage for organizational and cultural change that can have wide-reaching, positive impacts. Consider the following example.

Case 10.4. *The Chaplains in Need of Self-Care*

Approximately 6 months into a 9-month deployment, the BHO was asked to participate in a training for the chaplains. The chaplains were reporting a general level of stress and fatigue and requested training on self-care, with the intention of working together to build individual self-care plans. The chaplains engaged actively, sharing ideas specific to the unique and limited circumstances of the deployment. They easily recognized that while they were good at caring for others, they had been neglecting themselves. The training enabled the chaplains to implement strategies known to minimize deployment stress and vicarious traumas as well as help them model how to do the same for other soldiers.

CONCLUDING COMMENTS ABOUT SERVING IN AN EMERGING FIELD

Being assigned to an embedded or expeditionary mission takes providers out of their usual environments and networks that have well-established policies and practices that guide and reinforce behavior. EMH personnel work outside of these traditional medical settings, instead adapting and integrating into operational environments, and often facing novel situations, unavoidable multiple role relationships, and complex problems. Additionally, those serving in EMH positions tend to be more isolated from professional peers for consultation and problem solving new situations. These factors present situational and ethical challenges. It is critical that EMH personnel proactively take steps to support safe, ethical, and effective practice.

EMH providers can benefit from establishing a network of peers for consulting, learning, growing, and developing professionally. They should regularly engage with mental health professionals from both embedded and traditional mental health settings. Perhaps even more so when deployed, regardless of the time difference, it is important to call and consult with the rear operations, a friend/colleague or mentor in the same or an allied field. If a provider has access to the Internet, staying informed about research or taking advantage of online continuing education courses can maintain one's connection with the field of psychology as a whole. See Table 10.4 for additional recommendations.

TABLE 10.4. Developing as an EMH Professional

- Build network with EMH colleagues for consultation and support
- Rely on policy
- Find a mentor, be a mentor
- Maintain clinical currency and connections with MTF mental health community
- Rely on multiple contacts, cross-training, contingencies when unit members redeploy/are injured/killed

Serving in the emerging field of EMH presents opportunities for great impact and service to enhance units' operational performance as well as early prevention and treatment of mental health problems. As a field of practice, it is relatively small and young compared to traditional military mental health treatment settings. However, there is perhaps no better example than EMH of military medicine's primary mission to support operational readiness. Continuing development in policies, initial and continuation training, and other areas highlighted in this chapter are important steps for this growing community of practice.

REFERENCES

Brymer, M., Jacobs, A., Layne, C., Pynoos, R., Ruzek, J., Steinberg, et al. (2006). *Psychological First Aid, field operations guide* (2nd ed.). Washington, DC: National Center for PTSD. Retrieved from *www.nctsn.org/sites/default/files/resources//pfa_field_operations_guide.pdf*.

Department of the Army. (2011, November 17). *Army expanding successful embedded behavioral health program* [Press release].

Department of the Army. (2014, June 19). *Comprehensive soldier and family fitness* (Army Regulation 350-53). Washington, DC: Author

Department of Defense. (2011). *Command notification requirements to dispel stigma in providing mental health care to service members* (Department of Defense Instruction 6490.08). Washington, DC: Office of the Under Secretary of Defense for Personnel and Readiness.

Department of Defense. (2019, June 19). *Deployment health* (Department of Defense Instruction 6490.03). Washington, DC: Office of the Under Secretary of Defense for Personnel and Readiness.

Department of Defense Task Force on Mental Health. (2007). *An achievable vision: Report of the Department of Defense Task Force on Mental Health.* Falls Church, VA: Defense Health Board. Retrieved from *https://apps.dtic.mil/dtic/tr/fulltext/u2/a469411.pdf*.

Department of the Navy. (2016). *Combat and operational stress control* (MCTP 3-30E and NTTP 1-15M; revised version). Retrieved from *www.doctrine.usmc.mil*.

Johnson, W. B., Ralph, J., & Johnson, S. J. (2005). Managing multiple roles in embedded environments: The case of aircraft carrier psychology. *Professional Psychology: Research and Practice, 36,* 73–81.

Kennedy, C. H. (2012). Ethical dilemmas in clinical, operational, expeditionary, and combat environments. In C. H. Kennedy & E. A. Zillmer (Eds.). *Military psychology: Clinical and operational applications* (pp. 360–390). New York: Guilford Press.

Kennedy, C. H. (2020). *Military stress reactions: Rethinking trauma and PTSD.* New York: Guilford Press.

Langley, J. K. (2012, September). *Occupational burnout and retention of Air Force Distributed Common Ground System (DCGS) intelligence personnel.* Santa Monica, CA: RAND Corporation. Retrieved from *www.rand.org/content/dam/rand/pubs/rgs_dissertations/2012/RAND_RGSD306.pdf?gathStatIcon=true.*

Markway, B. (2014, March 16). Seven types of self-care activities for coping with stress. *Psychology Today.* Retrieved from *www.psychologytoday.com/blog/shyness-is-nice/201403/seven-types-self-care-activities-coping-stress.*

Moore, B. A., & Reger, G. M. (2007). Historical and contemporary perspectives of combat stress and the army combat stress control team. In C. R. Figley & W. P. Nash (Eds.), *Combat stress injury: Theory, research, and management* (pp. 161–181). Routledge Psychosocial Stress Series. New York: Routledge/Taylor & Francis Group.

Nash, W. P. (2006). *Operational Stress Control and Readiness (OSCAR): The United States Marine Corps initiative to deliver mental health services to operating forces.* Quantico, VA: Headquarters Marine Corps for Manpower and Reserve Affairs.

Naval Center for Combat & Operational Stress Control. (2020). *Embedded mental health guidebook: NECC: Coastal Riverine Force (CRF).* San Diego, CA: Author.

Office of the Command Surgeon, U.S. Forces Afghanistan, and Office of the Surgeon General, United States Army Medical Command. (2009, November 6). Mental *Health Advisory Team (MHAT-VI) report: Operation Enduring Freedom 2009 Afghanistan.* Retrieved from *https://armymedicine.health.mil/Reports.*

Office of the Secretary of the Air Force. (2020, October 13). *Flight and operational medicine program* (AFMAN 48-149). Washington, DC: Author.

Ogle, A. D., Rutland, J. B., Fedotova, A. V., Morrow, C., Barker, R., & Mason-Coyner, L. (2019). Initial job analysis of military embedded behavioral health services: Tasks and essential competencies, *Military Psychology, 31*(11), 1–12.

Penix, E. A., Kim, P. Y., Wilk, J. E., & Adler, A. B. (2019). Secondary traumatic stress in deployed healthcare staff. *Psychological Trauma: Theory, Research, Practice, and Policy, 11*(1), 1–9.

Pierce, K. E., Broderick, D., Johnston, S., & Holloway, K. J. (2020). Embedded mental health in the United States Marine Corps. *Military Medicine, 185*(9–10), e1499–e1505.

Psychological Health Center of Excellence. (2019). *Healthcare provider's practice guide for the utilization of behavioral health technicians (BHTs).* Retrieved from *www.pdhealth.mil/sites/default/files/images/docs/Provider%27s%20Practice%20Guide_4JUNE2019_508.pdf.*

RAND Corporation. (2020). *An evaluation of Task Force True North initiatives for the promotion of resilience and well-being within the Air Force.* Retrieved from *www.rand.org/pubs/research_reports/RR3190.html.*

Ritchie, E. (2001). Issues for military women in deployment: An overview. *Military Medicine, 166,* 10331037.

Russell, D. W., Whalen, R. J., Riviere, L. A., Clarke-Walper, K., Bliese, P. D., Keller, D. D., et al. (2014). Embedded behavioral health providers: An assessment with the Army National Guard. *Psychological Services, 11*(3), 265–272.

Schendel, C. L., & Kennedy, C. H. (2020). Consultation within the military setting. In C. A. Falender and E. P. Shafranske (Eds.), *Consultation in psychology: A competency-based approach* (pp. 301–318). Washington, DC: American Psychological Association.

Todd, S. (2008, June 1). "Babes in boyland." *Society of Air Force Psychologists Newsletter.*

Trail, T. E., Martin, L. T., Burgette, L. F., May, L. W. , Mahmud, A., Nanda, N., et al. (2017). *An evaluation of U.S. military non-medical counseling programs.* Santa Monica, CA: RAND Corporation. Retrieved from *www.rand. org/pubs/research_reports/RR1861.html.*

United States Central Command. (2020). *MOD Fifteen to USCENTCOM individual protection and individual-unit deployment policy.* Tampa, FL: Author.

U.S. Air Force, Office of the Air Force Director of Psychological Health. (2020). *Integrated operational support behavior health practice guide* [Unpublished document]. Falls Church, VA: Air Force Medical Readiness Agency.

U.S. Army Medical Command. (2014, August 17). *Embedded behavioral health operations anual* (OPORD 12–63, Embedded Behavioral Health Team Implementation). Fort Sam Houston, San Antonio, TX: Author.

U.S. Army Public Health Center. (2015, October). *Embedded behavioral health monitoring and surveillance within 22 Army Brigade combat teams July 2009 through September 2015* (Technical Report No. S.0022499–16). Aberdeen Proving Ground, MD: Author.

Military Applications
of Disaster Mental Health

Lyndse S. Anderson, Melisa S. Finley,
and Jessica Y. Combs

Disasters are considered events that have widespread and traumatic impact with the potential for significant loss and disruption for those affected. Formal definitions tend to vary; however, characteristics generally include "sudden onset, unpredictability, uncontrollability, huge magnitude of destruction, human loss and suffering greatly exceeding the coping capacity and resources of the affected community" (Math, Nirmala, Moirangthem, & Kumar, 2015, p. 263). Some estimates suggest that, on average, approximately 10% of the U.S. population will experience one or more major disasters in their lifetime (Goldstein et al., 2016). Military personnel are at high risk of being impacted by critical incidents or experiences that could be categorized as disasters given their unique roles and occupational demands in and outside of hazardous environments. Furthermore, service members may find themselves both directly affected by a crisis and acting as first responders. Given these anticipated occupational risks, military mental health providers continuously work to facilitate proactive psychoeducation, skill development, and resilience tools. In the event of a critical incident or disaster, early interventions aimed at reducing the potential for psychological casualty are provided to commands seeking to support their teams. This process largely mirrors other community and professional interventions used in response to disasters, collectively referred to as *disaster mental health* (DMH).

DMH was developed with the intent of preventing or reducing the long-term psychological impact of individuals both directly and indirectly

affected by disaster, regardless of the circumstances (i.e., natural, ecological, public health, etc.; Jacobs, Gray, Erickson, Gonzalez, & Quevillon, 2016; Halpern & Vermeulen, 2017). This active effort to anticipate psychological stressors and enhance resilience through proactive planning, training, and availability of resources has made the Department of Defense (DoD) an organizational model of executing responses aligned with disaster response (Wei et al., 2020; Nash & Watson, 2012). While there is some variance in training and implementation between each Service branch, the preparative tools and response models designed for critical stressors can be broadly categorized under the umbrella of DMH. Postdisaster military mental health roles may vary depending on the circumstance or operational need. Providers must be familiar with the broader theoretical foundations of DMH to ensure that regardless of the intervention delivered, it is rooted in the core principles that are supported by the field as a whole.

This chapter will provide military providers with an overview of core DMH concepts, trauma, current approaches in the military, and supported interventions. An overview of the differences and similarities seen across the tri-service mental health teams will be reviewed to include training, resource management, and field examples to aid as models of approaches to different scenarios, while maintaining the conceptual integrity of DMH approaches. This is not intended to be a comprehensive guide to DMH or replace necessary training, but rather, to demonstrate the value of DMH training among military mental health providers and available resources to enhance personal competence.

OVERVIEW OF DMH

Every year, disasters are the source of significant emotional, physical, and economic costs across the world (Goldstein et al., 2016). DMH encompasses a variety of interventions that occur both pre- and postdisaster aimed at reducing these costs with early roots in the studies of stress in the 1960s and 1970s (Yamashita, 2012). Distinctions are often made between natural (e.g., hurricane) and man-made (e.g., building collapse due to neglect) disasters, though these distinctions may be considered superficial to a degree as often disaster may occur as the result of some combination of both (Makwana, 2019). These distinctions are raised in part because of evidence that reactions and recovery may differ depending on what type of disaster is encountered (Math et al., 2015). In the case of man-made disasters, individuals can experience an increase in distress associated with the belief that the event could have been prevented. Natural or ecological disasters are notable for their tendency to rapidly overwhelm the resources of an entire community, creating a different source of distress and widespread barriers to resilience in the aftermath depending on an individual's proximity to these resource changes (Hamaoka et al., 2010; Morganstein & Ursano, 2020). Acts of intentional violence such as terrorism are typically differentiated as the most severe form of disaster in terms of mental health morbidity and are notable for responses divergent from other types of disaster (such as the desire to avenge), an important consideration for the military context (Math et al., 2015).

There are several unique elements that set DMH apart from typical mental health interventions. Disasters create rapidly evolving circumstances that may necessitate support in austere, dangerous, or unusual/ novel places. This requires flexibility and adaptation by professionals working in these settings as well as a high degree of self-awareness around one's own self-care needs through the taxing nature of caring for individuals through emergency circumstances (Halpern & Vermuelen, 2017). DMH also operates with an assumption of resilience and capability in survivors of a disaster (Brymer et al., 2006). This means that services are primarily directed toward otherwise healthy individuals who may not necessarily be seeking mental health assistance and will likely recover naturally from the challenges they encounter (Ford, Gusman, Friedman, Young, & Rusek, 1998), an important conceptual distinction from the clinical environment.

The environment in which DMH services are delivered typically lacks elements of control, predictability, or formality. Interventions aimed at addressing postdisaster stressors are often simple, but practical, interventions grounded within supported psychological principles. For example, providing survivors with blankets or water and assisting in directing them to a safe location while ensuring they have access to early and accurate information about the crisis may not seem like a mental health intervention; however, these actions are all associated with the psychological concept of safety and comfort (one of the eight core actions of Psychological First Aid [PFA]; see below), the most widely utilized early intervention in DMH; Brymer et al., 2006; Halpern & Vermuelen, 2017). The emphasis on practicality in early interventions can lead to the erroneous view of DMH as overly simple, with formal training or consultation regarded as being optional rather than required for the professionals delivering them. While traditional helping skills are valuable in DMH, they should not be considered sufficient or transferable without specialized training (Dailey & Lafauci Schutt, 2018).

Multiple elements are required to ensure efficacy in the provision of DMH. This includes predisaster planning and preparation, appropriately designed emergency response, conceptually sound interventions, and long-term referral infrastructure. DMH is typically viewed as a preventative and holistic mental health model that takes a "multidimensional community approach of health promotion, disaster prevention, preparedness, and mitigation" (Math et al., 2015, p. 261). Thus, DMH is not only the direct intervention, but also the planning and preparation prior to the disaster. It additionally encompasses the development of long-term infrastructure (referral networks) to support the remote aftermath for those who may go on to develop psychiatric conditions. Ford and colleagues (1998) address the importance of developing an organizational policy and team *before* disaster strikes to ensure that team members are identified and trained, that roles are established in the local and national response systems, and that "timely and phase-appropriate mental health services are provided to disaster survivors, families, workers, and organizations" (p. 3).

Providing any one of these elements without appropriate training and preparation could result in mishandling or even harm of the individuals being served. This includes the unintentional pathologizing of responses, inappropriate or overly invasive interventions, or lack of adequate resources for the most vulnerable individuals affected. A number of organizations such as the Red Cross, National Center for Post-Traumatic Stress Disorder and Child Traumatic Stress Network, and the American Psychological Society, have made training and resources in DMH both free and widely available (American Psychological Association, 2020), and competent and ethical practice is key (Flynn & Speier, 2014; Dailey & Lafauci Schutt, 2018).

ANTICIPATED RESPONSES VERSUS PSYCHOPATHOLOGY

A core element of DMH is the recognition of the natural resilience of individuals with the *expectation* that the majority of supported individuals served in postdisaster mental health are generally psychologically healthy individuals (Ford et al., 1998). One of the prevailing misconceptions about disaster is that a large majority of affected individuals will go on to develop posttraumatic stress disorder (PTSD). For example, a meta-analysis of studies reporting on the development of psychiatric disorders following a disaster found that the overall percentage of individuals experiencing PTSD postdisaster was 10% compared to 2% of nonexposed groups experiencing PTSD (Beaglehole et al., 2018). These rates are lower than previous meta-analyses that have historically reported a range of 20–25% but include delayed onset PTSD, less specific trauma exposure criteria, and typically do not include comparison groups (Utzon-Frank et al., 2014). Similar rates of PTSD, 9.1%, have been found among military personnel following near fatal operational mishaps (Berg, Grieger, & Spira, 2005). In this case, previous and subsequent life events played a seemingly more significant role in developing psychopathology than the singular disaster itself. This is consistent with other research suggesting that development of PTSD and other mental health disorders postdisaster is often due to a myriad of factors related to predisaster functioning and accessibility to postdisaster resources (Kennedy, 2020; Morganstein & Ursano, 2020).

Given that the majority of an impacted population is likely to experience only transient mental health phenomena, providers must learn to strike a balance between anticipating recovery and maintaining awareness of those likely to be most vulnerable to develop psychological sequelae. This is an important point to keep in mind when providing DMH services, particularly as those providing services are often clinical professionals with heightened awareness of dysfunction or pathology. A common way to conceptualize the distress individuals display during disaster is to classify it as a normal response to an abnormal circumstance (Ford et al., 1998). This conceptual frame is meant to reduce the potential for pathologizing anticipated and normative emotional and behavioral experiences that could be viewed as symptoms if not considered in the appropriate context and time frame. When providers are educated on the broad range of anticipated responses to a disaster, they are less likely to pathologize.

Potentially Traumatic Event, Resilience, and the Role of Pre-, Peri-, and Postdisaster Factors

Given the significant variation in long-term outcomes (Morganstein & Ursana, 2020), a disaster should be classified as a potentially traumatic event (PTE) for individuals impacted. A PTE is defined in the fifth edition of the *Diagnostic and Statistical Manual of Mental Disorders* (DSM-5) as "exposure to actual or threatened death, serious injury, or sexual violence" (American Psychiatric Association, 2013). In addition, a PTE is regarded as any experience that may result in feelings of terror, horror, helplessness, hopelessness, and/or perceived threat to safety or stability. Research has broadly demonstrated that most individuals impacted by a PTE are likely to exhibit a brief episode of subclinical symptoms in reaction to the event (Goldmann & Galea, 2014). Studies have consistently demonstrated that only a small percentage of individuals exhibit clinically significant symptoms or impairment characteristic of trauma-related stress disorders (Norris, Tracy, & Galea, 2008; Substance Abuse and Mental Health Services Administration [SAMHSA], 2014; Beaglehole et al., 2018). From a clinical treatment perspective, there are several paradigms to incorporate into conceptualization when supporting individuals impacted by PTEs, namely pre-, peri-, and postdisaster factors.

Predisaster factors are factors identified as existing before the event(s), either increasing or decreasing an individual's susceptibility for developing postdisaster symptomatology. These factors include: prior mental health difficulties, prior traumas, female gender, poor coping capacity, and being of middle age due to compounding life stressors and burdens associated with caring for others (Goldmann & Galea, 2013; Math et al., 2015). Mastery of effective coping skills prior to the event has been identified as a significant mitigating factor (SAMHSA, 2014). Peri-disaster factors define the potentially traumatizing event or disaster; that is, type of disaster, severity of event, duration of exposure, threat to life, death toll, loss of family members, and proximity to where the disaster occurred, and have been identified as the most predictive factor of postdisaster mental illness (Goldmann & Galea, 2014). Greater exposure has consistently served as the strongest predictor of increased risk. Postdisaster factors such as job loss, property damage, financial strain, marital stress, physical health conditions related to the disaster, and displacement additionally contribute to the potential for psychological casualty, particularly when there is a decrease in social support. Having early access to resources (i.e., medical, psychological, community, etc.) offers the greatest potential for mitigating these postdisaster casualties (Goldmann & Galea, 2014).

Anticipated Postdisaster Responses

The range of responses following a disaster considered normal fall on a broad continuum that includes emotional, physical, cognitive, and behavioral manifestations (see Table 11.1). Though potentially viewed as symptoms in a clinical context, even significant changes in functioning in the immediate aftermath of an event can be considered anticipated and normal. For example, hyperarousal or hypervigilance are common in individuals who have experienced trauma but are usually not followed by the development of PTSD (SAMHSA, 2014). Changes in behavior are often an extension of changes in biological and evolutionary response (i.e., expression/manifestation of anxiety, depression, and trauma expressed via avoidance, withdrawal, etc.) and may involve maladaptive attempts to achieve emotional regulation (SAMHSA, 2014). Cognitive changes often manifest as a result of an individual's just-world beliefs or core life assumptions being challenged or threatened through adverse events (SAMHSA, 2014). Individuals from various ethnic and cultural backgrounds have demonstrated increased likelihood to present for care to address physical symptoms in the wake of an adverse or traumatic event. Chief complaints in these cases typically include: sleep disturbances, gastrointestinal distress, cardiovascular abnormalities, neurological concerns, musculoskeletal complaints, respiratory difficulties, and dermatological disorders (SAMHSA, 2014).

Another paradigm to consider is the timing of an individual's response to the PTE, particularly the initial and delayed responses to the event. Conceptualizing postdisaster response in a temporal manner is an integral part of support formulation and monitoring for what could develop into symptoms over time. See Table 11.2 for potential delayed psychological responses.

TABLE 11.1. Potential Postdisaster Psychological Responses

Emotional	Physical	Cognitive	Behavioral
• Anger • Fear • Sadness • Sense of loss of control • Shame • Emotional dysregulation • Emotional numbing	• Sleep disturbance • Pervasive muscle tension • Being easily startled • Hyperarousal • Gastrointestinal distress • Cardiovascular abnormalities • Neurological concerns • Musculoskeletal complaints • Respiratory difficulties • Dermatological complaints	• Difficulties sustaining attention • Poor concentration • Increased cognitive errors	• High-risk behaviors • Self-injurious behaviors • Disordered eating • Compulsive behaviors such as gambling or overworking • Self-medicating

Note. Adapted from SAMHSA (2014).

Trauma-Related Disorders

Changes to psychological functioning during or after a disaster are categorized in phases marked as being acute or long-term (Math et al., 2015). Acute reactions are those that typically resolve within 3 months without explicit intervention. Several trauma treatment models conceptualize trauma as manifesting when the natural self-healing process is disrupted. Individuals with a disrupted self-healing process form the basis of the long-term manifestations when symptomology and negative impacts of major areas of functioning surpass 3 months (Math et al., 2015). In such cases, professional intervention and support may be indicated to facilitate recovery.

TABLE 11.2. Potential Postdisaster Responses: Initial, Severe, Delayed

Initial reactions	Severe responses	Delayed responses
• Exhaustion • Confusion • Sadness • Anxiety • Agitation • Emotional numbness • Dissociation • Physical arousal • Blunted affect	• Continuous distress without periods of relative calm or rest • Severe dissociation symptoms • Intense intrusive recollections that continue despite safety	• Persistent fatigue • Sleep disorders • Nightmares • Pervasive fear of recurrence • Anxiety focused on flashbacks • Depression • Avoidance of emotions, sensations, or activities that are associated with the trauma

Note. Adapted from SAMHSA (2014).

Individuals impacted by disaster may experience an acute stress reaction, a normal response to distress. Notably, the majority of individuals who experience acute stress reactions do not develop further impairment or PTSD (SAMHSA, 2014). However, disorders that may be seen in disaster-affected populations include adjustment disorders, acute stress disorder, PTSD, generalized anxiety disorder, major depressive disorder, somatic disorders, and substance misuse. When functioning in a mental health professional role in the wake of a disaster, it is pertinent that the disaster relief professional refrain from prematurely placing diagnostic labels on the individuals served. Per the National Child Traumatic Stress Network and National Center for PTSD (2006), pathologizing normal reactions does not serve the long-term well-being of individuals. Psychological screening aids in the identification of individuals with a more severe reaction, necessitating a higher level of care.

MILITARY DMH PROGRAMS

Acts of terrorism, combat action, or operational mishaps can create widespread exposure to traumatic and life-threatening events that have potential for direct psychological impact on service members (Nasky et al., 2009; Berg et al., 2005). While mitigated through training and preventative safety measures, operational casualties such as a downed aircraft, vehicle mishaps, or shipboard emergencies are risks inherent to military occupations, and DMH is a resource well suited for reducing the potential impact of these. What follows are some potential components of military DMH as well as delineation of the Services' different programs.

Psychoeduation

Psychoeducation in reference to stressful events typically includes information about common responses to stressful or traumatic events, a review of specific trauma-related disorders and their associated symptoms, suggestions for healthy coping strategies, and resources for seeking professional services. Psychoeducation is often included as a part of postdisaster interventions but can be delivered to individuals pretrauma, such as prior to a deployment, in an effort to prevent development of maladaptive stress reactions (Benedek & Elspeth, 2006). Psychoeducation is not a validated form of primary prevention or intervention for PTEs (Wessely et al., 2008; Skeffington, Rees, & Kane, 2013; Scholes, Turpin, & Mason, 2007; Turpin, Downs, & Mason, 2005). Hourani and colleagues (2011) concluded that "the strongest strategies to date appear to be those utilizing a combination of education, skills training, and stress reduction techniques to enhance resilience" (p. 729). Psychoeducation is an important component of all comprehensive intervention models.

Psychological Debriefing

Psychological debriefing has been used as a general term to describe various types of interventions that are delivered in the early or immediate aftermath of a traumatic event. Debriefing is typically a time-limited intervention following a crisis that encourages sharing about the trauma with the goal of preventing future psychological symptoms or problems (Bisson, McFarlane, Rose, Ruzek, & Watson, 2009). Psychological debriefing has proponents and opponents, given contradictory findings in the literature as to efficacy and potential harm (Howlett & Stein, 2016; Forneris et al., 2013; Rose, Bison, Churchill, & Wessely, 2002; Elhart, Dotson, & Smart, 2019). Because service members view briefings (inbriefs, after-action debriefs, outbriefs, etc.) as the norm and are accepting of them, there is a place for debriefings within military DMH; however, this must be done taking into consideration all of the available literature and the military culture. As with many topics, the use of psychological debriefing lacks strong empirical studies with the military population. See Kennedy (2020) for an in-depth review of psychological debriefing and below for use of debriefing in the Army's model.

Psychological First Aid

PFA is a DMH approach designed to provide intervention immediately following a traumatic incident in an effort to reduce initial distress and promote short- and long-term adaptive coping and functioning (Brymer et al., 2006). The PFA model is appropriate for individuals of all ages and cultural backgrounds. It is designed to be delivered in a flexible and culturally informed manner with adaptions to address working with specific populations, such as the homeless, those living in nursing homes, faith-based and community leaders, and public health workers (McCabe et al., 2011; Cullerton-Sen & Gerwitz, 2013; Brown & Hyer, 2008; Parker, Barnett, Everly, & Links, 2006; Mosley et al., 2008). PFA is also commonly used as a training component in military DMH programs and was adapted to help create combat and operational stress control first aid to provide intervention to military-specific personnel and military-specific traumatic events (Nash, Westphal, Watson, & Litz, 2010).

PFA can be delivered by mental health and other disaster response workers (Brymer et al., 2006) and includes eight core actions: specifically, contact and engagement, safety and comfort, stabilization, information gathering, practical assistance, connection with social support, information on coping, and linkage with collaborative services. The overall theme of these essential components is the provision of immediate support, information, and resources to those who initiate contact following a disaster or other traumatic incident. Experts across the DMH field have endorsed PFA as an essential component of providing mental health support following a traumatic event while noting the need for further research (Shultz & Forbes, 2014). While PFA is broadly supported as the preferred early intervention for postdisaster support, critics highlight that training programs have several shortcomings, such as lack of standardization, learning objectives that lack meaningful measurement, and lack of controlled evaluations measuring the effectiveness of PFA training (McCabe et al., 2014; Sijbrandij et al., 2020).

Air Force: DMH Program

The Air Force DMH Program (AFI 44-153, 2014) is considered a vital resource to all airmen and command teams in the behavioral health system. DMH teams are multidisciplinary and include at least the following members: DMH team chief, mental health personnel, religious support team, airmen and Family Readiness Center personnel, and community readiness consultant. Air Force DMH team members participate in quarterly trainings and exercises that cover such topics as burnout and secondary trauma, PFA, prevention, outreach, screening, triage, command consultation, ethical issues, needs assessment and surveillance, and education and referral services for individuals and groups. DMH teams are also trained to provide preventive preexposure preparation (PEP) to any group, unit, community, or individual that expects to encounter all-hazard incidents.[1]

Exercises are commonly utilized as a means to promote training of DMH team members and are typically facilitated at the wing and group command levels, involving all units across the base. During exercises, DMH teams are activated and role-play appropriate responses to incidents identified as part of the exercise. In addition to DMH teams participating as role-players in an exercise, alternate DMH team members are sometimes activated to stand by in the event there is a real-world incident or participants in the exercises have actual stress responses. For example, DMH team members may stand by during an active shooter exercise to support any personnel that may have a stress response, such as someone who becomes anxious due to a personal history/experience with a real-world active shooter incident. The following case example illustrates activation and implementation of an Air Force DMH team.

---

[1] Per AFI 44–153 (2014), an all-hazard incident is "any incident, natural, or manmade, serious enough to warrant action to protect the life, property, health, and safety of military members, dependents and civilians at risk, and minimize any disruptions to installation operations."

Case 11.1. The Car Accident

Two airmen and a sailor from the same unit were involved in a motor vehicle accident resulting in the deaths of the sailor and one of the airmen. One of the service members was driving a car and collided with the other two members who were on a motorcycle. All three were a part of an emergency response unit and, as a result, other members of their team were the first responders at the scene of the accident, resulting in the first responders witnessing the deaths of their friends and coworkers and being unable to save them. The unit commander requested DMH team support. Two different teams were activated in order to be present at two separate unit shifts. At the commander's call, DMH teams informed unit members of available services and resources and how to access them, and then conducted walkabouts[2] within the unit to provide general support to personnel, assess for any specific unit needs, and provide PFA. The majority of the members of this unit were between the ages of 18–25, and they exhibited a wide range of grief responses, particularly those who were a part of the team responding to the accident. A primary role of DMH team members was to be available to the units and their commanders for consultation and needs assessments in the weeks and months following the incident given that this response was largely grief-related. Seven members of the unit requested longer-term services, to include the surviving airman. Unit leadership sought out services for support as they managed the loss of their troops and tried to support the families and friends of the deceased.

Army: Traumatic Event Management

The Army's Traumatic Event Management (TEM) Program incorporates holistic approaches and support activities that are conducted before, during, and after a PTE to assist units. TEM aims to foster resilience and restore or enhance unit cohesion. TEM support is made up of both group and individual activities. Consultation and collaboration with identified leaders or key personnel are pertinent as TEM facilitators formulate the support plan of action, assess and ensure that basic needs are met (i.e., safety/security, food, water, clothing, sleep, communication, protection from ongoing threats, etc.), manage acute symptoms, monitor, and provide continued follow-up care (if needed). When the opportunity is afforded, before a PTE occurs, TEM facilitators work to develop relationships with

---

[2]Walkabouts are literally the act of a member of the team walking around the various work spaces of a unit in order to get a "pulse" of the unit as well as give individuals an opportunity to talk and pose questions that they might not otherwise ask in a group format. Walkabouts are commonly used in the military to establish rapport and allow service members to consult with a mental health provider without having to make a formal appointment to do so.

key personnel and define what constitutes a PTE. Facilitators guide the development of TEM standard operating procedures (SOPs) to encapsulate information resulting from the discussions. SOPs include what leadership actions to take after a PTE, and the identification and plan of activation for available resources.

In the wake of a PTE, TEM facilitators make an immediate assessment of support capability against time available and trained resources on hand. Initial assessments include determining the ability to function in the current environment and the magnitude and potential impact of stress reactions. Facilitators coordinate stabilization services as needed while instilling hope through the six R's: Reassuring normality, Rest, Replenish bodily needs, Restoring confidence, Remind of purpose, and Return to duty. PFA is provided continuously during and after PTEs. Where appropriate, TEM facilitators are expected to refer identified soldiers for appropriate clinical assessment, diagnosis, and treatment. The hallmark intervention for TEM is the leader-led after-action debriefing. These debriefings occur in group format and are for individuals impacted by the PTE(s). The Walter Reed Army Institute of Research promotes two forms of debriefing: event- or time-driven psychological debriefing executed in six phases. Phases include: introduction phase, review of ground rules, the event review, the reactions phase, self and buddy aid review, concluding with the resilience focus phase. During the debrief, participants are provided with an opportunity to share their perception of the event, the group is educated on the range of predictable reactions (i.e., immediate stress reactions), the importance of self and buddy care, and available resources. TEM is often implemented in the wake of disasters of various forms. However, one limitation of this approach is the lack of scientific data to support its efficacy.

Case 11.2. The Helicopter Crash

An Army Behavioral Health Officer (BHO) and her behavioral health technician (BHT) were assigned to an austere location serving as the sole behavioral health assets in support of 3,500 personnel, including U.S. military, contractors, and coalition forces. They were asked to respond to a unit that had suffered a Blackhawk (helicopter) crash, resulting in the deaths of two soldiers. She and the BHT had been performing routine walkabouts and psychoeducational briefs fairly regularly so all personnel were already familiar with them. To prepare to address the critical incident, the BHO recruited the assistance of the base chaplain in planning and orchestrating support activities, and joined forces with the affected unit's primary BHO. A multifaceted multiday support plan was created. In the immediate aftermath, the team relied on PFA principles promoting the opportunity for rest, security, and stabilization. This also allowed for the unit to engage in its own collective grieving process. Several psychological debriefs for identified subgroups of the unit (i.e., based on duties, responsibilities, and relational proximity to the crash victims) were conducted. Over the course of 5 days, this team executed three debriefs and ongoing check-in/support services. One week after the event, the team was present for the memorial service. The unit redeployed (i.e., returned home) 2 weeks after the event as originally scheduled. Follow-up with the unit was conducted by its primary BHO upon return to the States and then individually as needed.

Navy: Special Psychiatric Rapid Intervention Team

The Navy's Special Psychiatric Rapid Intervention Team (SPRINT) was first developed at Naval Hospital Portsmouth between 1975 and 1978 to address psychiatric symptoms and adverse military outcomes for individuals involved in a series of ship collisions and other mishaps at sea (McCaughey, 1987). With conceptual framing modeled off the combat stress support strategies at the time (proximity, immediacy, and expectancy; see Kennedy, 2020), the first SPRINT mission was mobilized to support survivors of the U.S. Coast Guard's ship the USCGC *Cuyahoga*. The team provided debriefing and encouraged group cohesion among survivors. They also advocated for return to duty to facilitate crew members' access to structure and purpose in their daily lives (Carlton, 1979). At the time of development, SPRINT was not guided by specific DMH intervention methodology but was instead developed as a Navy-specific model for preparing a team to mobilize and engage with a command in a consultative manner, which included an intervention phase.

The Navy presently has two primary SPRINT teams divided between Naval Medical Forces Atlantic and Naval Medical Forces Pacific. These teams frequently work together to determine how a response will be activated, but in general, affected or requesting commands will be supported by the team associated with the region that command is operationally associated with. In the event of a disaster, mishap, or potentially traumatic event, any U.S. Navy or U.S. Marine Corps command can request support.

The SPRINT teams are made up of military mental health providers who have been trained in the SPRINT model, command consultation, and PFA. This frequently means the inclusion of members from a variety of professional backgrounds, including psychologists, psychiatrists, psychiatric nurse practitioners, social workers, chaplains, and psychiatric technicians. The current training approach includes a half-day didactic experience to provide the foundational principles of the response structure and an introduction to PFA. Participation in group-based training vignettes, observation as a trainee on a mission, participation as a core team member on a mission, and qualification to act as a team lead are also core components of preparation for those who will serve on SPRINT missions. Team members assigned to the regional SPRINT engage in ongoing continuing education on DMH topics, debriefing of past missions for continued lessons learned, and maintaining practices consistent with evolving literature in the DMH field.

Case 11.3. The Maintenance Mishap

During flight prep, a last-minute maintenance check resulted in the death of a young and popular maintainer when he walked into an active propeller on the flight deck. Fellow service members were on scene and acted as first responders. Due to the trauma, grief affecting the entire unit, and concerns about the overall mental health of the crew, a SPRINT team was requested by the leadership. The team provided an in-brief with the command's senior leadership, an all-hands brief to introduce the team to the squadron, small group meetings that included psychoeducation, walk-abouts in the unit, and individual contacts from service members seeking support. Ultimately, five sailors from the unit identified themselves as having long-standing psychological distress that had been exacerbated by the recent events, and this group was connected with the local clinic. While SPRINT services were an element of support, ultimately a strong focus on coming together, avoiding blame, and allowing a significant pause in operations to appropriately grieve and pay respect to their fellow service member were the most valuable efforts at promoting a healthy unit in the aftermath of such a loss. Strong leadership and existing high unit cohesion and morale, in addition to the early intervention, resulted in no negative outcomes for any members of the unit.

While each Service conducts slightly different programs, mental health providers from the Services are able to easily adapt and work together. Take the following example of a mass shooting that affected service members and civilians from all Services.

Case 11.4. The Mass Shooting

In response to a mass shooting event, a Navy SPRINT with augments from the Army and Air Force was activated for rapid psychological support for more than 6,000 individuals, including active-duty and civilian personnel from all Services. The depth of grief, fear, distrust, and trauma responses among the survivors was immense, with many struggling from shock over the senselessness of the loss. Given the wide range of individuals affected, the team recognized a significant number of unique needs and worked to scaffold community leaders with supportive tools, action plans, and messaging that enhanced access for all individuals. Given the highly visible and publicized nature of the event, misinformation and frequent exposure via media coverage increased distress among those directly affected. Frequent, transparent, and centralized communication from senior leadership became a critical means for combatting this development. The response lasted 7 days and included the efforts of psychologists, psychiatrists, licensed clinical social workers, BHTs, and chaplains from the Navy, Air Force, and Army. The team also interfaced with the Fleet and Family Service Center and providers from the Employee Assistance Program given the large number of civilians affected. Collaboration across the various Services' support entities ensured consistency in response and helped to maximize the availability of resources. Upon completion of the initial response, the local military hospital took over for long-term monitoring and access to formal services. The rapid tri-service formation of an effective and cohesive DMH team for this mission highlighted the value of training that is built on a broader field of study, rather than Service-specific terminology.

Combat and Operational Stress Control (Tri-Service)

A close relative of DMH is combat and operational stress control (COSC), defined as a variety of programs and actions directed by military leadership to prevent, identify, and manage adverse combat and operational stress reactions (COSRs) in military personnel in combat and demanding operational environments (as outlined in the *U.S. Army Field Manual* 4-02.51; Department of the Army, 2006). These principles are similar to those of DMH but specific to the industrial/operational environment of the military and built around the idea that stress reactions are likely to occur and require proactive management to maintain unit health (vs. a response to an unexpected disaster). COSRs are considered all physiological, behavioral, and emotional reactions experienced as a direct result of the dangers and mission demands associated with operations in or outside combat environments, including participation in humanitarian and peacekeeping operations. COSC provides expeditionary support to commanders across the deployment and mission cycle through consultation, education, training, and prevention efforts. It aims to enhance mission performance, increase individual and unit resilience, conserve the fighting strength, and return service members to duty. This mission is executed through the enhancement of adaptive stress reactions, which in turn reduces the potential for COSRs to transform into behavioral health (BH) disorders.

A COSR is not a mental health diagnosis or disorder. As service members conduct their deployed missions, there is the possibility of experiencing a PTE. COSC interventions include nine functional areas of service: Unit Needs Assessment (UNA), consultation and education, triage, stabilization, TEM, BH treatment, restoration, reconditioning, and reconstitution support. These interventions incorporate fundamental PFA techniques tailored to mission, operational, and individual needs. Every Service branch in the DoD has a version of the COSC program. Having a framework that is widely distributed across the Services aids in creating shared language and interventions during joint Service responses.

COVID-19

As a real-time example of the utility of DMH, the COVID-19 pandemic has challenged us all. The world is currently grappling with one of the largest public health disasters in modern history, with U.S. deaths from COVID-19 having neared approximately 1,000,000 at the beginning of 2022 based on available estimation tools (*healthdata.org*). One study by Gobbi et al. (2020) reported that at least 50% of mental health patients surveyed worldwide reported an increase in preexisting psychiatric conditions during the COVID-19 pandemic. Similarly, providers surveyed frequently reported new symptoms in established patients and the need to update or change treatment course specifically as a result of pandemic-related stress (Gobbi et al., 2020). Other studies suggest that the COVID-19 pandemic may take the greatest psychological toll among those who did not have diagnosed disorders prior to the pandemic but have since come to report a significant increase in symptoms of anxiety and depression (Pan et al., 2020). The COVID-19 pandemic has additionally placed an unprecedented emotional strain on health care workers, and military mental health providers have deployed as a part of field hospitals and on hospital ships to support staff and patients.

Disaster preparedness models typically teach interventions planned around the beginning and end phases of a disaster, how to regroup during "blue sky" periods in preparation for the next wave of impact or hazard, how to increase coping behaviors, and how to focus on connection and companionship (Morganstein & Flynn, 2020). In the case of the COVID-19 pandemic, the shear length of the impact period of the disaster has only compounded the strain on individuals who may not be able to engage in typical coping practices and might be struggling through the social isolation required by quarantine periods and general viral transmission mitigation. Furthermore, the large majority of DMH interventions have been designed for in-person delivery. In the case of the COVID-19 pandemic, the risk and cost of disease transmission has had to be weighed against the value of in-person intervention.

Despite these challenges, DMH principles have remained relevant, imperative, and adaptable, demonstrating the importance of a conceptual framework rather than a singular intervention approach. Disaster organizations quickly rallied to provide resources that could be adapted for use specifically in environments limited by pandemic barriers. The International Federation of Red Cross (IFRC) and Red Crescent Societies published a guide for the provision of remote PFA and organizations such as the World Health Organization (WHO), Centers for Disease Control (CDC),

Substance Abuse and Mental Health Services Administration (SAMHSA), and many more produced infographics on healthy coping practices to manage anticipated stressors for mass distribution to the public (IFRC Psychosocial Support, 2020; WHO, 2020; CDC, 2020).

As conditions in the civilian health care sector worsened and health care workers experienced increasing loss and traumatic exposure from COVID-19, some civilian administrators turned to the military's combat stress management principles as a model to enhance resilience resources among their own medical teams (Wei et al., 2020). New York City and the Greater New York Public Health systems partnered with the DoD, U.S. Department of Veterans Affairs, and Uniformed Services University to create the Healing, Education, Resilience, and Opportunity (HERO-NY) initiative, which adapted DoD behavioral health curricula from the COSC program into a training model that could be deployed throughout their hospitals to reach as many frontline workers as possible and bring lasting change in the mental health resources provided to hospital staff during crises (Wei et al., 2020). COSC and DMH principles similarly aided providers at Naval Medical Center San Diego in rapidly establishing the Resiliency Support Team (ReST; Balboa Resiliency Support Team, 2020). This team developed a comprehensive plan to support health care workers in their hospital system through widespread and practical resource distribution, increased availability of mental health services specifically for frontline workers, daily meditation groups (offered remotely), a peer support program, and a publicly available website with coping resources, psychoeducational videos, and links to updates on the pandemic at both the local and national level.

National coverage of the COVID-19 outbreak on the *USS Theodore Roosevelt* demonstrated the first mass quarantine procedure implemented to mitigate a shipboard COVID-19 outbreak and ensure large unit health and military readiness (Malone, 2020). This additionally resulted in the first implementation of remote PFA by a Navy SPRINT. With thousands of individuals ushered into isolation, Naval Medical Forces Pacific deployed a SPRINT to augment the collective military resources mobilized in support of the crew (Sobocinski, 2020). This mission created a framework for supporting the many naval commands that required quarantine periods as part of their predeployment mitigation strategies prior to widespread vaccine access. These interventions incorporated both the broad principles of DMH and the military-specific frameworks of COSC applied in response to a public health stressor creating entirely novel stressors associated with operational planning.

COMMAND CONSULTATION

A critical element for military DMH is the role of consultant to the command (Milligan, Delaney, & Klam, 2016). When assistance is requested, commands expect to gain a team of experts who can assess the unique needs of their units and plan interventions accordingly. They also expect to gain information and recommendations from the team that can aid in the long-term support and recovery of their units even after the team has departed (Milligan et al., 2016). In the consultant role, providers integrate observations from their time with service members into feedback that is both empirically informed and helpful to military leadership. For example, unit cohesion is a known protective factor among service members who have endured traumatic exposure (Campbell-Sills et al., 2020; Kennedy, 2020). This is similarly aligned with the PFA aims of enhancing social connectedness as a means of resilience and disaster recovery (Halpern & Vermeulen, 2017). If a team recognizes that a military unit has significant morale issues or identifiable division among personnel that are creating barriers to connectedness, these areas might become a longer-term focus for leadership to support resilience.

Other areas that can be valuable to leadership include education on normal reactions to trauma, how to maximize use of available resources, maintaining awareness over those that may be most vulnerable in their units, and tools for enhancing resilience postdisaster. Experiencing a significant event characterized as a disaster does not guarantee a negative response trajectory by the individual(s) impacted, but initial reactions may seem symptomatic in some cases if not properly understood or characterized. This can lead to well-intended military leadership that is likely to be less familiar with what a normal stress reaction looks like, requesting more intrusive intervention than what is clinically or conceptually indicated. This is typically done out of an understandable desire to gain some control over an overwhelming circumstance or ensure that their people feel cared for and supported. It is imperative that military professionals responding to these events maintain awareness over anticipated responses and translate that into readily accessible information for military leaders. Translating the normal response and offering professional perspective on the appropriate level of intervention can ensure that leadership maintains a sense of responsiveness and engagement throughout the disaster without overreacting with what might be a counterproductive measure (e.g., command-directed evaluation).

Military personnel are typically well prepared for stressful scenarios in general; however, those with prior or subsequent life events that compound trauma or place strain on their coping abilities may be more vulnerable to lasting effects from a PTE (Berg et al., 2005; see Kennedy, 2020, for a full explanation of risk factors for stress reactions). Similarly, while it is well established that the majority of a population is unlikely to develop long-term psychiatric disorders as the result of a single disaster, the sum is not zero nor is it limited to PTSD. Concerns that are often overlooked but can develop as a result of disaster are substance use, suicidality, depression, and anxiety (Beaglehole et al., 2018; Kennedy, 2020), all of which pose a potential impact to military readiness if not addressed early on. In addition to preventative measures in the form of postdisaster early intervention, providers can support military leadership through education on the risks and early warning signs associated with psychiatric disorders. These can also serve as opportunities to discuss how to most effectively provide resources despite barriers such as stigma. For instance, reports of depression, PTSD, suicidal ideation, and interest in receiving care were 2 to 4 times higher among soldiers completing anonymous surveys versus a routine postdeployment health assessment (Warner et al., 2011). These types of data points, while derived from deployment research, can help to shape postdisaster resource distribution in a command that encourages the highest likelihood of use for those who need it.

A mental health consultant similarly assists commands in identifying available and appropriate resources. Teams connect with local mental health assets to ensure awareness of a possible influx in referrals for care, confirm the referral process, gather contact information, and include any pertinent information on accessing services that can be distributed directly to affected service members. Free and confidential resources such as Military OneSource (*militaryonesource.mil*) may be of particular importance in communities that are concerned about the impact of mental health care on their duty status or for whom local resources may be limited. As previously reviewed, military and partner organizations invest a high degree of resources and funding into the development of programs contributing to resilience development among service members (Bowles & Bates, 2010). These types of resources, when deemed appropriate for a given scenario, can be added to a command's plans for longer-term service member support. In the case of limited resources in austere or restricted environments, a DMH team will work to find creative ways to encourage lasting application of helpful coping practices that can continue after their departure (Milligan et al., 2016).

SUMMARY AND CONCLUSION

Military members represent a group of highly resilient and committed individuals who are regularly subject to high-stress scenarios that may benefit from a combination of pre- and post-event interventions informed by DMH. Military mental health providers may be called on to provide DMH support to a command regardless of their formal role or title. Actively seeking to expand one's knowledge on the broader concepts of DMH through specialized training and continuing education will prepare military providers to offer effective, individualized, and conceptually informed intervention when appropriate. Even in the case of limited prior DMH experience, utilization of consultation, free professional resources, and "just-in-time" training can significantly improve knowledge and skills for providers called to emergent scenarios requiring immediate response (Benedek & Elspeth, 2006; Reeves, 2002).

Despite continued criticism regarding the limitations in empirical validation of DMH interventions, data continue to improve knowledge of which interventions are best supported by existing research and which are contraindicated. In the case of early interventions recommended for use during DMH responses, PFA has emerged with the greatest support for large-scale training and utilization across a variety of contexts. As a result, while training approaches and DMH programs vary between civilian and military entities as well as military branches, core concepts and training content have evolved into a generally consistent message, thus allowing for quick integration of resources during crisis. DMH principles prove highly adaptable in part due to reliance on informed concept, rather than pre-scribed interventions.

Historical examples of mental health responses from a variety of different disasters (natural, health-related, man-made, etc.) across both military and civilian settings in the form of case studies, vignettes, and other educational resources serve as helpful learning tools to demonstrate adaptations that may be required and helpful across various circumstances. With broad applications to military readiness, DMH should be considered a foundational skill set among all mental health professionals working with the military. As military medical infrastructure moves toward integration of the tri-services under the Defense Health Agency, there may be additional value in establishing DMH training and resources that further serve the mission of rapid integration and consistency of services during emergency response.

REFERENCES

American Psychiatric Association. (2013). *Diagnostic and statistical manual of mental disorders* (5th ed.). Arlington, VA: Author.

American Psychological Associations. (2020). *APA's disaster mental health history*. Retrieved from *www.apa.org/practice/programs/dmhi/history*.

Balboa Resiliency Support Team (ReST). (2020). Retrieved from *https://balboar-est.com*.

Beaglehole, B., Mulder, R. T., Frampton, C. M., Boden, J. M., Newton-Howes, G., & Bell, C. J. (2018). Psychological distress and psychiatric disorder after natural disasters: Systematic review and meta-analysis. *British Journal of Psychiatry, 213*(6), 716–722.

Benedek, D. M., & Elspeth, C. R. (2006). "Just-in-time" mental health training and surveillance for the project HOPE mission. *Military Medicine, 171*(10), 63–65. Retrieved from *https://fgul.idm.oclc.org/scholarly-journals/just-time-mental-health-training-surveillance/docview/217069198/se-2?accountid=10868*.

Berg, J. S., Grieger, T. A., & Spira, J. L. (2005). Psychiatric symptoms and cognitive appraisal following the near sinking of a research submarine. *Military Medicine, 170*(1), 44–47. Retrieved from *https://fgul.idm.oclc.org/scholarly-journals/psychiatric-symptoms-cognitive-appraisal/docview/217060797/se-2?accountid=10868.*

Bisson, J. I., McFarlane, A. C., Rose, S., Ruzek, J. I., & Watson, P. J. (2009). Psychological debriefing for adults. *Effective Treatments for PTSD: Practice Guidelines from the International Society for Traumatic Stress Studies, 2,* 83–105.

Bowles, S. V., & Bates, M. J. (2010). Military organizations and programs contributing to resilience building. *Military Medicine, 175*(6), 382–385.

Brown, L. M., & Hyer, K. (2008). *Psychological first aid: Field Operations guide for nursing homes.* Available at *http://amh.fmhi.usf.edu/pfanh.pdf.*

Brymer, M., Layne, C., Jacobs, A., Pynoos, R., Ruzek, J., Steinberg, A., et al. (2006). *Psychological first aid field operations guide* (2nd ed.). Washington, DC: National Center for PTSD and National Child Traumatic Stress Network. Retrieved June 1, 2020, from *www.nctsn.org/content/psychological-first-aid.*

Campbell-Sills, L., Flynn, P. J., Choi, K. W., Ng, T., Aliaga, P. A., Broshek, C., et al. (2020). Unit cohesion during deployment and post-deployment mental health: Is cohesion an individual- or unit-level buffer for combat-exposed soldiers? *Psychological Medicine,* 1–11.

Carlton, T. G. (1979). SPRINT: A psychiatric contingency response team in action. *U.S. Navy Medicine, 70.*

Centers for Disease Control and Prevention. (2020, March 28). *COVID-19 cases, deaths, and trends in the US: CDC COVID data tracker.* Retrieved from *https://covid.cdc.gov/covid-data-tracker/#cases_casesper100klast7days.*

Cullerton-Sen, C., & Gerwitz, A. (2013). Psychological First Aid for families experiencing homelessness. Minneapolis, MN: Ambit Network and the National Child Traumatic Stress Network. Retrieved from *www.trauma-informed-california.org/wp-content/uploads/2012/02/PFA_Families_homelessness.pdf.*

Dailey, S. F., & Lafauci Schutt, J. M. (2018, January). *Disaster mental health: Ethical issues for counselors.* Retrieved from *www.counseling.org/docs/default-source/ethics/ethics-columns/ethics_january_2018_disaster-mental-health.pdf?sfvrsn=ba25522c_4.*

Department of the Air Force. (2014). *Disaster mental health response and combat and operational stress control* (Department of Air Force Instruction 44-153). Arlington, VA: Author.

Department of the Army. (2006, July). *U.S. Army field manual: Combat and operational stress control* (4-02.51, FM8-51). Washington, DC: Author.

Elhart, M. A., Dotson, J., & Smart, D. (2019). Psychological debriefing of hospital emergency personnel: Review of critical incident stress debriefing. *International Journal of Nursing Student Scholarship, 6.*

Flynn, B.W., & Speier, A. H. (2014, August). Disaster behavioral health: Legal and ethical considerations in a rapidly changing field. *Current Psychiatry Reports, 16*(8), 457.

Ford, J. D., Gusman, F. D., Friedman, M. J., Young, B. H., & Ruzek, J. I. (1998).

Disaster mental health services: A guidebook for clinicians and administrators. Washington, DC: National Center for PTSD.

Forneris, C. A., Gartlehner, G., Brownley, K. A., Gaynes, B. N., Sonis, J., Coker-Schwimmer, E., et al. (2013). Interventions to prevent post-traumatic stress disorder: A systematic review. *American Journal of Preventive Medicine, 44*(6), 635–650.

Gobbi, S., Płomecka, M. B., Ashraf, Z., Radziński, P., Neckels, R., Lazzeri, S., et al. (2020). Worsening of preexisting psychiatric conditions during the COVID-19 pandemic. *Frontiers in Psychiatry, 11.*

Goldmann, E., & Galea, S. (2014). Mental health consequences of disasters. *Annual Review of Public Health, 35,* 169–183.

Goldstein, R. B., Smith, S. M., Chou, S. P., Saha, T. D., Jung, J., Zhang, H., et al. (2016). The epidemiology of DSM-5 posttraumatic stress disorder in the United States: Results from the National Epidemiologic Survey on Alcohol and Related Conditions-III. *Social Psychiatry and Psychiatric Epidemiology, 51*(8), 1137–1148.

Halpern, J., & Vermeulen, K. (2017). *Disaster mental health interventions: Core principles and practices.* New York: Routledge.

Hamaoka, D. A., Kilgore, J. A., Carlton, J., Benedek, D. M., & Ursano, R. J. (2010). Military and civilian disaster response and resilience: From gene to policy. *Military Medicine, 175*(Suppl. 7), 32–36.

Hourani, L. L., Council, C. L., Hubal, R. C., & Strange, L. B. (2011). Approaches to the primary prevention of posttraumatic stress disorder in the military: A review of the stress control literature. *Military Medicine, 176*(7), 721–730.

Howlett, J. R., & Stein, M. B. (2016). Prevention of trauma and stressor-related disorders: A review. *Neuropsychopharmacology, 41*(1), 357–369.

International Federation of Red Cross and Red Crescent Societies. (2020, March). Remote Psychological First Aid during a COVID-19 outbreak: Final guidance note. Retrieved from *https://pscentre.org/?resource=remote-psychological-first-aid-during-covid-19-may-2020.*

Jacobs, G. A., Gray, B. L., Erickson, S. E., Gonzalez, E. D., & Quevillon, R. P. (2016). Disaster mental health and community-based psychological first aid: Concepts and education/training. *Journal of Clinical Psychology, 72*(12), 1307–1317.

Kennedy, C. H. (2020). *Military stress reactions: Rethinking trauma and PTSD.* New York: Guilford Press.

Makwana N. (2019). Disaster and its impact on mental health: A narrative review. *Journal of Family Medicine and Primary Care, 8*(10), 3090–3095.

Malone, J. D. (2020). *USS Theodore Roosevelt,* COVID-19, and ships: Lessons learned. *JAMA Network Open, 3*(10), e2022095.

Math, S. B., Nirmala, M. C., Moirangthem, S., & Kumar, N. C. (2015). Disaster management: Mental health perspective. *Indian Journal of Psychological Medicine, 37*(3), 261–271.

McCabe, O. L., Everly, G. S., Brown, L. M., Wendelboe, A. M., Hamid, N. H. A., Tallchief, V. L., et al. (2014). Psychological First Aid: A consensus-derived, empirically supported, competency-based training model. *American Journal of Public Health, 104*(4), 621–628.

McCabe, O. L., Perry, C., Azur, M., Taylor, H. G., Bailey, M., & Links, J. M.

(2011). Psychological First-Aid training for paraprofessionals: A systems-based model for enhancing capacity of rural emergency responses. *Prehospital and Disaster Medicine, 26*(4), 251–258.

McCaughey, B. G. (1987). U.S. Navy Special Psychiatric Rapid Intervention Team (SPRINT). *Military Medicine, 152*(3), 133–135.

Milligan, J., Delaney, E. M., & Klam, W. P. (2016). Responding to trauma at sea: A case study in Psychological First Aid, unique occupational stressors, and resiliency self-care. *Military Medicine, 181*(11), e1692–e1695.

Morganstein, J., & Flynn, B. (2020). Supporting healthcare professionals in times of disaster: Reflections on "at-risk employees." *The Exchange.* Retrieved from *https://files.asprtracie.hhs.gov/documents/supporting-healthcare-professionals-in-times-of-disaster-at-risk-employees.pdf.*

Morganstein, J. C., & Ursano, R. J. (2020). Ecological disasters and mental health: Causes, consequences, and interventions. *Frontiers in Psychiatry, 11,* 1.

Mosley, A. M., McCabe, O. L., Everly Jr., G. S., Gwon, H. S., Kaminsky, M. J., Links, J. M., et al. (2008). The tower of ivory meets the house of worship: Psychological First Aid training for the faith community. *Call for Papers, 9*(3), 171–180.

Nash, W. P., & Watson, P. J. (2012). Review of VA/DOD clinical practice guideline on management of acute stress and interventions to prevent posttraumatic stress disorder. *Journal of Rehabilitation Research and Development, 49*(5), 637–648.

Nash, W. P., Westphal, R. J., Watson, P., & Litz, B. T. (2010). *Combat and operational stress first-aid: Caregiver training manual.* Washington, DC: Department of the Navy, Bureau of Medicine and Surgery

Nasky, K. M., Hines, N. N., & Simmer, E. (2009). The *USS Cole* bombing: Analysis of pre-existing factors as predictors for development of post-traumatic stress or depressive disorders. *Military Medicine, 174*(7), 689–694.

Norris, F. H., Tracy, M., & Galea, S. (2008). Looking for resilience: Understanding the longitudinal trajectories of responses to stress. *Social Science Medicine, 68*(2), 190–198.

Pan, K. Y., Kok, A., Eikelenboom, M., Horsfall, M., Hörg, F., Luteijn, R. A., et al. (2020). The mental health impact of the COVID-19 pandemic on people with and without depressive, anxiety, or obsessive–compulsive disorders: A longitudinal study of three Dutch case-control cohorts. *Lancet Psychiatry, 8*(2), 121–129.

Parker, C. L., Barnett, D. J., Everly Jr., G. S., & Links, J. M. (2006). Establishing evidence-informed core intervention competencies in psychological first aid for public health personnel. *International Journal of Emergency Mental Health, 8*(2), 83–-92.

Reeves, J. J. (2002). Perspectives on disaster mental health intervention from the *USNS Comfort. Military Medicine, 167*(9), 90–92.

Rose, S. C., Bisson, J., Churchill, R., & Wessely, S. (2002). Psychological debriefing for preventing posttraumatic stress disorder (PTSD). *Cochrane Database of Systematic Reviews, 2.*

Scholes, C., Turpin, G., & Mason, S. (2007). A randomised controlled trial to assess the effectiveness of providing self-help information to people with symptoms of acute stress disorder following a traumatic injury. *Behaviour Research and Therapy, 45*(11), 2527–2536.

Shultz, J. M., & Forbes, D. (2014). Psychological First Aid: Rapid proliferation and the search for evidence. *Disaster Health, 2*(1), 3–12.

Sijbrandij, M., Horn, R., Esliker, R., O'May, F., Reiffers, R., Ruttenberg, L., et al. (2020). The effect of Psychological First Aid training on knowledge and understanding about psychosocial support principles: A cluster-randomized controlled trial. *International Journal of Environmental Research and Public Health, 17*(2), 484.

Skeffington, P. M., Rees, C. S., & Kane, R. (2013). The primary prevention of PTSD: A systematic review. *Journal of Trauma & Dissociation: The Official Journal of the International Society for the Study of Dissociation (ISSD), 14*(4), 404–422.

Sobocinski, A. B. (2020, July 14). A SPRINT to Guam: Psychological first aid in the COVID-19 pandemic. Retrieved from *www.navy.mil/Press-Office/News-Stories/Article/2284362/a-sprint-to-guam-psychological-first-aid-in-the-covid-19-pandemic*.

Substance Abuse and Mental Health Services Administration. (2014). *Trauma-informed care in behavioral health services* (Chapter 3). Treatment Improvement Protocol Series 57. Retrieved from *www.ncbi.nlm.nih.gov/books/NBK207201*.

Substance Abuse and Mental Health Services Administration. (2022, January 31). Coronavirus (COVID-19) resources. Retrieved from *www.samhsa.gov/coronavirus*.

Turpin, G., Downs, M., & Mason, S. (2005). Effectiveness of providing self-help information following acute traumatic injury: Randomised controlled trial. *The British Journal of Psychiatry, 187*(1), 76–82.

Utzon-Frank, N., Breinegaard, N., Bertelsen, M., Borritz, M., Eller, N. H., Nordentoft, M., et al. (2014). Occurrence of delayed-onset post-traumatic stress disorder: A systematic review and meta-analysis of prospective studies. *Scandinavian Journal of Work, Environment, & Health, 40*, 215–229.

Warner, C. H., Appenzeller, G. N., Grieger, T., Belenkiy, S., Breitbach, J., Parker, J., et al. (2011, October). Importance of anonymity to encourage honest reporting in mental health screening after combat deployment. *Archives of General Psychiatry, 68*(10), 1065–1071.

Wei, E. K., Segall, J., Linn-Walton, R., Eros-Sarnyai, M., Fattal, O., Toukolehto, O., et al. (2020). Combat stress management and resilience: Adapting Department of Defense combat lessons learned to civilian healthcare during the COVID-19 pandemic. *Health Security, 18*(5).

Wessely, S., Bryant, R. A., Greenberg, N., Earnshaw, M., Sharpley, J., & Hughes, J. H. (2008). Does psychoeducation help prevent posttraumatic psychological distress? *Psychiatry: Interpersonal and Biological Processes, 71*(4), 287–302.

World Health Organization. (2022, January 31). The coronavirus disease (COVID-19) pandemic. Retrieved from *www.who.int/emergencies/diseases/novel-coronavirus-2019*.

Introduction to Operational Psychology

Thomas J. Williams, James J. Picano,
Robert R. Roland, and L. Morgan Banks

This chapter provides an introduction to operational psychology, a relatively new and emerging role for military psychologists providing support to national security, military decision making, and military operations (Kennedy & Williams, 2011; Staal & DeVries, 2020; Staal & Harvey, 2019c; Williams, Picano, Roland, & Bartone, 2012). Psychology as a profession has long benefited from its contributions in time of national threats, with growth, relevance, and expansions of scope of practice resting on the contributions to national security threats and their aftermath. In fact, the conceptual basis for the profession of psychology's contributions to society rest on the foundation of psychological assessment and testing in support of our nation's mobilization during World War I (National Research Council, 1991), World War II, the Cold War, and the Global War on Terrorism (see, e.g., Christie & Montiel, 2013; also Chapter 1, this volume).

Few areas of psychology rest at the crossroads of science and society, in both practice and application, as does the practice of operational psychology. Operational psychology involves the application of the scientific principles and practices of psychology that involve services and consultation in support of national security (e.g., counterintelligence operations, direct and indirect assessments, insider threat detection), military intelligence (e.g., consultant to interrogations), law enforcement activities (e.g., interrogation support, hostage negotiation), and/or programs (e.g., assessment and selection; Williams et al., 2012, p. 38).

This introduction to operational psychology places both the science and profession into the context of contemporary contributions of psychological applications that serve society and the individuals within it. Operational psychology does not promulgate or promote national security or

military policies; it focuses on actions, activities, and outcomes designed to serve society in preserving the security and well-being of our nation, from all foreign threats, many of which today are more complex than in the past. What is important for psychologists practicing in this area is that their contributions today are built on the foundation of what makes psychology so rewarding: serving society and the people within it (Mangelsdorff, 2006).

American psychologists have provided direct support to the military since the beginning of the 20th century, and over the past two decades have answered the call to help advance the security of our society. They have done so by meeting the challenge and demonstrating contributions and value-added dimensions offered by operational psychologists. Similar to military organizations that have transformed to remain responsive and relevant to changing circumstances and requirements, threats, and opportunities; so too have military psychologists adapted, evolving existing methods and developing new processes in order to provide meaningful, relevant, and effective support to operational and strategic military commanders (for a review, see Staal & Harvey, 2019c).

The 9/11 terrorist attacks demonstrated and highlighted the changing nature of what has been referred to as asymmetric warfare and the challenge this type of warfare poses for our society and for our military commanders (Williams, 2003). Although contributions by operational psychologists pre-date those terrorist attacks (e.g., profiling enemy commanders), it was within this changing realm and reality of new threats to our society that the field of *operational psychology* was propelled forward to assist military commanders (Adams, 2001; Williams & Johnson, 2006).

Operational psychology offers a broader use of the science and practice of our field than the more traditional clinical delivery of services to individual clients or patients. Essentially, it provides psychological consultation on human behavior in support of national security. In fact, the ability to work in this area is now a significant draw for many early career psychologists. Their interest is primarily the opportunity to work in this field in order to serve society, contribute to national security, and leverage the science of psychology to advance that protection. Within this context, operational psychology provides consulting psychology services in a national security environment—with many of the processes and ethical issues very similar to those of more traditional consulting psychologists.

Prior to the 9/11 terrorist attacks, few sources identified operational psychology as their focus; with early use anticipating the type of support described in this chapter (Staal & Stephenson, 2013). In a study completed by a National Aeronautics and Space Administration (NASA) psychologist on the operational psychology aspects of preparing for space travel, Holland and Curtis (1998) focused on the psychological activities associated with crew member assessment, composition, training, preparation, interventions, well-being, family issues (Pincus et al., 2001; Knapp & Newman,

1993), and repatriation activities. Another aspect of operational psychology has been the support provided by Naval Operational Medicine Institute involving human factors and performance, biostatistics, psychometrics, selection, testing, and training to promote operational effectiveness and safety in Navy fleet and Fleet Marine Force activities (Naval Operational Medicine Institute, 2002).

Both of these perspectives provide grounding for the current practice of operational psychology, primarily in the areas of assessment and selection, offering perspectives that help to reveal the full potential for what operational psychology offers along a spectrum of support, ranging from assessment and selection to national security and military commander support, and extending into space exploration. Kennedy and Williams (2011) offer a more complete representation of other contributions of psychologists serving in operational roles.

OPERATIONAL PSYCHOLOGY DEFINED

This chapter focuses on operational psychology, the actions by military psychologists who support the employment and/or sustainment of military forces (and in particular military commanders) to attain operational and strategic goals in a theater of war or theater of operations. They do so by leveraging and applying their psychological expertise in designing and implementing assessment and selection programs in support of special populations and high-risk missions; in helping to identify enemy capabilities, personalities, and intentions; in facilitating and supporting intelligence operations; and in providing an operationally focused level of consulting support focused on psychological resiliency of the force.

Implied within this definition is the need for operational psychologists to maintain both mental agility and flexibility in understanding and applying the tools of their profession to support the operational art of warfare. It also implies the need to maintain the ability to anticipate the strategic objectives and the relationship of the ends, ways, and means (see, e.g., Joint Publication (JP) 3-0, p. II-4), the demands of supported commanders, and the anticipation of how to apply psychological expertise to those demands to either enhance military effectiveness or mitigate risks. Reduced to its essentials, like a commander's operational art, an operational psychologist must answer three important questions:

1. How might an operational psychologist leverage his or her psychological expertise to contribute to the commander's intended military condition that he or she seeks to produce to achieve the strategic goal? (*Ends*)
2. Of the identified sequence of actions that is most likely to produce

the condition, what psychological resources or products might be brought to bear to support that condition? (*Ways*)

3. How might the operational psychologist contribute to helping the commander use the psychological resources (e.g., psychological profiles, enemy forces capitulation assessments, etc.) that can be applied to help accomplish the desired sequence of actions. (*Means*) (See, e.g., Field Manual (FM) 100-5, p. 10; FM 3-0, 1-26.)

It is an accepted dictum that "all military operations have a psychological effect on all parties concerned—friendly, neutral, and hostile" (JP 3-0, pp. III-19, 24). Recognizing this, and as an example, commanders integrate psychological operations (PSYOP) campaigns into their joint force planning at all levels with the intent to influence the emotions, motives, decision making, and ultimately the behavior of their adversaries (cf. JP 3-0). Thus, PSYOP campaigns are used to either reinforce or induce collective favorable foreign attitudes and behavior (see Figure 12.1). Consequently, operational psychologists must maintain situational awareness of the focus and intent of PSYOP campaigns since both depend on insights into the attitudes and behaviors of specific targets or potential adversaries within the psychological domain.

One important role that an operational psychologist provides involves consultative support based on our knowledge of human behavior to combatant commanders by focusing on an opposing adversary's individual emotions, motives, decision making, and behaviors in order to support the Joint Force commander's strategy, operational design, and tactical action (Schneider & Post, 2003). The effectiveness of these products will often depend on the individual's experience, expertise in developing these products, the situational awareness of the enemy dispositions, and perhaps most importantly, how well these products support the commander's concept of operations.

Planning for the provision of operational psychology support requires several important considerations in order to remain responsive and relevant to operational military commanders. The areas in which operational psychologists assist will vary by military service, agency, or mission. These contributions include support to: assessment and selection (A&S; see Chapter 13, this volume); security clearance evaluations (see Chapter 14, this volume); intelligence support (interrogation, indirect assessment, counterintelligence [CI] support); operations support;[1] operations debriefing

---

[1] Also called Red Teaming, an independent group that a commander establishes to challenge planning assumptions and think critically and creatively, to avoid false mind-sets and/or inaccurate analogies in framing a problem. Red Cells are subsets of Red Teams and perform threat emulation to carefully assess friendly operations from an adversary's point of view (JP 5-0, p. III-76).

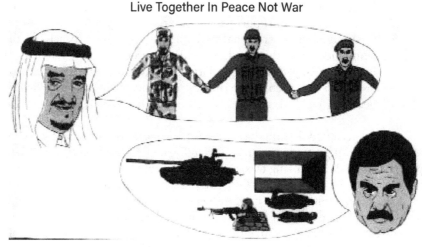

"We are all brothers . . .
neighbor Arabs. . . .
We want peace."

FIGURE 12.1. PSYOP leaflet example. This illustrated Gulf War PSYOP leaflet portrays King Fahd of Saudi Arabia as wanting all Arabs to live together in peace as brothers, while Saddam Hussein thinks of Kuwait, war, and death. (From 4th Psychological Operations Battalion, Fort Bragg, North Carolina.)

(assisting in gathering information from operational personnel to obtain their perspectives after the missions); risk assessment of individuals); industrial/organizational (I/O) support (psychological operations, public affairs operations [PAO] support; military deception support); survival, evasion, resistance, escape (SERE) support (see Chapter 15, this volume); command consultation; education and training (leader development, performance enhancement, platform instruction); crisis negotiation (see Chapter 16, this volume); and aviation psychology (see Kennedy & Kay, 2013). When planned for and implemented, the products of an operational psychologist can serve as a powerful force multiplier for the commander and the mission supported.

The operational psychologist and commander's roles and responsibilities interface at a critical juncture often referred to as the human dimension of warfare. As such, it involves leadership, the individuals who are led, and their morale. The morale of the force is considered the most important intangible element of the human dimension (see, e.g., FM 22-100, § 2-26, 3-36). To the operational psychologist, it serves as the domain in which strong emotions serve as the wellspring for battlefield courage, resiliency, and hardiness to face terror and hardship on the battlefield. Every effective commander understands that morale is the essential human element and seeks to find ways to promote it in his or her forces while denying or undermining it in the enemy. It is within this realm of the human dimension where one faces the great physical, emotional, and mental strain of war and where operational and combat stress reactions occur (see, e.g., Banks & James, 2007; Reger & Moore, 2006).

Those operational and combat stress reactions to combat were captured by S.L.A. Marshall (1947), a military officer who served as the Chief Military Historian for the Army in World War II. Marshall went about the war zone interviewing surviving members of units in the aftermath of intense battles. While in the past military psychologists would have focused primarily on what actions promote high morale and resilience for his or her own or allied troops, Marshall's observations help to highlight how operational psychologists need expertise in identifying what factors will contribute to the lessening or demise of morale in those enemy forces or adversaries who engage our forces. Therefore, operational psychologists leverage battlefield stress information and seek an understanding of how various attributes will impact the military's morale and will to fight, both ours and the enemies (see, e.g., Watson, 1997).

Hoge and colleagues 2004 (see also Friedman, 2004) made an important contribution toward understanding the terrible toll wrought by this human interface with the stress of warfare. This study provides an important assessment of the extent to which combat operations in Iraq and Afghanistan contributed to an increased risk of mental health problems in service members and identified some of the perceived barriers to those service members receiving care (see also Pincus, House, Christenson, & Adler, 2001). Importantly, psychologists serving in and supporting these operations will need to understand and appreciate the need to operationalize their "mental health" services as they also provide support to intelligence operations (cf. Helmus & Glenn, 2005).

SUPPORT TO INTELLIGENCE OPERATIONS

To become optimally effective as a force multiplier, operational psychologists must carefully attend to five main areas related to understanding and contributing to intelligence operations.

1. Operational psychologists must develop and maintain a good understanding of strategic-level military intelligence assets and resources that are available and how to leverage their psychological expertise in applying information developed from the intelligence cycle that supports

the commander's intent. Implied is that the operational psychologist will have the appropriate-level security clearances (i.e., Top Secret) along with access and necessary "read-on" to sensitive compartmented information (SCI) programs that would allow that access (see, e.g., Intelligence Community Directive 704, Technical Amendment; Director of National Intelligence, 2019; Director of Central Intelligence Agency, 1998).

2. The operational psychologist must become integrated early into the intelligence and operational planning cells as well as understand how to integrate operational psychology processes and procedures with national-level intelligence assets supporting military operations (see, e.g., Jones, 2001). As noted above, this requires the appropriate security clearances and understanding of the operational cycle in campaign planning (see, e.g., JP 1-02 and FM 100-7, especially pp. 5-17 through 5-19; see also Army Techniques Publications (ATP) 3-93, 2014).

3. Operational psychologists must serve as a primary asset of the J2 or Intelligence section to ensure, where applicable, integration of operational psychology products and processes with ongoing intelligence initiatives, access to the classified information necessary to fulfill the requirements identified above, and to ensure they remain accessible and integrated into the various elements of the intelligence operations.

4. The operational psychologist must maintain situational awareness of campaign planning to ensure optimal responsiveness in providing information in a timely manner on those personalities or issues most critical for success. Therefore, attending the operational updates provided to a commander is critical if the operational psychologist is to maintain the appropriate situational awareness for the priorities of the commander.

5. The fifth area of expertise for an operational psychologist involves the need to develop expertise in completing indirect assessments (see, e.g., Neller, 2019). In this important area, the operational psychologist can assist the commander in helping to sift through intelligence reports to identify vulnerabilities or tendencies in the personalities and idiosyncrasies of enemy commanders (Liddell Hart, 1967, pp. 207–221). As an example, during World War II, William Langer, head of Research and Analysis for the Office of Strategic Services (OSS), employed the services of both his brother, OSS psychologist Walter Langer (1972), and psychiatrist Henry Murray (1943), of the Harvard Psychological Clinic, to develop a psychological profile of Adolph Hitler. It is interesting to note that Murray's (1943) profile predicted Hitler would commit suicide at the war's end.

One need only explore several other open-source documents to begin to develop an understanding of what potential the operational psychologist offers in this area. For example, in former President Jimmy Carter's (1982) book *Keeping Faith,* he praises the intelligence community for providing him with a "psychological analyses" of Egyptian President Anwar al-Sadat and Israeli Prime Minister Menachem Begin as he began the negotiation for the Camp David Accords:

> I was poring over psychological analyses of two of the protagonists which had been prepared by a team of experts within our intelligence community. This team could write definitive biographies of any important world leader, using information derived from a detailed scrutiny of events, public statements, writings, known medical histories, and interviews with personal acquaintances of the leaders under study. . . . What made them national leaders? What was the root of their ambition? What events during past years had helped to shape their characters? . . . Likely reaction to intense pressure in a time of crisis? Strengths and weaknesses? . . . Whom did they really trust? . . . I was certain they were preparing for our summit conference in a similar manner. (in Carter, 1982, p. 320)

INDIRECT ASSESSMENT

Given the importance of indirect assessments in the repertoire of the operational psychologist, some elaboration is warranted here. Indirect assessments of personality have a long history, and there are several valuable sources that provide samples of both techniques and approaches (e.g., see Freud's (1910/1964) seminal study of Leonardo da Vinci), but perhaps the most valuable is the overview offered by Jerrold Post (2004). Post (2004) provides the details behind the indirect psychological profiles that he helped develop that Jimmy Carter described in *Keeping Faith* and how these were instrumental in helping Carter and various U.S. government leaders anticipate and predict the next moves of those with whom they negotiated. There are several other sources for using this approach, but most are directed at political leaders as opposed to military leaders (see, e.g., Alexander, 1988, 1990; Brickfield, 2001; Elms, 1988, 1994; Feldman & Valenty, 2001). This technique is similar to the commonly accepted indirect assessments that allow law enforcement behavioral profilers to discern offenders' behavioral and personality characteristics (Ault & Reese, 1980; Jackson & Bekerian, 1997; Jackson, van den Eshof, & De Kleuver, 1997; Douglas, Ressler, et al., 1986; Silke, 2001; see Chapter 16, this volume) and other psychological studies that focus on the personality, character, and leadership characteristics of presidents (Rubenzer & Faschingbauer, 2004). However, the use of profiling techniques has not been without controversy and Alison, West, and Goodwill (2004) have proposed a strategy to pragmatically address some of the concerns.

Another related technique for indirect assessments that offers some promise and opportunity for extrapolation is one described by Ritzler and

Singer (1998). They used self-statements culled from the autobiography of Nazi war criminal Rudolph Hoess (1959) to illustrate a method of "MMPI by proxy" that was integrated and compared to a Rorschach completed with Hoess when he was a war crimes trial prisoner in Nuremburg shortly after World War II. Ritzler and Singer (1998) demonstrated good reliability in completing personality assessments by proxy using a technique of self-expression (i.e., the Rorschach) with one of self-report (i.e., the Minnesota Multiphasic Personality Inventory [MMPI]); noting that such techniques offer a reliable way to "deepen one's understanding of personality functioning" (p. 212).

Another valuable area of indirect assessment support is focused on determining how psychological factors contribute in counterespionage activities. For example, an increased understanding of human nature, needs, and motives can prove valuable in determining who is vulnerable for recruitment or betrayal in counterintelligence operations (see, e.g., Marbes, 1986; Olson, 2001; Williams et al., 2012).

By extrapolating from these techniques, an operational psychologist might also assess reports of enemy morale and provide an evaluation of likely capitulation or surrender probabilities using an understanding of both cultural and psychological characteristics of enemy forces and their "will to fight" (see, e.g., Wong, Kolditz, Millen, & Potter, 2003, Watson, 1997; Kecskemeti, 1958). Military operational psychologists must remain aware that in war, our opponents will be *thinking, creative,* and *adaptive.* This is ever more the case with asymmetric approaches to war since our opponents must find indirect ways to counter our strengths as a military. An operational psychologist might extrapolate from these techniques to assess how the enemy's reported or observed patterns of behavior or conduct do or do not adhere to their known doctrine, as well as assess the influence of any cultural factors on the psychology of enemy commanders or forces and their known alliances. In using this information, the operational psychologist can then assist and facilitate the commander's *probing of the enemy commander's mind.* The use of that information may then make an operationally relevant contribution in the identification of the all-important enemy psychological balance and disposition, to include the center of gravity along with likely enemy courses of action. Consequently, operational psychologists play an important role in helping commanders understand both their adversary's and their own way of thinking (cf. Williams, 2003).

The history of warfare is replete with examples of how effectively opposing commanders use their understanding of human nature and personalities to mount effective deception plans, playing off the psychological advantage to gain a military outcome (Latimer, 2001; Smith, 1995; Strosnider, 2002; Sun Tzu, 1971). In 1747, Frederick the Great captured

well the importance of helping a commander see the situation through the eyes of the enemy:

> A general in all of his projects should not think so much about what he wishes to do as what his enemy will do; that he should never underestimate his enemy, but he should put himself in his place to appreciate difficulties and hindrances the enemy could interpose; that his plans will be deranged at the slightest event if he has not foreseen everything and if he has not devised means with which to surmount the obstacles. (Heinl, 1988, p. 102)

Therefore, another important focus for the operational psychologist involves remaining cognizant of how deception plans might facilitate indirect assessments of the most likely reactions of an opponent commander's personality that is identified and assessed in support of the campaign plan. These assessments might then facilitate the development of either "divisive" deception plans to undermine or compromise the efficiencies of enemy commanders or "consolidative" deception plans to then promote and facilitate military operations, but in an area where their expenditure of force and resources will have less effect.

The operational psychologist will also need to be prepared to help identify operationally relevant aspects of enemy commanders' personalities across the spectrum of tactical, operational, and strategic levels of war, alerting the commander to any identified vulnerabilities or likely reactions to requests for surrenders, the *will to fight* if only certain units or positions are targeted, and the centers of gravity for leadership and morale (see, e.g., JP 3-0, p. III-30; Wong et al., 2003). As Eisenhower (1959) once shared, "In war nothing is more important to a commander than the facts concerning the strengths, dispositions, and intentions of his opponent, and the proper interpretation of these facts." In a very real sense, an operational psychologist can contribute to "effects-based" operations in helping commanders sift through various commander intents in response to selected actions to counter those intents (see, e.g., Fayette, 2001). Indeed, the human mind has been described as the "last dimension of future battlefields" (Hall, 1998, p. 1).

At first appearance, this may seem to dramatically shift the skill set for operationally focused military psychologists. However, what it really suggests is that a military psychologist attending military education programs (e.g., intermediate-level military education, such as the Command and Staff College for the Army) has a responsibility to learn and understand the military organization he or she operates within and the likely enemies he or she may face. It is exactly the comprehensive understanding of human behavior, combined with understanding of the military organization, that makes operational psychologists valuable assets.

ASSESSMENT AND SELECTION

One of the most famous constellations of applying the science and practice of psychology to support a nation at war is described in the now classic *The Assessment of Men* (OSS, 1948; see Handler, 2001, for an overview). During World War II, a group of academic psychologists were brought together to develop a method for personnel assessment and selection to carry out counterintelligence, spying, and espionage operations in support of military operations (OSS, 1948). Given that A&S is currently the best-established and predominant function of military operational psychologists, there are numerous contemporary examples of how military psychologists either develop and/or provide assistance to A&S programs for special populations (e.g., military aviators, submariners, drill instructors, leaders), high-risk missions, or entry into U.S. Special Forces (Harrell, 1945; Maranto & Ernesto, 2002; Picano, Roland, Rollins, & Williams, 2002).

Operational psychologists are instrumental in setting up and running programs and processes for military members who volunteer for nonstandard, high-risk assignments (Picano et al., 2002; Picano, Williams, Roland, & Long, 2011; Harvey, 2019; Thompson, Morrow, & Staal, 2019). In doing so, they ensure the right attributes are assessed in a manner that is both predictive of success and of value to those military members completing the assessment and selection processes. They also ensure that these processes provide valuable self-assessment opportunities to promote increased self-awareness, hardiness, and resiliency in those who are successful. Chapter 13 (this volume) expounds on A&S of high-risk operational military personnel, to include required competencies of these personnel, components of A&S programs, and predictors of personnel success.

PRISONERS OF WAR: SURVIVAL, PREPARATION, PROCESSING, AND INTERROGATIONS

Few who saw them will ever forget the vivid images of abuses inflicted on Iraqi prisoners of war at Abu Ghraib prison that were released in April/May 2004. Many were quick to point out the parallel between Zimbardo's (1971) prison study using college students in a basement at Stanford University (Haney, Banks, & Zimbardo, 1973; Zimbardo, Haney, Banks, & Jaffe, 1975), in which normal college students assigned to be guards began to behave cruelly toward those students who were assigned to be prisoners. For this, and other reasons, it is critical that operational psychologists recognize the psychological dynamics of captivity, for both captors and those held captive, and the various interrogation techniques that are employed (see, e.g., Greene & Banks, 2009; Stanton, 1969 for important overviews), along with the ethical and legal boundaries for participation in these activities (see, e.g., Brandon et al., 2019a; Brandon, Kleinman, & Arthur, 2019b). This is an area where operational psychologists draw heavily from their background in social psychological processes, to include diffusion of responsibility, the interplay between personal accountability and moral disengagement for one's actions, dehumanization of enemy combatants, social modeling, and group conformity pressures, to name a few. There are a number of other important areas for operational psychologists to understand, including the clinical issues and professional responsibilities for clinical interventions with victims of torture (see, e.g., Pope & Garcia-Peltoniemi, 1991); working through interpreters (Miller, Martell, Pazdirek, Caruth, & Lopez, 2005); as well as increasing one's understanding of cross-cultural issues (see, e.g., Hong, Morris, Chiu, & Benet-Martinez, 2000; Stuart, 2004; Betancourt, 2004).

The Department of the Army's investigation report (Taguba, 2004), James and Freeman (2008), and Bartone (2004) provide a cogent analysis of some of the contextual/situational factors that they believe influenced behavior in the Abu Ghraib prisoner situations. Bartone (2004) identified the situational/contextual factors as: ambiguity with chain of command/leadership; laissez-faire attitude of the leadership toward what was happening within the prison; a lack of training of the prison guards; lack of discipline; and the psychological stressors of being in constant danger over an extended period of time, with reduced quality of life.

Staal (2019) provides a resource for operational psychologists in addressing behavioral science consultation to military interrogations, the history of the development of Behavioral Science Consultation Teams (BSCTs), a review of the training of psychologists as members of BSCTs (DoDI 2310.09; Department of Defense Instruction [DoDI], 2019), concerns raised by the American Psychological Association (APA) in the Hoffman Report (a controversial report on psychologists' involvement in wartime interrogations, with disparate opinions as to the legitimacy of the process and findings; APA, 2015) about the role of psychologists in national security settings, and national security policies developed early on to ensure legal and ethical practices (Dunivin, Banks, Staal, & Stephenson, 2011). The DoD recently issued an instruction that provides policy, assigns responsibilities, and specifically describes the purpose and roles of Behavioral Science Support (BSS) personnel in detainee operations and in support of intelligence interrogations (DoDI 2310.09). This is an important document for any military psychologist supporting detainee operations or intelligence interrogations, either directly or indirectly, to comply with applicable U.S. laws, the law of war (e.g., Geneva Conventions of 1949), and applicable policies and directives in supporting these types of operations. This document also establishes and defines BSS personnel qualifications, distinguishes operational support from medical operations, and "establishes a DoD-wide process to collect integrate, and analyze information on the utilization and effectiveness of BSS" procedures (DoDI 2310.09, p. 1).

The recent controversies surrounding interrogations highlight the importance for operational psychologists to familiarize themselves with the Law of Land Warfare and the provisions of the Geneva Conventions (see, e.g., FM 27-10) as well as important regulations governing the handling of prisoners of war or detainees (see, e.g., Army Regulation (AR) 190-8 and FM 34-52, especially Chapter 6). One role for operational psychologists is to help develop unit training for support to interrogations and interrogation processes that might include instruction on the psychological processes and motivations that are activated during detention; increasing awareness of possible resistance techniques (see, e.g., FM 34-52); as well as recognizing and making evident their ethical and professional responsibilities (as both a psychologist and professional military officer) to help provide supervision and accountability to the command for activities they observe or suspect are occurring (see also Wedgewood, 2004).

Taylor (1991; see especially pp. 494–496) and Hunter (1991) have also addressed several important issues of relevance for operational psychologists. In particular, Taylor (1991) points out that few individuals are resilient enough to resist an intense and prolonged interrogation, noting that the state of health, strength of purpose, psychological hardiness, and understanding of strategy being used by the interrogators all contribute. Thus, operational psychologists make a valuable contribution by helping train unit members about the stress and strain of captivity.

As terrorist organizations expand their net of potential captives, many of whom are nonmilitary, there is an increasing need for the readiness and preparation of both military and interagency operational psychologists to meet this need. Therefore, an operational psychologist needs to understand the dynamics of captivity, the psychological processes that occur within captives, the interpersonal dynamics activated between captives and their captors (Leo & Drizin, 2010; Surmon-Böhr, Alison, Christiansen, & Alison, 2020), lessons learned from safe, ethical interrogations (Duke, Wood, Magee, Escobar, 2018; Staal, 2019), and what preventive measures there are to promote hardiness and resiliency within captives. For example, Hunter (1991) provides an excellent overview of the common psychological and psychosocial sequelae and difficulties, postcaptivity, for former captives and their families. In addition, military psychologists have long played a vital role in SERE training and in the development of appropriate education and assessment programs (see Chapter 15, this volume).

An important area for the operational psychologist is to identify and set clear practice boundaries between operational support activities versus medical treatment activities (cf. Staal & Harvey, 2019b; Williams & Kennedy, 2011) in order to prevent role confusion and ethical dilemmas (see

Chapter 17, this volume). However, at times, emergencies arise that make this difficult. Consider the following example.

Case 12.1. The Detainee with a Medical Emergency

An operational psychologist was monitoring the intelligence interrogation of a civilian High-Value Detainee (HVD). Just as the interrogation was commencing with the interrogator asking the HVD to share his name, the HVD suddenly began sweating profusely, started trembling and shaking, displayed shortness of breath, and grabbed his chest complaining of chest pain. The interrogator turned to the operational psychologist, who advised stopping the interrogation immediately and obtaining a medical evaluation. The brigade surgeon was contacted by the psychologist and summoned to medically evaluate the HVD; with an estimated arrival in 20 minutes. Given the isolated nature of the forward-deployed combat setting, there was no ambulance to call and the brigade surgeon was the most available medical professional with the expertise to medically evaluate the HVD to determine his status. Given the travel time before the arrival of the physician and the absence of any other CPR-trained personnel at this remote location, the brigade surgeon requested that the operational psychologist stay with the HVD, lay him down, try to help him relax and determine if he had a history of a heart condition and/or panic attacks. The HVD confirmed that he had no history of a heart condition, only a history of panic attacks. The brigade surgeon's medical assessment resulted in the detainee being transferred to a location with onsite medical personnel for further evaluation.

Another such area where a potential blending of roles may occur is when an operational psychologist participates in the recovery of detained personnel, prisoners of war, or those held captive by terrorists. As the individual is freed from captivity, the operational psychologist may provide immediate crisis intervention with the recovered personnel and remain with them until they are transferred to an appropriate medical treatment facility (MTF)–based mental health provider. This also activates the requirement for the MTF–based mental health provider to ensure he or she is competent in postrecovery interventions given that the provider may have occasion to interact with recovered personnel at some point in his or her career.

The Joint Personnel Recovery Agency (JPRA) is the DoD proponent for repatriation activities. Operational psychologists should familiarize themselves with several Department of Defense Directives (DoDD) and Instructions (DoDI), as well as Joint Publications (JP), that are particularly relevant; they are listed in Table 12.1.

Hayes (2003) provides an overview of Joint–SERE training issues, noting the 17 subject areas taught by all DoD-approved SERE courses and addressing the Level C SERE policy differences among the three Services.

TABLE 12.1. Recommended Department of Defense Directives, Instructions, and Joint Publications

Number	Title (publication year)	Directive/instruction/ joint publication
DoDD 2310.4	*Repatriation of Prisoners of War (POW), Hostages, Peacetime Government Detainees, and Other Missing or Isolated Personnel* (2000)	Directive
DoDD 2310.1E	*DoD Detainee Program* (2014)	Directive
DoDD 1300.7	*Training and Education to Support the Code of Conduct* (2000)	Directive
DoDD 5110.10	*Defense POW/MIA Accounting Agency* (DPAA, 2017)	Directive
DoDI 1300.21	*Code of Conduct Training and Education* (2001)	Instruction
DoDI 2310.5	*Accounting for Missing Persons* (2000)	Instruction
DoDI 2310.6	*Non-Conventional Assisted Recovery in the Department of Defense* (2000)	Instruction
DoDI 2310.9	*Behavioral Science Support (BSS) for Detainee Operations and Intelligence Interrogations* (September 5, 2019)	Instruction
JP 3-0	*Joint Operations* (October 22, 2018)	Joint publication
JP 3-50.3	*Administrative Processing of DoD Individuals Who Have Returned from Isolated Territory* (especially Appendix A; September 6, 1996)	Joint publication
JP 5-0	*Joint Planning* (December 1, 2020)	Joint publication

Note. Full citations for the specific publications noted in this table are listed in the references.

Given the increasing threats of hostage taking and terrorist activities, psychologists who anticipate providing services to recovered personnel (military or civilian) should ensure they are familiar with postcaptive psychological treatments. For a comprehensive review of the operational psychologist's role in SERE training, see Chapter 15, this volume.

TERRORISM/COUNTERTERRORISM: OPERATIONAL SUPPORT

The 9/11 Commission report (National Commission on Terrorist Attacks, 2004) helped bring greater awareness to the multifaceted danger and challenge posed by Al-Qaeda and terrorism. That report offers an important overview of the psychology of terrorists in general and, specifically, the psychology of Al-Qaeda terrorists that killed over 3,000 Americans.

Military psychologists who support operational activities focused on terrorist groups need to explore their psychological vulnerabilities and appeal to those who are recruited into terrorism (see, e.g., Staal & Myers, 2019). This offers valuable explanations for why certain individuals (or groups) are vulnerable to recruitment into terrorist groups (Staal & Myers, 2019). Understanding historical accounts of state-sponsored, political, and nationalistic terrorism can be obtained from reviews of how certain psychological and biographical attributes—especially loyalty, indoctrination, and disillusionment—play such an important role in the recruitment of terrorists (Zillmer, 2012). The terrorist threat to society represents a significant challenge for operational psychologists to remain sensitive to the complex interplay of the personality, situational, and religious dynamics of terrorist groups; how these psychological processes combine to form a dangerous elixir of hate, purpose, and action that demands our vigilance and action around the world.

There has long been a growing concern that terrorists or other nations seeking world recognition will achieve their goal of obtaining and using weapons of mass destruction (WMD), including nuclear materials and/or biological or chemical agents (Gunaratna, 2002). This threat has been a concern and focus for psychologists for many years (see, e.g., White, 1986, especially pp. 9–33 detailing the toll this threat poses on our feelings and our children). A now more uncertain and unknown threat lurks in the shadows of terrorism. As the world has confronted a reality of a pandemic, the significant impact on every nation brings to light the potential psychological effects of an attack using nuclear, biological, or chemical agents (Zhang & Gronvall, 2020). As the full effects of the pandemic are not likely to be realized for years to come, it is useful to reflect on a prior overview of psychological variables, effects, changes, and chronic reactions associated with exposure to ionizing radiation and its potential effect on military manpower (see, e.g., Mickley & Bogo, 1991).

CRISIS NEGOTIATION

Crisis negotiation offers the potential to create another natural tension between the mental health and operational roles important to an operational psychologist. On the one hand, very few psychologists receive training in formal negotiation or mediation, although success could mean life or death for a hostage. In asymmetric warfare, decisions made about how to handle any given situation on a tactical level offer the potential to have strategic-level implications. Therefore, several important sources are worth considering as background for this important topic. For example, Fuselier (1988, 1991) provides an overview of support that mental health professionals can provide to a police hostage negotiation team. An operational psychologist should strive to become familiar with several negotiation or mediation models to ensure adaptability and readiness for different challenges he or she will confront in hostage negotiations (see, e.g., Pruitt, 1986, pp. 35–50; Fisher & Ury, 1981; Rubin, 1986; Wells, 2015). Chapter 16, this volume, reviews communication-based psychological strategies for crisis negotiation consultation, presents current models, provides tips specific to consulting to negotiations when a current or former military member is the hostage taker or barricaded subject, presents the roles of the consulting operational psychologist, and addresses ethical issues specific to crisis negotiation consultation. Competent operational psychologists have the potential to counter a too often leveled criticism that "mental health professionals may have something to offer in the hostage situation, but probably less than the field commanders might hope for" (Poythress, 1980, p. 32).

ETHICAL AND LEGAL CONSIDERATIONS
FOR OPERATIONAL PSYCHOLOGISTS

The four primary ethical dilemmas for operational psychologists have been identified as mixed agency, competence, multiple relationships, and informed consent. These are reviewed in depth in Chapter 17 (this volume). The varied and innovative roles and responsibilities in which operational psychologists engage prompt ethical and legal considerations that are best addressed in the realm of professional competencies (American Psychological Association, 2002). Kaslow (2004) offers a model for clinically based professional competency that is easily adapted to promote a legal and ethical competency-based practice model for operational psychologists. For example, competence is defined as "an individual's capability and demonstrated ability to understand and do certain tasks in an appropriate and effective manner consistent with expectations for a person qualified by education and training in a particular profession or specialty thereof" (Kaslow, 2004, p. 775).

It is also important for operational psychologists to understand and develop competence in multicultural assessments (cf. Glover & Friedman, 2015; see also Staal & Bluestein, 2019; Chapter 17, this volume). Dana (2002) has identified several important considerations for becoming competent in multicultural assessments: (1) recognition that it is a multifaceted construct; (2) respect for how cultural differences are predicated on increased self-awareness, personal experiences, and knowledge of the other cultures; (3) ability to offer simultaneous interpretations of standard and multicultural assessments that strengthens both approaches; (4) increased need for awareness of possible bias in research methods (e.g., comparative research studies and assessment methods); (5) increased need to understand cross-cultural equivalence and psychometric issues in testing; and (6) a recommendation for initial supervision of multicultural assessments.

Since operational psychologists may find themselves challenged to

provide support in new operational areas without clearly delineated ethical or legal parameters, a foundation for a competency-based ethical and legal decision-making model is imperative. Toward that end, the operational psychologist will often have to use his or her professional judgment to assess situations and make decisions about what to do or not to do; maintain a self-awareness of how to use self-reflective practice to modify one's decision, as appropriate; carry out his or her actions in accord with the ethical principles, standards, guidelines, and values of the profession with the understanding that competency is context dependent, and with the execution of that competency, they vary depending on the setting and environment (Kaslow, 2004; Epstein & Hundert, 2002; Staal & Harvey, 2019a; Williams & Kennedy, 2011).

Today's threats to national security and increased contributions of military psychologists offer operational psychologists many different settings and environments within which to exercise their ethical and legal decision-making process (see, e.g., Staal & Harvey, 2019b). There is growing recognition and increased awareness of the need for an expanded view of ethical principles that recognizes the complex interplay of cultural factors, beliefs, religions, and political systems (Fisher, 2004; Kennedy & Williams, 2011; Pettifor, 2004). In this volatile and uncertain world, operational psychologists will find they must consider how to resolve ethical dilemmas across diverse cultural and political contexts (Fisher, 2004; Staal & Harvey, 2019b; Williams & Kennedy, 2011).

These ethical issues, and the diverse cultural and political contexts within which operational psychologists may provide national security consultations worldwide, raise the importance of both training and the profession's "service to society" obligations. Consequently, LoCicero and colleagues (2016) raise the concern that clinical psychology graduate students may need more training in the proper duties of psychologists in military settings or in the ethical guidance offered by international treaties within the context of "do no harm." The complexity of the context of that potential "do no harm" is revealed by the findings of Thornewill, DeMatteo, and Heilbrun (2020). They surveyed over 1,100 psychologists engaged in treatment-focused and non-treatment-focused activities as well as over 500 members of the general public. Findings revealed that the general public is more accepting of psychologists' involvement in activities in national security settings (i.e., activities highlighted in the Hoffman Independent Review) than psychologists. As a psychologist's profession is one that strives to serve the interests of society, it is important not to discount the views of the general public and their more positive perceptions of psychologists serving in national security settings.

These settings may place psychologists in roles that place them at odds with their treatment- and practice-based ethics (cf. LoCicero et al., 2016; see also Staal & Harvey, 2019b; Williams & Kennedy, 2011). When psychologists provide consultations in support of national security, the thoughtful analysis of the consultation, in the context of the aspirational goals and intent of the ethics code using a good decision-making model (cf. Williams & Kennedy, 2011), can resolve almost all of the issues. In doing so, the differing roles and responsibilities that psychologists confront in completing forensic assessments versus patient care seemingly offer a basis to initiate the resolution of this conflict (Williams & Kennedy, 2011; see also, e.g., Alison et al., 2004).

Those roles and responsibilities have been specifically addressed in multiple ways (see, e.g., Dunivin et al., 2011; Staal & Harvey, 2019b; Kennedy & Williams, 2011). Military operational units have implemented training programs to ensure that those military psychologists who transition into becoming operational psychologists have the competencies to support military operations, are familiar with the roles and responsibilities (e.g., those outlined in DoDI 2310.09), and are able to ensure the development of professional psychological practice guidelines in the particular areas of practice (cf. Bush, 2019) that have been introduced above.

It is perhaps fair to say that as psychologists respond to the national security threats, the scope of practice for an operational psychologist may not fall readily or neatly within the realm of the profession's currently established treatment-focused ethics code (Staal & Harvey, 2019b; Williams & Kennedy, 2011). Accordingly, this increases the responsibility and need for operational psychologists to promote optimal behavior and regulate their own professional behavior within a reflective, decision-making model with a moral framework (see, e.g., Kennedy & Williams, 2011; Pettifor, 2004; Pack-Brown & Williams, 2003).

As an initial step in approaching this complex issue, Ewing and Gelles (2003) provided several examples and offered an excellent discussion of ethical dilemmas in the nontraditional roles psychologists increasingly find themselves in when providing professional consultations. Staal and Harvey (2019c) and Kennedy and Williams (2011) address these issues in more depth across several traditional and nontraditional roles (see also Staal & DeVries, 2020). In light of these new challenges and opportunities, this introduction to operational psychology is intended to initiate the identification and articulation of the needed competencies for success, to include the knowledge, skills, and attitudes necessary for the ethical and legal professional practice in this increasingly important domain of military psychology.

REFERENCES

Adams, T. K. (2001). Future warfare and the decline of human decisionmaking. *Parameters, 31*(4), 57–71.

Alexander, I. E. (1988). Personality, psychological assessment, and psychobiography. *Journal of Personality, 56,* 265–294.

Alexander, I. E. (1990). *Personology: Method and content in personality assessment and psychobiography.* Durham, NC: Duke University Press.

Alison, L, West, A., & Goodwill, A. (2004). The academic and the practitioner: Pragmatists' views of offender profiling. *Psychology, Public Policy, and Law, 10*(1/2), 71–101.

American Psychological Association (2002). Ethical principles of psychologists and code of conduct. *American Psychologist, 57,* 1060–1073.

Ault, R. L., Jr., & Reese, J. T. (1980, March). A psychological assessment of crime profiling. *FBI Law Enforcement Bulletin,* 1–4.

Banks, L. M., & James, L. C. (2007). Warfare, terrorism, and psychology. In B. Bongar, L. M. Brown, L. E. Beutler, J. N. Breckenridge, & P. G. Zimbardo (Eds.), *Psychology of terrorism* (pp. 216–222). New York: Oxford University Press.

Bartone, P. T. (2004). Understanding prisoner abuse at Abu Ghraib: Psychological considerations and leadership implications. *The Military Psychologist, 20*(2), 12–16.

Betancourt, J. R. (2004). Cultural competence—Marginal or mainstream movement? *New England Journal of Medicine, 351*(10), 953–955.

Brandon, S. E., Arthur, J. C., Ray, D. G., Meissner, C. A., Kleinman, S. M., Russano, M. B., et al. (2019a). The High-Value Detainee Interrogation Group (HIG): Inception, evolution, and outcomes. In M. A. Staal & S. C. Harvey (Eds.), *Operational psychology: A new field to support national security and public safety* (pp. 263–285). Santa Barbara, CA: Praeger.

Brandon, S. E., Kleinman, S. M., & Arthur, J. C. (2019b). A scientific perspective on the 2006 U.S. Army Field Manual 2-22.3. In M. A. Staal & S. C. Harvey (Eds.), *Operational psychology: A new field to support national security and public safety* (pp. 287–325). Santa Barbara, CA: Praeger.

Brickfield, F. X. (2001). The impact of stroke on world leaders. *Military Medicine, 166*(3), 231–232.

Bush, S. S. (2019). Use of practice guidelines and position statements in ethical decision making. *American Psychologist, 74*(9), 1151–1162.

Carter, J. (1982). *Keeping faith.* New York: Bantam.

Christie, D. J., & Montiel, C. J. (2013). Contributions of psychology to war and peace. *American Psychologist, 68*(7), 502–513.

Dana, R. H. (2002). Introduction to special series: Multicultural assessment: Teaching methods and competence evaluations. *Journal of Personality Assessment, 79*(2), 195–199.

Department of the Army. (1956, July 18). Field Manual (FM) 2710: *Law of land warfare.* Arlington, VA: Author. Retrieved from *www.benning.army.mil/ infantry/DoctrineSupplement/ATP3–21.8/PDFs/fm27_10.pdf.*

Department of the Army. (1987, May 8). Field Manual (FM) 34-52: *Intelligence interrogation.* Arlington, VA: Author. Retrieved from *www.loc.gov/rr/frd/ Military_Law/pdf/intel_interrogation_may-1987.pdf.*

Department of the Army. (1986, May 5). Field Manual (FM) 100-5: *Operations.* Arlington, VA: Author. Retrieved from *https://archive.org/details/FM100– 51968.*

Department of the Army. (1995, May 31). Field Manual (FM) 100-7: *Decisive force: The Army in theater operations.* Arlington, VA: Author. Retrieved from *https://archive.org/details/milmanual-fm-100–7-decisive-force.*

Department of the Army. (1997, October 1). Army Regulation (AR) 190-8: Enemy prisoners of war, retained personnel, civilian internees and other detainees. Arlington, VA: Author. Also Department of the Navy (OPNAVINST 346.6), Department of the Air Force (AFJI 31-304), and Department of the Marine Corps (MCO 3461.1). Retrieved from *https://armypubs.army.mil/epubs/DR_pubs/DR_a/pdf/web/r190_8.pdf.*

Department of the Army. (1999, August 31). Field Manual (FM) 22-100: *Army leadership: Be, know, do.* Arlington, VA: Author. Retrieved from *https://archive.org/details/milmanual-fm-22–100-army-leadership-be-know-do.*

Department of the Army. (2014, November 26). *Theater Army operations* (Techniques Publication No. 3-93). Arlington, VA: Author.

Department of the Army. (2017, December 6). Field Manual (FM) 3-0, C1: *Operations.* Arlington, VA: Author. Retrieved from *https://armypubs.army.mil/epubs/DR_pubs/DR_a/ARN6503-FM_3–0-001-WEB-8.pdf.*

Department of Defense. (1996, September 6). Joint Publication 3-50.3, Appendix A: *Administrative processing of DoD individuals who have returned from isolated territory.* Arlington, VA: Author.

Department of Defense. (2000a). *Accounting for missing persons* (Department of Defense 2310.5). Retrieved from *https://biotech.law.lsu.edu/blaw/dodd/corres/pdf/i23105_013100/i23105p.pdf.*

Department of Defense. (2000b). *Non-conventional assisted recovery in the Department of Defense* (Department of Defense Instruction 2310.6). Retrieved from *https://biotech.law.lsu.edu/blaw/dodd/corres/pdf/i23106_101300/i23106p.pdf.*

Department of Defense. (2000c). *Repatriation of prisoners of war (POW), hostages, peacetime government detainees, and other missing or isolated personnel* (Department of Defense Directive 2310.4). Retrieved from *https://biotech.law.lsu.edu/blaw/dodd/corres/pdf/i23104_112100/i23104p.pdf.*

Department of Defense. (2000d). *Training and education to support the code of conduct* (Department of Defense Directive 1300.7). Retrieved from *www.dpaa.mil/portals/85/Documents/LawsDirectives/dodd_1300_7.pdf.*

Department of Defense. (2001). *Code of Conduct (CoC) training and education* (Department of Defense Instruction 1300.21). Retrieved from *https://biotech.law.lsu.edu/blaw/dodd/corres/pdf/i130021_010801/i130021p.pdf.*

Department of Defense. (2014, August 19). *Department of Defense Detainee Program* (Department of Defense Directive 2310.1E). Retrieved from *www.loc.gov/rr/frd/Military_Law/pdf/LOAC-Documentary-Supp-2015_Ch31.pdf.*

Department of Defense. (2017). *Defense Prisoner of War/Missing in Action Office (DPMO)* (Department of Defense Directive 5110.10). Retrieved from *www.esd.whs.mil/Portals/54/Documents/DD/issuances/dodd/511010_dodd_2017.pdf.*

Department of Defense. (2018, October 22). Joint Publication 3-0: *Joint Operations.* Arlington, VA: Author.

Department of Defense. (2019). *Behavioral science support (BSS) for detainee operations and intelligence interrogations* (Department of Defense Instruction 2310.09). Retrieved from *www.esd.whs.mil/Portals/54/Documents/DD/issuances/dodi/231009p.PDF?ver=2019–09–05–085854–810.*

Director of Central Intelligence Agency. (1998, July). *Personnel security standards and procedures governing eligibility for access to sensitive compartmented information* (Directive No. 6/4). Langley, VA: Author. Retrieved from *https://fas.org/irp/offdocs/dcid6–4/dcid6–4.pdf.*

Director of National Intelligence. (2018). *Personnel security standards and procedures governing eligibility for access to sensitive compartmented information* (Intelligence Community Directive 704, Technical Amendment). Retrieved from *https://fas.org/irp/dni/icd/icd-704.pdf.*

Douglas, J. E., Ressler, R. K., et al., (1986). Criminal profiling from crime scene analysis. *Behavioral Sciences and the Law, 4*(4), 401–421.

Duke, M. C., Wood, J. M., Magee, J., & Escobar, H. (2018). The effectiveness of Army Field Manual interrogation approaches for deducing information and building rapport. *Law and Human Behavior, 42*(5), 442–457.

Dunivin, D., Banks, L. M., Staal, M. A. , & Stephenson, J. A. (2011). Behavioral science consultation to interrogation and debriefing operations: Ethical considerations. In C. H. Kennedy & T. J. Williams (Eds.), *Ethical practice in operational psychology: Military and national intelligence applications* (pp. 85–106). Washington, DC: American Psychological Association.

Eisenhower, D. D. (1959). Remarks at the cornerstone-laying ceremony for the Central Intelligence Agency Building, Langley, VA. Retrieved from *www.presidency.ucsb.edu/documents/remarks-the-cornerstone-laying-ceremony-for-the-central-intelligence-agency-building.*

Elms, A. C. (1988). *Freud as Leonardo: Why the first psychobiography went wrong. Journal of Personality, 56,* 19–40.

Elms, A. C. (1994). *Uncovering lives: The uneasy alliance of biography and psychology.* New York: Oxford University Press.

Epstein, R. M., & Hundert, E. M. (2002). Defining and assessing professional competence. *Journal of the American Medical Association, 287,* 226–235.

Ewing, C. P., & Gelles, M. G. (2003). Ethical concerns in forensic consultation regarding national safety and security. *Journal of Threat Assessment, 2*(3), 95–107.

Fayette, D. F. (2001). Effects-based operations. Retrieved November 8, 2004, from *www.afflhorizons.com/briefs/june01/IF00015.html.*

Feldman, O., & Valenty, L. O. (2001). *Profiling political leaders: Cross-cultural studies of personality and behavior.* Westport, CT: Praeger.

Fisher, C. B. (2004). Challenges in constructing a cross-national ethics code for psychologists. *European Psychologist, 9*(4), 273–277.

Fisher, R., & Ury, W. (1981). *Getting to yes: How to negotiate agreement without giving in.* Boston: Houghton Mifflin.

Freud, S. (1910/1964). *Leonardo da Vinci and a memory of his childhood* (A. Tyson, Trans.). New York: Norton.

Friedman, M. J. (2004). Acknowledging the psychiatric cost of war. *New England Journal of Medicine, 351*(1), 75–77.

Fuselier, G. D. (1988, April). Hostage negotiation consultant: Emerging role for the clinical psychologist. *Professional Psychology: Research & Practice, 19*(2), 175–179.

Fuselier, G. D. (1991). Hostage negotiation: Issues and applications. In Reuvan, G. & A.D. Mangelsdorff (Eds.), *Handbook of military psychology* (pp. 711–724). Chichester, UK: John Wiley & Sons.

Glover, J., & Friedman, H. L. (2015). An approach to understanding and applying culture. In J. Glover & H. L. Friedman (Eds.), *Transcultural competence: Navigating cultural differences in the global community* (pp. 17–27). Washington, DC: American Psychological Association.

Greene, C. H., & Banks, L. (2009). Ethical guideline evolution in psychological support to interrogation operations. *Consulting Psychology Journal: Practice and Research, 61*(1), 25–32.

Gunaratna, R. (2002). *Inside al Qaeda: Global network of terror.* New York: Columbia University Press.

Hall, W. M. (1998). *Thinking and planning: Vision 2010* (Report No. 98–6). Arlington, VA: Institute of Land Warfare.

Handler, L. (2001) Assessment of men: Personality assessment goes to war by the Office of Strategic Services assessment staff. *Journal of Personality Assessment, 76*(3), 558–578.

Haney, C., Banks, W. C., & Zimbardo, P. G. (1973). Interpersonal dynamics in a simulated prison. *International Journal of Criminology and Penology, 1,* 69–97.

Harrell, T. W. (1945). Applications of psychology in the American Army. *Psychological Bulletin, 42*(1), 453–460.

Harvey, S. C. (2019). Operational psychology consultation within special operations units. In M. A. Staal & S. C. Harvey (Eds.), *Operational psychology: A new field to support national security and public safety* (pp. 79–100). Santa Barbara, CA: Praeger.

Hayes, M. W. (2003, April 7). *A Joint Level-C survival, evasion, resistance, and escape (SERE) program for the Armed Forces.* Carlisle Barracks, PA: Strategy Research Project, U.S. Army War College.

Heinl, R. D. (1988). Frederick the Great in instructions for his generals. In *Dictionary of Military and Naval Quotations* (p. iii) Annapolis, MD: United States Naval Institute.

Helmus, T. C., & Glenn, R. W. (2005). *Steeling the mind: Combat stress reactions and their implications for urban warfare.* Santa Monica: RAND Corporation. Retrieved from *www.rand.org/pubs/monographs/MG191.html.*

Hoess, R. (1959). *Commandant of Auschwitz: The autobiography of Rudolf Hoess.* New York: World.

Hoge, C. W., Castro, C. A., Messer, S. C., McGuirk, D., Cotting, D. I., & Koffman, R. L. (2004). Combat duty in Iraq and Afghanistan, mental health problems, and barriers to care. *New England Journal of Medicine, 351*(1), 13–22.

Holland, A. W., & Curtis, K. (1998). Operational psychology countermeasures during the Lunar-Mars Life Support Test Project. *Life Support Biosphere Science: Journal of Earth Space, 5*(4), 445–452.

Hong, Y., Morris, M. W., Chiu, C., & Benet-Martinez, V. (2000). Multicultural minds: A dynamic constructivist approach to culture and cognition. *American Psychologist, 55,* 709–720.

Hunter, E. D. (1991). Prisoners of war: Readjustment and rehabilitation. In R. Gal & A. D. Mangelsdorff (Eds.), *Handbook of military psychology* (pp. 741–757). Chichester, UK: John Wiley & Sons.

Jackson, J., & Bekerian, D. (Eds.). (1997). *Offender profiling: Theory, research, and practice.* Chicester, UK: John Wiley & Sons.

Jackson, J., van den Eshof, P., & De Kleuver, E. (1997). A research approach to offender profiling. In J. Jackson & D. Bekerian (Eds.), *Offender profiling: Theory, research, and practice* (pp. 107–132). Chichester, UK: John Wiley & Sons.

James, L. C., & Freeman, G. A. (Collaborator). (2008). *Fixing hell: An army psychologist confronts Abu Ghraib.* New York: Grand Central Publishing/ Hachette Book Group.

Jones, G. (2001). Working with the CIA. *Parameters, 31*(4), 28–29.

Kaslow, N. J. (2004). Competencies in professional psychology. *American Psychologist, 59*(8), 774–781.

Kecskemeti, P. (1958). *Strategic surrender: The politics of victory and defeat.* Stanford, CA: Stanford University Press.

Kennedy, C. H., & Kay, G. (2013). *Aeromedical psychology.* Aldershot, UK: Ashgate.

Kennedy, C. H., & Williams, T. J. (2011). *Ethical practice in operational psychology: Military and national intelligence applications.* Washington, DC: American Psychological Association.

Knapp, T. S., & Newman, S. J. (1993). Variables related to the psychological well being of Army wives during the stress of an extended military separation. *Military Medicine, 158,* 77–80.

Langer, W. C. (1972). *The mind of Adolph Hitler: The secret wartime report.* New York: Basic Books.

Latimer, J. (2001). *Deception in war: The art of the bluff, the value of deceit, and the most thrilling episodes of cunning in military history, from the Trojan Horse to the Gulf War.* Woodstock, NY: Overlook.

Leo, R. A., & Drizin, S. A. (2010). The three errors: Pathways to false confession and wrongful conviction. In D. G. Lassiter & C. A. Meissner (Eds.), *Police interrogations and false confessions: Current research, practice, and policy recommendations* (pp. 9–30). Washington, DC: American Psychological Association.

Liddell Hart, B. H. (1967). *Strategy.* New York: Signet.

LoCicero, A., Marlin, R. P., Jull-Patterson, D., Sweeney, N. M., Gray, B. L., & Boyd, J. W. (2016, November). Enabling torture: APA, clinical psychology training and the failure to disobey. *Peace and Conflict: Journal of Peace Psychology, 22*(4), 345–355.

Mangelsdorff, A. D. (Ed.). (2006). *Psychology in the service of national security.* Washington, DC: American Psychological Association.

Maranto, D., & Ernesto, M. (2002). *Developing effective selection procedures for screening security personnel.* Washington, DC: American Psychological Association.

Marbes, W. (1986, Summer). Psychology of treason. *Studies in Intelligence, 30*(2), 1–11.

Marshall, S. L. A. (1947). *Men against fire: The problem of battle command in future war.* New York: Morrow.

Mickley, G. A., & Bogo, V. (1991). Radiological factors and their effects on military performance. In R. Gal & A. D. Mangelsdorff (Eds.), *Handbook of military psychology* (pp. 365–385). Chichester, UK: John Wiley & Sons.

Miller, K. E., Martell, Z. L., Pazdirek, L., Caruth, M., & Lopez, D. (2005). The role of interpreters in psychotherapy with refugees: An exploratory model. *American Journal of Orthopsychiatry, 75*(1), 27–39.

Murray, H. A. (1943, October). *Analysis of the personality of Adolph Hitler: With predictions of his future behavior and suggestions for dealing with him now and after Germany's surrender* (Office of Strategic Studies Confidential Report copy 11 of 30). Washington, DC: Office of Strategic Services.

National Commission on Terrorist Attacks Upon the United States. (2004). *The 9/11 Commission Report.* New York: W.W. Norton.

National Research Council. (1991). *Performance assessment for the workplace* (Vol. I). Washington, DC: National Academies Press.

Naval Operational Medicine Institute. (2002). *Operational psychology— Code 41.* Retrieved May 28, 2004, from *www.nomi.med.navy.mil/text/ directorates/41page.thm.*

Neller, D. J. (2019). Foundations of indirect assessment. In M. A. Staal & S. C. Harvey (Eds.), *Operational psychology: A new field to support national security and public safety* (pp. 211–240). Santa Barbara, CA: Praeger.

Olson, J. M. (2001). The Ten Commandants of counterintelligence. *Studies in Intelligence.* Retrieved from *www.cia.gov/csi/studies/fall_winter_2001/articles08html.*

OSS Assessment Staff. (1948). *Assessment of men.* New York: Rinehart.

Pack-Brown, S., & Williams, S. (2003). *Ethics in a multicultural context.* Thousand Oaks, CA: SAGE.

Pettifor, J. L. (2004). Professional ethics across national boundaries, *European Psychologist, 9*(4), 264–272.

Picano, J. J., Roland, R. R., Rollins, K. D., & Williams, T. J. (2002). Personality correlates of staff and peer ratings in operational assessment. *Proceedings of the Annual Conference of The International Military Testing Association, Australia,* pp. 191–195.

Picano, J. J., Williams, T. J., Roland, R., & Long, C. (2011). Operational psychologists in support of assessment and selection: Ethical considerations. In C. H. Kennedy & T. J. Williams (Eds.), *Ethical practice in operational psychology: Military and national intelligence applications* (pp. 29–49). Washington, DC: American Psychological Association.

Pincus, S. H., House, R., Christenson, J., & Adler, L. E. (2001). *The emotional cycle of deployment: A military family perspective.* Retrieved from *http:// call.army.smil.mil/products/trngqtr/tq2–02/pincus.htm.*

Pope, K. S., & Garcia-Peltoniemi, R. E. (1991). Responding to victims of torture: Clinical issues, professional responsibilities, and useful resources. *Professional Psychology: Research and Practice, 22*(4), 269–276.

Post, J. (2004). *Leaders and their followers in a dangerous world: The psychology of political behavior.* Ithaca, NY: Cornell University Press.

Poythress, N. G. (1980). Optimizing the use and misuse of psychologists in a hostage situation. *Police Chief, 47*(8), 30–32

Pruitt, D. G. (1986). Achieving integrative agreements in negotiation. In R. K. White (Ed.), *Psychology and the prevention of nuclear war* (pp. 463–489). New York: New York University Press.

Reger, G. M., & Moore, B. A. (2006). Combat operational stress control in Iraq: Lessons learned during Operation Iraqi Freedom. *Military Psychology, 18*(4), 297–307.

Ritzler, B., & Singer, M. (1998). MMPI-2 by proxy and the Rorschach: A demonstration assessment of the commandant of Auschwitz. *Journal of Personality Assessment, 71*(2), 212–227.

Rubenzer, S. J., & Faschingbauer, T. R. (2004). *Personality, character, and leadership in the White House: Psychologists assess the presidents.* Washington, DC: Brassey's.

Rubin, J. Z. (1986). Some roles and functions of a mediator. In R. K. White (Ed.), *Psychology and the prevention of nuclear war* (pp. 490–510). New York: New York University Press.

Schneider, B. R., & Post, J. M. (2003). *Know thy enemy: Profiles of adversary leaders and their strategic cultures.* Maxwell Air Force Base, AL: USAF Counterproliferation Center. Retrieved from *www.airuniversity.af.edu/Portals/10/CSDS/Books/knowthyenemy3.pdf.*

Silke, A. (2001). Chasing ghosts: Offender profiling and terrorism. In D. P. Farrington, C. R. Hollin, & M. McMurran (Eds.), *Sex and violence: The psychology of crime and risk assessment* (pp. 242–258). New York: Routledge.

Smith, J. D. D. (1995). *Stopping wars: Defining the obstacles to cease-fire.* Boulder, CO: Westview Press.

Staal, M. A. (2019). Behavioral science consultation to military interrogations. In M. A. Staal & S. C. Harvey. *Operational psychology: A new field to support national security and public safety* (pp. 241–260). Santa Barbara, CA: Praeger.

Staal, M. A., & Bluestein, B. (2019). Cross-cultural issues in operational psychology. In M. A. Staal & S. C. Harvey (Eds.), *Operational psychology: A new field to support national security and public safety* (pp. 17–33). Santa Barbara, CA: Praeger.

Staal, M. A., & DeVries, M. R. (2020). Military operational psychology. *Psychological Services, 17*(2), 195–198.

Staal, M. A., & Harvey, S. C. (2019a). History, goals, and applications of operational psychology. In M. A. Staal & S. C. Harvey (Eds.), *Operational psychology: A new field to support national security and public safety* (pp. 3–16). Santa Barbara, CA: Praeger.

Staal, M. A., & Harvey, S. C. (2019b). The ethics of operational psychology. In M. A. Staal & S. C. Harvey (Eds.), *Operational psychology: A new field to support national security and public safety* (pp. 35–51). Santa Barbara, CA: Praeger.

Staal, M. A., & Harvey, S. C. (Eds.). (2019c). *Operational psychology: A new field to support national security and public safety.* Santa Barbara, CA: Praeger.

Staal, M. A., & Myers, C. (2019). Psychology of terrorism and self-radicalization. In M. A. Staal & S. C. Harvey (Eds.), *Operational psychology: A new field to support national security and public safety* (pp. 327–347). Santa Barbara, CA: Praeger.

Staal, M. A., & Stephenson, J. A. (2013). Operational psychology post-9/11: A decade of evolution. *Military Psychology, 25*(2), 93–104.

Stanton, G. (1969, Fall). Defense against communist interrogation organizations. *Studies in Intelligence, 13*(4), 49–74.

Strosnider, W. R. (2002, April 9). *Deception and the future battlefield: Information superiority at risk.* Carlisle Barracks, PA: Strategy Research Project, U.S. Army War College.

Stuart, R. B. (2004). Twelve practical suggestions for achieving multicultural competence. *Professional Psychology: Research and Practice, 35*(1), 3–9.

Sun Tzu. (1971). *The art of war* (S. B. Griffith, Trans.). New York: Oxford University Press.

Surmon-Böhr, F., Alison, L., Christiansen, P., & Alison, E. (2020). The right to silence and the permission to talk: Motivational interviewing and high-value detainees. *American Psychologist, 75*(7), 1011–1021.

Taguba, A. M. (2004). *Article 15-6 Investigation of the 800th Military Police Brigade Report*. Retrieved May 17, 2004, from *www.agonist.org/annex/taguba. html*.

Taylor, A. J. W. (1991). Individual and group behaviour in extreme situations and environments. In R. Gal & A. D. Mangelsdorff (Eds.), *Handbook of military psychology* (pp. 491–501). Chichester, UK: John Wiley & Sons.

Thompson, B., Morrow, C. E., & Staal, M. A. (2019). Personnel suitability screening. In M. A. Staal & S. C. Harvey (Eds.), *Operational psychology: A new field to support national security and public safety* (pp. 55–78). Santa Barbara, CA: Praeger.

Thornewill, A., DeMatteo, D., & Heilbrun, K. (2020). In the immediate wake of Hoffman's Independent Review: Psychologist and general public perceptions. *American Psychologist, 75*(5), 694–707.

Trail, T. E., Sims, C. S., & Tankard, M. (2019). *Today's Army spouse survey: How Army families address life's challenges*. Santa Monica, CA: RAND Corporation. Retrieved from *www.rand.org/pubs/research_reports/RR3224.html*.

Watson, B. A. (1997). *When soldiers quit: Studies in military disintegration*. Westport, CT: Praeger.

Wedgewood, R. (2004, May 23). The steps we can take to prevent another Abu Ghraib. *The Washington Post*, p. B5.

Wells, S. (2015). Hostage negotiation and communication skills in a terrorist environment. In J. Pearse (Ed.), *Investigating terrorism: Current political, legal and psychological issues* (pp. 144–166). Hoboken, NJ: Wiley-Blackwell.

White, R. K. (Ed.). (1986). *Psychology and the prevention of nuclear war*. New York: New York University Press.

Williams, T. J. (2003). Strategic leader readiness and competencies for asymmetric warfare. *Parameters, 33*(2), 19–35.

Williams, T. J., & Johnson, W. B. (2006). Introduction to special issue: Operational psychology and clinical practice in operational environments. *Military Psychology, 18*(4), 261–268.

Williams, T. J., & Kennedy, C. H. (2011). Operational psychology: Proactive ethics in a challenging world. In C. H. Kennedy & T. J. Williams (Eds.), *Ethical practice in operational psychology: Military and national intelligence applications* (pp. 125–140). Washington, DC: American Psychological Association.

Williams, T. J., Picano, J., Roland, R. R., & Bartone, P. T. (2012). Operational psychology: Science, foundation, and applications. In J. Lawrence & M. Mathews (Eds.), *Military psychology* (pp. 37–49). New York: Oxford University Press.

Wong, L., Kolditz, T. A., Millen, R. A., & Potter, T. M. (2003). *Why they fight: Combat motivation in the Iraq War*. Carlisle Barracks, PA: U.S. Army War College, Strategic Studies Institute.

Zhang, L. & Gronvall, G. K. (2020, August). Red Teaming the biological sciences for deliberate threats. *Terrorism and Political Violence 32*(6), 1225–1244.

Zillmer, E. A. (2012). The psychology of terrorists: Nazi perpetrators, the Baader–Meinhof Gang, war crimes in Bosnia, suicide bombers, the Taliban, and Al Qaeda. In C. H. Kennedy & E. A. Zillmer (Eds.), *Military psychology: Clinical and operational applications* (2nd ed., pp. 331–359). New York: Guilford Press.

Zimbardo, P. G. (1971). *The psychological power and pathology of imprisonment.* A statement prepared for the U.S. House of Representatives Committee on the Judiciary (Subcommittee No. 3; Robert Kastenmeyer, Chairman; Hearings on Prison Reform).

Zimbardo, P. G., Haney, C., Banks, W. C., & Jaffe, D. (1975). The psychology of imprisonment: Privation, power, and pathology. In D. Rosenhan & P. London (Eds.), *Theory and research in abnormal psychology* (2nd ed., pp. 270–287). New York: Holt, Rinehardt, & Winston.

CHAPTER 13

Assessment and Selection of High-Risk Operational Personnel
Key Competencies of High-Risk Operators

James J. Picano, Robert R. Roland,
and Thomas J. Williams

The assessment and selection (A&S) of military personnel for high-risk jobs and special mission units is a central role of psychologists working in operational military settings (Staal & Stephenson, 2006; Williams, Picano, Roland, & Banks, 2006). High-risk operational personnel engage in physically and psychologically demanding missions under conditions of extreme threat, isolation, and complexity (Picano, Roland, Williams, & Bartone, 2017). High-risk operational personnel are distinguished from other military and operational personnel by the specific mission profiles and operational and environmental demands they ordinarily encounter in the execution of their duties. These are outlined in Table 13.1.

Missions performed by high-risk operational personnel are typically critical and sensitive, often involving national security, and carry dire consequences for failure including death and national embarrassment. These personnel operate in dynamic and often novel tactical environments involving unknown and uncontrollable situations, have little logistical support or backup, and confront situations for which standard "textbook" solutions are insufficient. The complexity, instability, and unpredictability of these missions and environments place high adaptive performance demands on individuals who must operate in them.

According to this framework, high-risk operational personnel include, but are not limited to, Special Operations Forces (SOF) personnel, clandestine intelligence operatives, astronauts, and certain tactical law enforcement

TABLE 13.1. Occupational Demands of High-Risk Operational Jobs

Mission demands

- Nonroutine, nonstandard, or unconventional tactics
- Dire consequences for failure

Operational/environmental demands

- Unpredictable and uncontrollable factors, highly dynamic
- Extreme or harsh, hostile, and nonpermissive areas
- Various cultural settings
- High autonomy with no or very limited logistical and/or tactical support

personnel, such as police special operations personnel. Others have used the term *high-demand, high-attrition* (HDHA; Lytell et al., 2018) to refer to similar occupational groups in the U.S. Air Force with high rates of training attrition, such as pararescue jumpers (PJ) and explosive ordnance disposal (EOD). Within the U.S. Marine Corps, reconnaissance is an example of an HDHA specialty (Nowicki, 2017). The mission and environmental demands we outline differentiate high-risk operational personnel from others whose jobs have high psychological competency demands, but with a lesser degree of mission and environmental challenge, such as nuclear power plant operators, airline pilots, air traffic controllers, and most emergency services personnel, as well as others in *high-reliability* occupations (Flin, 2001).

Mission characteristics and operating environments demand individuals who possess specialized technical skills and psychological competencies well beyond those of their peers. Given this, high-risk operational personnel for the most demanding missions and operating environments undergo rigorous A&S procedures in order to determine their suitability for high-risk military assignment. These programs incorporate multiple methods to evaluate the degree to which applicants possess the competencies required for successful training and job performance. Identifying necessary competencies for this successful training and job performance is critical to the design and success of these efforts.

KEY COMPETENCIES OF HIGH-RISK OPERATIVES

The psychological competencies required of personnel who perform high-risk missions were reviewed in order to identify key or core psychological competencies required for successful performance (Picano, Williams, & Roland, 2012). Though not exhaustive, the review encompassed a wide range of high-risk operational personnel: clandestine intelligence operatives (Fiske, Hanfmann, MacKinnon, Miller, & Murray, 1997; see also Office of Strategic Services Assessment Staff, 1948); U.S. Army Special Forces soldiers (SFAS; Kilcullen, Mael, Goodwin, & Zazanis, 1999); U.S. Air Force Special Duty aircrew (Patterson, Brockway, & Greene, 2004); U.S. SOF personnel (Christian, Picano, Roland, & Williams, 2010); U.S. astronauts (Galarza & Holland, 1996): Norwegian Naval Special Forces (NSF; Hartmann, Sunde, Kristensen, & Martinussen, 2003); and undercover law enforcement officers (Girodo, 1997). These accounts spanned generations of selection efforts from World War II to the present day, and included military, nonmilitary, and non-U.S. selection efforts.

In order to distill the key psychological competencies of high-risk operational personnel, the results were organized according to 20 different competencies that emerged from a survey conducted of subject matter experts (SMEs) in the development of an assessment program for a U.S. Department of Defense (DoD) special mission unit in the Global War on Terror (Picano et al., 2012). Four competencies emerged as essential across high-risk operational personnel over time (from World War II to the present day) and across jobs: *stress tolerance, adaptability, cooperation with others,* and *overall physical fitness and stamina.*

All of the accounts reviewed emphasized some aspect of *stress tolerance,* such as staying calm under pressure, effective performance under stress, and emotional control. In addition, *adaptability,* the ability to adapt to changing demands or circumstances, emerged across all of the samples. A third critical competency, labeled *cooperation,* included labels such as "teamwork," "team orientation," or "effective group interactions." It reflects the degree to which individuals are able to subordinate their own needs for the sake of the team or group and work cooperatively with others. Perhaps because high-risk operational occupations by definition involve extreme and unusual environmental and physical challenges, all of the accounts reviewed stressed *physical fitness and stamina.*

Three other competencies were identified that were included by most (all but one) of the reports: *judgment, motivation,* and *initiative.* Exercising good judgment and reasoning in decision making emerged in most of the different accounts reviewed. Likewise, nearly all of the descriptions emphasized the need for high intrinsic motivation, self-direction, and commitment to the mission and organization. Finally, initiative, often described in terms of ambition and achievement drive, appeared in nearly all of the accounts reviewed. As a result, seven competencies were identified that were considered to be key competencies for high-risk operational personnel. Table 13.2 enumerates these seven key competencies along with sample descriptors and other labels applied to similar descriptors.

These competencies are not sufficient for characterizing any one particular group, since differences among specific mission sets and operational communities require additional unique competencies. Additionally, these competencies are broad, and more specific subcompetencies typically

TABLE 13.2. **Key Competencies for High-Risk Operational Personnel**

Competency	Descriptors	Similar or related terms
Stress tolerance	• Be emotionally resilient, sturdy • Tolerate difficulties and frustrations well • Be effective in an emergency or during periods of stress	Resilience, stress resistance, emotional stability
Cooperation	• Puts group goals ahead of individual goals • Supports team efforts • Contributes to group effectiveness	Teamwork, team orientation, interpersonal effectiveness
Adaptability	• Acts promptly to changing demands • Modifies plans in response to changing demands • Generates novel solutions to problems	Innovativeness, flexibility, resourcefulness
Physical ability	• Possess stamina and endurance • Physically fit • Rugged, able to tolerate harsh environments and conditions	Stamina, fitness
Judgment	• Accurately and quickly assesses risks, outcomes, and repercussions in problem-solving situations • Demonstrates sound judgment under pressure • Assess risks, likely outcomes, and possible repercussions in problem-solving situations	Decision making, reasoning, problem solving, critical thinking
Motivation	• Self-motivated and directed • Motivated by challenges (intrinsic motivation) • Mission (specific) orientation and interest	Self-direction, perseverance, determination
Initiative	• Displays initiative • Ambitious • Motivated to advance, achieve	Drive, energy, achievement orientation

emerge from job or competency analyses. Thus, these are viewed as key competencies that are necessary, if not sufficient, for all high-risk operational personnel. The seven competency areas identified serve as a useful beginning in developing a competency model for high-risk operational personnel selection.

A recent project examined the causes of training attrition among a family of U.S. Air Force Special Operations/combat support positions collectively viewed as HDHA jobs (Lytell et al., 2018). Among those are some that fit the definition of high-risk operational jobs as previously defined in this chapter, for example, a PJ and EOD. Other specialties included are combat control; survival, resistance, escape, evasion (SERE); Special Operations Weather Team; and Tactical Air Control Party (TACP). These specialties have a high degree of training attrition, generally around 50%, but for some, that rate is as high as 75%. Attrition rates for other specialized military training programs provide some context for the magnitude of this attrition. For example, attrition for U.S. Air Force Undergraduate Pilot Training (UPT) is under 10% (Akers, 2020), whereas attrition for the training of U.S. Navy air traffic controllers runs about 30% (Brown et al., 2019).

In addition to quantitative analysis of important predictors of training success (discussed below), Lytell and colleagues conducted qualitative analyses to identify gaps in screening and assessment of important knowledge, skills, abilities, and other characteristics (KSAOs) that might be important to training success. They performed SME interviews with U.S. Air Force operational psychologists and training instructors from the six Air Force HDHA specialty areas, as well as with SMEs on high-risk operational jobs outside of the Air Force, such as U.S. Army Special Forces, and FBI and U.S. Customs and Border Protection special operations units. Five KSAOs across the HDHA specialties were critical to training success:

- *Physical fitness.* Performs and excels in physically demanding tasks.
- *Persistence.* Continues effort, even under adverse conditions and/ or failure.
- *Teamwork.* Facilitates cooperation and positively contributes to morale and mission effectiveness.
- *Stress tolerance.* Remains composed under pressure (e.g., demanding workload; dangerous or emergency situations).
- *Critical thinking.* Identifies and analyzes problems; seeks out appropriate information, weighs relevance and accuracy of information; recognizes assumptions.

These characteristics align fairly well with those initially identified for high-risk operatives. Some differences are apparent, for example, the competency area of *adaptability* does not appear in this listing. However, upon deeper inspection of the descriptors in their report, this competency appears to be subsumed under *critical thinking* in the HDHA competency model with descriptors such as *rapidly adapts to new information* and *when necessary, comes up with creative solutions (e.g., under resource constraints)*. Likewise, the HDHA model gives prominence to *perseverance,* which did not appear among the most prevalent characteristics in the initial review, although it did appear as an important subcompetency in the domain of motivation, initiative, and drive (Picano et al., 2012). These differences might relate to the fact that not all HDHA specialties studied fit the conceptualization of high-risk operational jobs (e.g., SERE), and some differences might therefore be expected. More likely, differences result from varying levels of abstraction in the definition of the competency area with some captured broadly, comprising multiple, related subcompetencies, and others framed more narrowly. This can sometimes make direct comparisons difficult even among similarly named competencies. Another issue is that some competencies have different labels, although the descriptors suggest that they are very similar. This is known as the "jangle" fallacy and was first described by Kelley (1927). Note, for example, the similarities in our descriptors for *judgment* and those in the HDHA model for *critical thinking*, and our use of the term *cooperation (with others)* and the HDHA use of the label *teamwork*. Overall, there is considerable overlap in these two competency models, and a comparison illustrates how key competencies can cut across a family of related jobs with unusually high performance demands in different operational communities.

Another body of work demonstrates how differences among specific mission sets within the same operational job can drive the importance of specific competencies for selection in a competency model. Barrett, Holland, and Vessey (2015) conducted an extensive job analysis to identify the psychological and behavioral competencies important for NASA astronauts in a variety of mission sets involving current and projected future space missions. The mission types they considered differed on important spaceflight mission and environmental parameters, such as the size of the vehicle/habitat, mission duration, and the length of a communications delay (owing to distance from Earth). Four mission types were considered and were analogous to 6-month and 12-month missions in low Earth orbit (LEO), such as on the International Space Station, and two deep space exploration missions including deep space sorties up to 12 months in duration, and a 3-year planetary expedition (e.g., Mars exploration mission).

Interviews with a core group of SMEs, including astronauts who had flown long-duration missions, resulted in a list of 18 competencies that were relevant to the different spaceflight missions. Additional SMEs were recruited to rate the criticality of these competencies for each mission. This allowed for identification of key competencies for all astronauts regardless of mission flown, as well as the identification of specific competencies critical for a particular mission.

A number of familiar competencies for high-risk operational personnel ranked highly across all four mission profiles: *teamwork, adaptability/ stress tolerance, judgment,* and *motivation.* A perhaps less familiar one, *self-care,* described as monitoring oneself and pacing work/rest/personal time to maintain reserves, was also rated as critical across all four mission profiles. These five competencies likely comprise the core competencies of a long-duration mission astronaut. However, when the SMEs considered longer-duration missions, and especially those in which communications delay became an important mission parameter, *small-group living*, that is, tolerance of others' differences including cultural differences, respect for others' personal needs and boundaries, and respect for common living areas, increased in importance. So, too, did competencies related to increased autonomy and independence, such as solving technical issues independently and with limited resources, and working autonomously without dependence on ground input.

The results of this job analysis highlight the importance of understanding how the specific competencies in a competency model for a particular high-risk operational job can vary in importance according to the unique operational demands for the types of missions that organization performs. While key competencies for a particular job can drive the A&S of an operator, the pattern of strengths and weaknesses of those competencies can make someone more or less suitable for a particular mission in that organization.

These two reports illustrate a couple of important points. Despite similarities across high-risk jobs, there is probably not a "one-size-fits-all" competency model. Second, when judging the suitability of an applicant within a selection program, there is probably no such thing as a "plug and play" operator for all mission sets in a given organization. This latter point speaks to the importance of postselection efforts by operational psychologists to develop and train competencies in personnel, and to consult with commanders on the suitability of individuals for assignment to a specific mission.

A&S PROGRAM COMPONENTS

Personnel who perform jobs with high performance demands usually undergo some type of psychological screening to ensure that they are suitable for the work. For those in positions where public safety is concerned, such as the high reliability jobs mentioned earlier, this might involve psychological tests and/or interviews to ensure applicants are stable and free from psychiatric disorder or psychopathology. Generally speaking, as the performance demands of the job increase, so, too, does the intensity of the screening and selection effort.

Case 13.1. The Law Enforcement Officer
with Posttraumatic Symptoms

Two operational psychologists were contracted to help evaluate applicants for a specialized U.S. government tactical law enforcement unit, which drew on qualified officers within the larger organization. The A&S course consisted of a week of demanding physical and tactical activities, as well as an evaluation by the psychologist. There were no formal entry medical standards for the unit, but a competency analysis for the job identified high-stress tolerance as a critical competency. One applicant, an experienced officer, also happened to be a former active-duty military officer with combat deployments to Iraq. During the interview with the psychologist, he disclosed that he was still experiencing posttraumatic stress symptoms (e.g., nightmares and sleep difficulties) as well as some postconcussive symptoms (e.g., difficulty concentrating) from the explosion of an improvised explosive device (IED) during his deployment nearly a year earlier. The psychologist encouraged the applicant to seek treatment for his issues, and when asked directly by the applicant if his disclosure would disqualify him, the psychologist told the applicant that he would not recommend him for assignment to the unit, because he was currently vulnerable to operational stress. The nature of the deployments that the unit engaged in (including combat zones) would present an unacceptable risk to the individual's health and performance, and mission safety and success.

Assessing and selecting high-demand military operational personnel involves two stages: selecting out and selecting in (Suedfeld & Steel, 2000). In the selecting (or screening) out phase, the assessment of psychological and emotional stability—that is, freedom from psychopathology and a minimal risk of developing psychological problems in the future—is of central concern (as demonstrated in Case 13.1 above). Screening out procedures typically involve records reviews, psychological testing, and interviews. For some specialized high-demand military positions (e.g., sniper training), screening out may be the only psychological selection process used. On the other hand, selecting in involves the use of multiple selection methods to find the best-suited candidates for the nature of the work.

Personnel who perform high-risk operational missions are typically subjected to the most rigorous A&S procedures. These A&S courses are designed to assess special skills, aptitude, trainability, and sustained performance under stress using multiple methods with high fidelity to the particular operational environment. They are both physically and psychologically depleting, using physical pressures such as sleep and food restriction, heavy loads, and demanding physical events (e.g., obstacle courses, ruck marches) to both test fitness and induce stress. They often extend for several weeks. Candidates who attend these A&S programs have already passed multiple gates, including technical (military skills), medical, security, and psychological screens. In some cases, especially for the most elite units, they have been through other demanding A&S programs along the way.

The content and structure of these A&S courses are informed by the competencies that must be addressed. Most follow a typical assessment center model, which use multiple methods and measures such as detailed psychological evaluations (cognitive ability and personality tests; psychological interviews), situational tests (team and individual, usually under high-stress conditions), and physical performance/fitness events. The use of simulation tasks (or situational tests) and other performance events closely follows the assessment center model, with tasks typically designed specifically to assess the unique job demands and competencies required for the specific position. The content of these tasks and situations mimics the operational demands of the job with as much fidelity as possible. Scores for the various competencies across the assessment are aggregated and an overall assessment of suitability is determined using an individual (subjective) or mechanistic (statistical) approach, or more typically, some combination of the two (Picano et al., 2017).

Among the most common constructs measured in A&S programs for high-risk operational personnel are physical ability (especially in highly physical courses); cognitive ability (or g); and personality functioning often using standardized, omnibus measures, sometimes with scales mapped to particular competencies. Personality assessment often involves appraisal of psychopathology, which is an important "select out" criterion. For many high-risk jobs, there are specific medical and psychiatric standards that applicants must meet. The absence of psychopathology (frequently operationalized as a formal psychiatric diagnosis) is often a critical medical standard. Most psychiatric disorders bring some degree of individual instability that can be unpredictable or exacerbated under stress and can jeopardize personal or team safety, impact team cohesion (in the case of certain personality disorders), and present an unacceptable risk to mission success.

Examining the more consistent findings among these constructs that predict successful completion of these rigorous A&S programs can provide an empirical way of identifying and validating important competencies required of high-risk operational personnel and add to our understanding of those from qualitative descriptions.

PREDICTORS OF SUCCESSFUL COMPLETION IN A&S PROGRAMS FOR HIGH-RISK OPERATIONAL PERSONNEL

Physical and cognitive ability are the most consistent and significant predictors of success in A&S programs for high-risk operational personnel. Personality traits tend to be rather inconsistent predictors of success, with some more recent notable exceptions highlighted below.

Physical Ability

High-risk operational personnel engage in high-intensity operations in challenging physical environments, with tactical and logistical autonomy often requiring them to carry heavy loads for long periods. A&S courses for high-risk operational personnel simulate these physically demanding operational environments and include taxing physical events (such as obstacle courses, ruck marches, swims, etc.) and challenging performance standards to test physical ability and stamina. It comes as no surprise that baseline physical fitness, typically measured by performance on standard military physical fitness tests prior to attending the course, consistently emerges as one of the strongest, if not the strongest, predictor of successful completion of A&S programs for high-risk operational personnel including U.S. Army Special Forces (SFAS; Beal, 2010; Eskreis-Winkler, Shulman, Beal, & Duckworth, 2014; Farina et al., 2019; Tiplitzky, 1991); U.S. Navy SEALs (Taylor et al., 2006); and special duty law enforcement personnel (Orr, Caust, Hinton, & Pope, 2018). Physical fitness was the strongest predictor of training success among recruits in U.S. Air Force HDHA specialties (Lytell et al., 2018) and in the U.S. Marine Corps Basic Reconnaissance Course (Nowicki, 2017).

Case 13.2. The Special Forces Officer Who Was Suitable but Unfit

An Army Special Forces Captain volunteered for assignment to a special mission unit. The A&S course for this unit is intensely rigorous. A physical fitness test score is the best predictor of successful completion of the course. In order to minimize attrition for applicants, volunteers for this course are provided with a suggested physical training regimen prior to attending the course with recommended times, distances, and carrying loads for various training activities (e.g., ruck marches). The Captain reported to the course straight off a prolonged deployment to Afghanistan, where he was assigned to a remote outpost with little opportunity to complete the physical preparation. He was not even in his customary level of physical fitness (had routinely "maxed" his physical fitness tests). Upon initial screening evaluation prior to the onset of the assessment course, the operational psychologist found him highly suited for assignment to the unit. However, given his current physical fitness status, she concluded that he was not likely to successfully complete the course. She briefed this to the unit A&S commander who decided to drop the applicant from the assessment course, but offered him the possibility of attending the next A&S course, scheduled 6 months later.

High levels of physical fitness may exert an effect on selection and training success in multiple ways. Obviously, higher levels of precourse fitness result in better performance on important physical events in A&S courses (Lytell et al., 2018), but physical fitness also buffers stress responses in extreme military training (Taylor et al., 2008). Thus, it is plausible that physical fitness confers additional protection against the depleting effect of stress on performance in other events in these demanding A&S courses. As the case example illustrates, physical fitness is the most, if not only, modifiable predictor of success in A&S programs for high-risk operational personnel.

Cognitive Ability

Cognitive ability has consistently proven to be one of the strongest predictors of future job performance and training success across many different types of occupations (Schmitt, 2014; Schmidt & Hunter, 1998). Testing of general mental ability, or g (otherwise referred to as GMA), is a central component of the psychological evaluations in A&S programs for high-risk operational personnel (Christian et al., 2010). In such programs, cognitive ability has repeatedly been shown to predict selection for SFAS (Beale, 2010; Eskreis-Winkler et al., 2018; Hazlett & Sanders, 1999), U.S. Navy SEALs (Taylor et al., 2006), and special operations law enforcement personnel (Soccorso, Picano, Moncata, & Miller, 2019). In addition, Armed Services Vocational Aptitude Battery (ASVAB) test scores at entry into military service predict completion of PJ training (Chappelle et al., 2018; Chappelle, Skinner, Thompson, Schultz, & Hayden, 2017) and in HDHA U.S. Air Force specialties more generally (Lytell et al., 2018). The General Technical (GT) score from the ASVAB at entry also predicts successful completion of the U.S Marine Corps Basic Reconnaissance Course (Nowicki, 2017).

Consistent with theoretical assumptions about cognitive ability, applicants for high-stress occupational jobs who score higher in GMA may simply be better at performing the novel problem-solving tasks and situations confronting them in A&S programs. However, sustained military operations, those carried out with limited or no rest/sleep for greater than a 36-hour period, degrade cognitive functioning and can lead to problems in performance (Vrijkotte, Roelands, Meeusen, & Pattyn, 2016). Chronic partial sleep restriction also leads to cognitive decrements in laboratory studies (e.g., Van Dongen, Rogers, & Dinges, 2003). A&S courses leverage both of these conditions to increase performance demands on candidates. In addition, the extended stress experienced in A&S courses likely results in cognitive performance problems, as has been shown in extended high-stress military training (SERE; Harris, Hancock, & Harris, 2005). It is plausible that individuals who demonstrate higher GMA are not only better able to solve the complex novel problems confronting them in these A&S courses, but are also more "cognitively resilient" to the depleting effects of stress, fatigue, and food and sleep restriction in A&S programs because they possess a greater *cognitive reserve capacity,* which acts to ameliorate impairments in cognitive functioning resulting from this depletion (Stern & Barulli, 2019). Scores on intelligence measures or tests of GMA serve as good proxy measures of cognitive reserve capacity. Thus, individual variance in cognitive reserve capacity may partially account for the observed relationship between GMA scores and performance success in rigorous A&S courses.

Personality

The prevailing model of personality organizes personality traits into five broad domains: *emotional stability,* which includes resilience and freedom from negative emotionality; *extraversion* comprising sociability, drive, and positive emotion; *openness,* including intellectual curiosity, broad-mindedness, and aesthetic interests; *agreeableness,* including compassion, cooperation with others, and friendliness; and *conscientiousness,* including orderliness, dependability, integrity, and industriousness (Digman & Takemoto-Chock, 1981). An important meta-analysis of studies of personality in the workplace established that personality played an important predictive role in work and training performance (Barrick & Mount, 1991). Facets of conscientiousness, and to a lesser extent emotional stability, relate to a number of different job performance criteria, whereas openness to experience appears important to training success, and agreeableness tends to be important to occupations in which teamwork is critical for job success (Mount, Barrick, & Stewart, 1998; Woo, Chernyshenko, Stark, & Conz, 2014). With respect to military populations, a meta-analysis of 20 independent military samples who were administered the Self-Description Inventory, a self-report measure of the five-factor model of personality, showed emotional stability and conscientiousness to be the most important and consistent predictors of military work-related outcomes (Darr, 2011). As expected, high-risk operational personnel differ from the general population and other comparison groups on Big Five dimensions and score higher in the domains of emotional stability and conscientiousness (Picano et al., 2012).

Evidence has been less consistent for the predictive effects of personality traits in A&S for high-risk military operational personnel. Many of the studies reviewed previously failed to show differences between successfully selected individuals and failures in A&S courses for high-risk operational personnel or failed to increment beyond physical and cognitive ability (Picano et al., 2012). Recently, Chappelle and colleagues showed that personality constructs (many loading in the areas of emotional stability and conscientiousness) significantly differentiated successful graduates from PJ training, and added variance in prediction models beyond cognitive test results (Chappelle et al., 2017; Chappelle et al., 2018). Personality traits mapped primarily to emotional stability (e.g., optimism) and conscientious (responsibility) assessed using a psychometrically advanced measure specifically developed for military applications (Tailored Adaptive Personality Assessment System or TAPAS) differentiated those who passed the SFAS selection course (Nye et al., 2014). However, the TAPAS was not useful in predicting training success across U.S. Air Force HDHA specialties, including PJ (Lytell et al., 2018).

Investigators have turned to other personality constructs related to important competencies identified for high-risk operational personnel; chief among them are dispositional resilience (e.g., hardiness) and grit. *Hardiness* has been shown to relate to a number of positive outcomes in military personnel under stressful conditions, including deployment (Orme & Kehoe, 2014). It is reasonable to predict that individuals high in hardiness would be more likely to be successful in the highly stressful and resource-depleting conditions of A&S courses for high-risk operational personnel. Hardiness predicted successful completion of SFAS (Bartone, Roland, Picano, & Williams, 2008) and Norwegian border patrol military personnel (Johnsen et al., 2013). More recently, hardiness predicted success in an A&S course for U.S. special tactical law enforcement officers (Soccorso et al., 2019). In related work, resilience as conceptualized by the Connor-Davidson Resilience Scale (CD-RISC) was also found to predict successful completion of SFAS (Farina et al., 2019).

Another important construct to emerge in recent years is *grit*. Grit is a dispositional tendency to pursue long-term goals with sustained interest and effort over a prolonged period, and is thought to be a rather narrow facet of the larger personality domain of conscientiousness (Duckworth, Peterson, Matthews, & Kelly, 2007). Grit has proven to be a robust predictor of successful completion of SFAS. In an initial study, grit predicted completion of SFAS, and this effect held when other important predictors such as GMA, physical fitness, and age were controlled (Eskries-Winkler et al., 2014). In a more recent study, grit again predicted completion of SFAS (Farina et al., 2019).

CONCLUSIONS

Relatively little is published about the A&S of high-risk operational personnel owing largely to security concerns for both the missions and methods. The accumulated evidence from both job analyses and empirical studies representing multiple job specialties with high mission and environmental adaptive demands continues to highlight the importance of several key competencies to selection and training success from our earlier reviews.

Stress tolerance (resilience), motivation, initiative, teamwork, adaptability, judgment (including *reasoning* and *problem-solving under pressure*), and *stamina and physical ability* comprise these key competency areas. These should be part of any comprehensive competency assessment model in selection programs for individuals in high-risk and high-demand jobs. As a whole, our review suggests that successful performance in high-risk operational jobs requires individuals who are smart, physically fit, resilient, motivated and persistent, team-oriented, and highly responsive to changes in the surrounding operational environment and circumstances. These findings are based almost entirely on the results of assessment and training course outcomes. Studies of on-the-job performance for high-risk operators are rare. This may reflect both the realistic limitations in time and resources for operational psychologists to conduct such analyses, and the likelihood that security requirements preclude public dissemination of such findings from many high-risk operational organizations (Christian et al., 2010).

The consistency with which these competencies emerge in studies of individuals in jobs with extraordinary adaptive demands suggests that they may reflect something more fundamental about human adaptation beyond job fitness. Indeed, the staff of the Office of Strategic Services (OSS) concluded that their competencies tapped the "total potentialities of the candidate for meeting the challenges of life" (Fiske et al., 1997, p. 217). Elsewhere, we discussed how the constructs to predict job suitability in high-risk operators (viz., cognitive ability, physical fitness, personality effectiveness, and psychological and physical health) tap into a broader, latent construct that evolutionary biologists and psychologists term a *general fitness factor* (*F-factor*; Miller, 2000; see also Sefcek & Figueredo, 2010). According to this theory, one hypothetical factor, fitness factor, explains the shared variance indicated by small but robust correlations observed in population studies among measures of physical health, mental health (psychopathology), GMA or *g*, and the general factor of personality (GFP). Measures of these broader constructs, such as those used in A&S courses (e.g., intelligence tests, personality tests, and medical and physical fitness tests), serve as genetic *fitness indicators*. Thus, our competencies and the measures that are used to assess them in A&S programs may tap a more fundamental dimension of *general adaptive capacity*.

Finally, it is important to note that the competency model presented here emerged almost entirely from military job specialties for which only men were eligible in the past. Little is known about whether these or other competencies apply to women's success in these roles (a point also made by Lytell et al., 2018). As the integration of women into these career fields continues, further information will become available as to what, if any, differences in the predictors of women's success are.

REFERENCES

Akers, C. M. (2020). Undergraduate Pilot Training attrition: An analysis of individual and class composition component factors. *Theses and Dissertations,* 3749. Wright-Patterson Air Force Base, OH: Air Force Institute of Technology, AFIT Scholar. Retrieved from *https://scholar.afit.edu/etd/3749.*

Barrett, J. D., Holland, A. W., & Vessey, W. B. (2015). *Identifying the "right stuff": An exploration focused astronaut job analysis.* Philadelphia: 30th Annual Conference of the Society for Industrial and Organizational Psychology.

Barrick, M. R., & Mount, M. K. (1991). The Big Five personality dimensions and job performance: A meta-analysis. *Personnel Psychology, 44,* 1–26.

Bartone, P. T., Roland, R. R., Picano, J. J., & Williams, T. J. (2008). Psychological hardiness predicts success in U.S. Army Special Forces candidates. *International Journal of Selection and Assessment, 16*(1), 7818.

Beal, S. A. (2010). *The roles of perseverance, cognitive ability, and physical fitness in U.S. Army Special Forces assessment and selection* (Research Report 1927). Fort Belvoir, VA: United States Army Research Institute for the Behavioral and Social Sciences.

Brown, N. L., Foroughi, C. K., Coyne, J. T., Sibley, C., Olson, T., & Myrick, S. (2019). Predicting attrition and performance in Navy and Marine Corps Air Traffic Control School. *Proceedings of the Human Factors and Ergonomics Society Annual Meeting, 63*(1), 863–867.

Chappelle, W., Skinner, E., Thompson, W., Schultz, R., & Hayden, R. (2017). *Assessing the utility of noncognitive aptitudes as additional predictors of graduation from U.S. Air Force Pararescue Training.* USAFSAM/FHOH Wright-Patterson AFB United States.

Chappelle, W., Thompson, W., Ouenpraseuth, S., Spencer, H., Goodman, T., Sanford, E., et al. (2018). *Pre-training cognitive and non-cognitive psychological predictors of U.S. Air Force pararescue training outcomes* (No. AFRL-SA-WP-TR-2018–0016). Wright-Patterson Air Force Base, OH: U.S. Air Force School of Aerospace Medicine.

Christian, J. R., Picano, J. J., Roland, R. R., & Williams, T. J. (2010). Guiding principles for selecting high-risk operational personnel. In P. T. Bartone, B. H. Johnsen, J. Eid, M. Violanti, & J. C. Laberg (Eds.), *Enhancing human performance in security operations: International law enforcement perspectives* (pp. 121–142). Springfield, IL: Charles C. Thomas.

Darr, W. (2011). Military personality research: A meta-analysis of the Self Description Inventory. *Military Psychology, 23*(3), 272–296.

Digman, J. M., & Takemoto-Chock, N. K. (1981). Factors in the natural language of personality: Re-analysis, comparison, and interpretation of six major studies. *Multivariate Behavioral Research, 16,* 149–170.

Duckworth, A. L., Peterson, C., Matthews, M. D., & Kelly, D. R. (2007). Grit: Perseverance and passion for long-term goals. *Journal of Personality and Social Psychology, 92*(6), 1087–1101.

Eskreis-Winkler, L., Shulman, E. P., Beal, S. A. & Duckworth, A. L. (2014). The grit effect: Predicting retention in the military, the workplace, school and marriage. *Frontiers in Psychology, 5,* 1–12.

Farina, E. K., Thompson, L. A., Knapik, J. J., Pasiakos, S. M., McClung, J. P., & Lieberman, H. R. (2019). Physical performance, demographic, psychological, and physiological predictors of success in the U.S. Army Special Forces Assessment and Selection Course. *Physiology & Behavior, 210,* 112647.

Fiske, D. W., Hanfmann, E., MacKinnon, D. W., Miller, J. G., & Murray, H. A. (1997). *Selection of personnel for clandestine operations: Assessment of men.* Laguna Hills, CA: Aegean Park Press.

Flin, R. (2001). Selecting the right stuff: Personality and high-reliability occupations. In R. Hogan & B. R. Roberts (Eds.), *Personality psychology in the workplace* (pp. 253–275). Washington, DC: American Psychological Association.

Galarza, L., & Holland, A. (1996). *Critical astronaut proficiencies required for long-duration spaceflight* (SAE Technical Paper 1999-01-2097). Washington, DC: Society of Automotive Engineers.

Girodo, M. (1997). Undercover agent assessment centers: Crafting vice and virtue for imposters. *Journal of Social Behavior and Personality, 12*(5), 237–260.

Harris, W. C., Hancock, P. A., & Harris, S. C. (2005). Information processing changes following extended stress. *Military Psychology, 17*(2), 115–128.

Hartmann, E., Sunde, T., Kristensen, W., & Martinussen, M. (2003). Psychological measures as predictors of training performance. *Journal of Personality Assessment, 80,* 87–98.

Hazlett, G. A., & Sanders, M. (1999). Cognitive and personality assessment in Special Forces assessment and selection. *Special Warfare, 12*(4), 14–20.

Johnsen, B. H., Bartone, P., Sandvik, A. M., Gjeldnes, R., Morken, A. M., Hystad, S. W., et al. (2013). Psychological hardiness predicts success in a Norwegian armed forces border patrol selection course. *International Journal of Selection and Assessment, 21*(4), 368–375.

Kelley, T. L. (1927). *Interpretation of educational measurements.* Oxford, UK: World Book.

Kilcullen, R. N., Mael, F. A., Goodwin, G. F., & Zazanis, M. M. (1999). Predicting U.S. Army Special Forces field performance. *Human Performance in Extreme Environments, 4,* 53–63.

Lytell, M. C., Robson, S., Schulker, D., Krueger, T. C., Matthews, M., Mariano, L. T., et al. (2018). *Training success for U.S. Air Force Special Operations and combat support specialties: An analysis of recruiting, screening, and development processes* (RR-2002-AF). Santa Monica, CA: RAND Corporation.

Miller, G. F. (2000). Mental traits as fitness indicators: Expanding evolutionary psychology's adaptationism. In D. LeCroy & P. Moller (Eds.), *Evolutionary approaches to human reproductive behavior.* In *Annals of the New York Academy of Sciences* (No. 907, pp. 62–74).

Mount, M. K., Barrick, M. R., & Stewart, G. L. (1998). Five-factor model of personality and performance in jobs involving interpersonal interactions. *Human Performance, 11,* 145–165.

Nowicki, A. C. (2017). *United States Marine Corps basic reconnaissance course: Predictors of success.* Monterey, CA: Naval Postgraduate School.

Nye, C. D., Beal, S. A., Drasgow, F., Dressel, J. D., White, L. A., & Stark, S. (2014). *Assessing the Tailored Adaptive Personality Assessment System for Army*

Special Operations Forces *personnel*. Fort Belvoir, VA: U.S. Army Research Institute for the Behavioral and Social Sciences.

Office of Strategic Services Assessment Staff. (1948). *Assessment of men: Selection of personnel for the Office of Strategic Services*. New York: Rinehart.

Orme, G. J., & Kehoe, E. J. (2014). Hardiness as a predictor of mental health and well-being of Australian Army reservists on and after stability operations, *Military Medicine, 179*, 404–412.

Orr, R. M., Caust, E. L., Hinton, B., & Pope, R. (2018). Selecting the best of the best: Associations between anthropometric and fitness assessment results and success in police specialist selection. *International Journal of Exercise Science, 11*(4), 785.

Patterson, J. C., Brockway, J., & Greene, C. (2004). *Evaluation of an Air Force Special Duty assessment and selection program* (Contract F41624-00-6/1001/0001). San Antonio, TX: Conceptual MindWorks.

Picano, J. J., Roland, R. R., Williams, T. J., & Bartone, P. T. (2017) Assessment of elite operational personnel. In S. Bowles & P. Bartone (Eds.), *Handbook of military psychology* (pp. 277–289). Cham, Switzerland: Springer.

Picano, J. J., Williams, T. J., & Roland, R. R. (2012). Assessment and selection of high-risk operational personnel. In C. H. Kennedy & E. A. Zillmer (Eds.), *Military psychology: Clinical and operational applications* (2nd ed., pp. 50–72). New York: Guilford Press.

Schmidt, J. E., & Hunter, F. L. (1998). The validity and utility of selection methods in personnel psychology: practical and theoretical implications of 85 years of research findings. *Psychological Bulletin, 24*, 262–274.

Schmitt, N. (2014). Personality and cognitive ability as predictors of effective performance at work. *Annual Review of Organizational Psychology and Organizational Behavior, 1*, 45–65.

Sefcek, J. A., & Figueredo, A. J. (2010). A life-history model of human fitness indicators. *Biodemography and Social Biology, 56*, 42–66.

Soccorso, C. N., Picano, J. J., Moncata, S. J., & Miller, C. D. (2019). Psychological hardiness predicts successful selection in a law enforcement special operations assessment and selection course. *International Journal of Selection and Assessment, 27*(3), 291–295.

Staal, M. A., & Stephenson, J. A. (2006). Operational psychology: An emerging subdiscipline. *Military Psychology, 18*(4), 269–282.

Stern, Y., & Barulli, D. (2019). Cognitive reserve. In S. T. Dekosky & S. Asthana (Eds.), *Handbook of clinical neurology: Vol. 167. Geriatric neurology* (pp. 181–190). Amsterdam: Elsevier.

Suedfeld, P., & Steel, G. D. (2000). The environmental psychology of capsule habitats. *Annual Review of Psychology, 51*, 227–253.

Taylor, M. K., Markham, A. E., Reis, J. P., Padilla, G. A., Potterat, E. G., Drummond, S., et al. (2008). Physical fitness influences stress reactions to extreme military training. *Military Medicine, 173*(8), 738–742.

Taylor, M. K., Miller, A., Mills, L., Potterat, E., Padilla, G. A., & Hoffman, R. (2006). *Predictors of success in Basic Underwater Demolition/SEAL (BUDIS) Training—Part 1: What do we know and where do we go from here?* (Technical Document No. 06–3). San Diego, CA: Naval Health Research Center.

Tiplitzky, M. L. (1991). *Physical performance predictors of success in Special*

Forces assessment and selection (Research Report 1606). Fort Belvoir, VA: United States Army Research Institute for the Behavioral and Social Sciences.

Van Dongen, H. P., Rogers, N. L., & Dinges, D. F. (2003). Sleep debt: Theoretical and empirical issues. *Sleep and Biological Rhythms, 1*(1), 5–13.

Vrijkotte, S., Roelands, B., Meeusen, R., & Pattyn, N. (2016). Sustained military operations and cognitive performance. *Aerospace Medicine and Human Performance, 87*(8), 718–727.

Williams, T. J., Picano, J. J., Roland, R. R., & Banks, L. M. (2006). Introduction to operational psychology. In C. H. Kennedy & E. A. Zillmer (Eds.), *Military psychology: Clinical and operational applications* (pp. 193–214). New York: Guilford Press.

Woo, S. E., Chernyshenko, O. S., Stark, S. E., & Conz, G. (2014). Validity of six openness facets in predicting work behaviors: A meta-analysis. *Journal of Personality Assessment, 96*(1), 76–86.

CHAPTER 14

Security Clearance Evaluations

Carrie H. Kennedy and Sally Harvey

Meeting the qualifications for a security clearance, as well as maintaining those same qualifications over time, is a fundamental requirement for many military jobs, given that the business of the military is national security. Because the primary issue at stake in deciding to grant someone a clearance is essentially an attempt to predict the behavior of an individual with access to classified information and/or materiel, military psychologists necessarily play a critical role in the security clearance process. Specifically, military psychologists address security clearances in three contexts:

1. The conduct of a formal security clearance mental health evaluation at the request of the granting agency, due to concerns related to an individual's mental health history (initial clearance) or current mental health status (maintenance of the clearance) and consequent concerns about stability, judgment, reliability, and/or trustworthiness,
2. When questioned by the granting agency regarding a prior or existing patient, or
3. As a general recommendation in the course of fitness-for-duty evaluations.

This chapter will review the mental health professional's role in the context of these three scenarios as well as review the fundamental components of a comprehensive security clearance evaluation. It is important to note that the role of the psychologist is to provide a targeted assessment of the individual's capacity to meet the requirements for a security clearance (the aforementioned stability, judgment, reliability, and trustworthiness), not to render an opinion as to whether the individual should be granted a clearance. This determination is entirely up to the granting agency and its decision is based on multiple sources of information, of which the mental health professional's input is but one.

COMPONENTS OF THE SECURITY CLEARANCE EVALUATION

Security clearance evaluations are akin to forensic evaluations and must be viewed with this standard in mind (Young, Harvey, & Staal, 2011). Consequently, when conducting a formal security clearance evaluation, there is no traditional doctor–patient relationship and these evaluations are routinely performed by both clinical psychologists and operational psychologists (see Chapter 12, this volume; Myers & Trent, 2019), depending on the setting. Recognizing that not all evaluations are performed by military or government mental health professionals, the Office of the Director of National Intelligence (ODNI, 2017) describes those who perform these evaluations as "a duly qualified mental health professional (e.g., clinical psychologist or psychiatrist) employed by, or acceptable to and approved by the U.S. Government" (p. 19). Regardless of whether the evaluation is being conducted within a military treatment facility or an operational command or by a uniformed, government or civilian psychologist, the process is the same and includes informed consent, clinical interview, psychometric assessment, and record/collateral information review.

Informed Consent

While the entire security clearance process is highly invasive, as it pertains to personal privacy, it is important to remember that the process is also voluntary.[1] A security clearance evaluation is only conducted because an agency is asking to obtain or maintain a clearance for the individual in question. An individual who has not already consented to the process with the granting agency will not be referred for an evaluation. Prior to arrival at the appointment, the individual will have already provided an authorization for release of medical information, which includes the disclosure of the answers to four mental health-related questions (Standard Form 86; U.S. Office of Personnel Management, 2017):

---

[1] Refusal to participate in the process will necessarily result in the agency being unable to disposition the clearance request. Per the U.S. Office of Personnel Management (2017), "Providing the information is voluntary. If you do not provide each item of requested information, however, we will not be able to complete your investigation, which will adversely affect your eligibility for a national security position, eligibility for access to classified information, or logical or physical access."

1. Does the person under investigation have a condition[2] that could impair his or her judgment, reliability, or trustworthiness?
2. If so, describe the nature of the condition and the extent and duration of the impairment or treatment.
3. What is the prognosis?
4. Dates of treatment?

This authorization however does not negate the need for the mental health professional to obtain informed consent prior to the evaluation, though that informed consent should be tailored to the context of the evaluation. The psychologist should take care to ensure that the service member understands that he or she is not entitled to a copy of the evaluation and will receive no feedback from the psychologist, that the service member is aware of the potential outcomes of the evaluation, that there is no traditional doctor–patient relationship, and that the service member is aware that he or she has waived the HIPAA Privacy Rule as it pertains to disclosure. The service member should also be reminded that the evaluation is voluntary and that he or she is able to decline participation.

Clinical Interview

The clinical interview conducted for the purposes of a security clearance evaluation is similar to that conducted for the purpose of a fitness-for-duty evaluation (see Chapter 2, this volume for a discussion of these components). However, other, nonroutine areas of psychological functioning should be included. The psychologist should consider the Security Executive Agent Directive 4 (SEAD 4) National Security Adjudicative Guidelines (ODNI, 2017) when conducting the evaluation and focus on those areas of particular importance to mental health functioning and related behavior. The adjudicative guidelines include:

Guideline A: Allegiance to the United States
Guideline B: Foreign Influence
Guideline C: Foreign Preference
Guideline D: Sexual Behavior
Guideline E: Personal Conduct
Guideline F: Financial Considerations
Guideline G: Alcohol Consumption
Guideline H: Drug Involvement and Substance Misuse

---

[2]It is important to note that the ODNI adjudicative guidelines (2017) do not treat the word "condition" in the same manner as most mental health professionals. Question 1 is not asking if the individual has a formal diagnosis, but rather any circumstance that raises concerns about stability, judgment, reliability, or trustworthiness.

Guideline I: Psychological Conditions
Guideline J: Criminal Conduct
Guideline K: Handling Protected Information
Guideline L: Outside Activities
Guideline M: Use of Information Technology

This list comprises many factors that are addressed in any standard psychological evaluation, as well as others that might not necessarily be a focus of a traditional mental health assessment but are pertinent to this type of evaluation. As it pertains to the mental health evaluation, Guidelines D–J should be considered integral components. Let's consider these briefly.

Guideline D: Sexual Behavior

Sexual behavior is usually not the primary focus of a traditional fitness-for-duty evaluation, but for the purposes of a security clearance evaluation, the presence of problematic or risky sexual behavior is a significant issue, and the topic should be addressed during each evaluation.[3] Issues such as pornography habits and preferences, involvement with prostitutes, impulse control and judgment as it relates to sexual decisionmaking, and the like are important areas to cover. Per the ODNI adjudicative guidelines, in addition to obvious problems related to criminal sexual behavior, concerns revolve around "a pattern of compulsive, self-destructive, or high-risk sexual behavior that the individual is unable to stop" and/or "sexual behavior that causes an individual to be vulnerable to coercion, exploitation, or duress" (2017, p. 12). Schendel and Kennedy (2020) provide an example of an Army Sergeant (SGT) with long-standing transvestic fetishism, which would normally not preclude a security clearance, except that he attempted to hide it (e.g., making him "vulnerable to coercion, exploitation, or duress"). The SGT went so far as to physically threaten his coworkers, family, and friends who were interviewed as a part of the clearance process if they disclosed it, raising obvious concerns about his judgment, reliability, and trustworthiness.

Guideline E: Personal Conduct

Under Guideline E, the primary concern is any behavior that raises questions about "an individual's reliability, trustworthiness, and ability to protect classified or sensitive information" (pp. 12–13). This covers a wide range of behavior, ranging from a pattern of rule violations to a history of violence. The reader is directed to the adjudicative guidelines (pp. 12–15) for a comprehensive discussion. However, of particular interest to a mental

---

[3]Note that the adjudicative guidelines expressly state that "no adverse inference . . . may be raised solely on the basis of the sexual orientation of the individual" (p. 12).

health professional conducting a security clearance evaluation is that the provision of false or misleading information or the omission of relevant information to any professional involved in the security clearance determination, to include the mental health professional, is considered personal conduct that is contrary to granting or maintaining a security clearance. In the course of conducting the evaluation, should the mental health professional learn that the service member has not been forthright regarding his or her mental health history, this would be considered a "condition" that would be reported to the requesting/granting agency.

Guideline F: Financial Considerations

While the background investigation will assess for illegal financial issues, significant debt, tax issues, etc., the security clearance evaluation should consider mental health issues relevant to finances. These may include signs consistent with such mental health conditions as a personality disorder (e.g., a pattern of taking financial advantage of others or pathologic entitlement), manic episodes with significant spending, an impulse control problem (e.g., a pattern of grossly irresponsible spending), or an addictive problem, such as a gambling disorder or compulsive shopping that have resulted in significant financial issues. Using gambling as an example, problem or pathological gambling places an individual at great risk of doing something potentially reckless to satisfy debts, and gambling debts can accumulate quickly. In one study of primarily enlisted service members in gambling treatment, average gambling debt was \$11,407 (SD = \$17,746) and average gambling losses were \$24,154 (SD = \$33,125; Kennedy, Cook, Poole, Brunson, & Jones, 2005). Consider the following case.

Case 14.1. The Soldier Who Badly Needed Money

The soldier was a Sergeant First Class with a security clearance and access to a classified program. He had recently been placing bets on sporting events, which got quickly out of control. Over the course of 3 months, he depleted his life savings and was approximately \$20,000 in debt. He began aggressively chasing his losses, compounding his debt, borrowing money from disreputable sources, and becoming increasingly desperate. He decided to take classified information from his workspace and try to find a buyer. Fortunately, safeguards within the program alerted the chain of command to irregularities, and his attempted theft was thwarted.

Finances are not normally considered a routine part of a mental health evaluation, but the way that people make financial decisions, their financial situation, their financial priorities, and the way in which they approach debt and spending can be valuable pieces of information. These all relate to personality characteristics or mental health disorders that can be key to the conceptualization of any security clearance evaluation.

Guideline G: Alcohol Consumption

The alcohol portion of the security clearance evaluation is similar to that of a standard substance use evaluation (see Chapter 7, this volume), with an additional focus on drinking habits in those who do not meet criteria for a disorder. Alcohol consumption, given its widespread use, legality, and judgment-impairing properties, is clearly a concern for those with security clearances. The adjudicative guidelines state, "Excessive alcohol consumption often leads to the exercise of questionable judgment or the failure to control impulses, and can raise questions about an individual's reliability and trustworthiness" (p. 16). Thus, the evaluating psychologist will need to assess not just for the presence of a disorder, but of the service member's drinking habits overall and how they make decisions regarding when and where to drink and how much they drink on those occasions. For example, in a typical alcohol evaluation, a service member's decision to arrange for a designated driver because there is a plan to become intoxicated may be considered responsible drinking. For an individual with a clearance, a decision to become intoxicated at all may be an issue. Per the guidelines, "Binge consumption of alcohol to the point of impaired judgment, regardless of whether the individual is diagnosed with alcohol use disorder" is considered a condition that raises a security concern. For the security clearance evaluation, any irresponsible drinking would prompt a "yes" response to the following question: Does the person under investigation have a condition that could impair his or her judgment, reliability, or trustworthiness? Consider the following case depicting the dangers of intoxication.

Case 14.2. The Sailor Who Exhibited Poor Judgment

The sailor's ship pulled into port in a foreign country, and he was granted liberty to go into town. Like all of the other sailors, he had been onboard for a long time and really wanted to get off the ship and relax. This sailor had a security clearance and was privy to certain classified planned operations of the ship. He entered a local bar with a plan to have no more than two beers. Shortly after he sat down, an attractive local woman approached him and they drank for several hours. By the time he left the bar, he had revealed all of the ship's upcoming movements to her. He realized what he had done the next morning and reported himself to the ship's security officer.

Guideline H: Drug Involvement and Substance Misuse

Like the alcohol portion of the evaluation, assessing for other substance concerns is standard (see Chapter 7, this volume) and should include assessment related to the use of illegal drugs, misuse of prescription/nonprescription medications, or any other substance that can "cause physical or mental impairment" (p. 17), as well as a history of treatment or other intervention.

The concerns about the use of mind-altering substances are that "such behavior may lead to physical or psychological impairment and because it raises questions about a person's ability or willingness to comply with laws, rules, and regulations" (p. 17). Like the alcohol section above, any findings in this area would prompt a "yes" response to the following question: Does the person under investigation have a condition that could impair his or her judgment, reliability, or trustworthiness? See Case 14.5 for an example.

Guideline I: Psychological Conditions

Per the adjudicative guidelines, "Certain emotional, mental, and personality conditions can impair judgment, reliability, or trustworthiness. A formal diagnosis of a disorder is not required for there to be a concern under this guideline" (p. 19). In addition to judgment, reliability, and trustworthiness concerns cited throughout the guidelines, stability is added as an extra dimension here, with the assumption that any instability threatens judgment, reliability, and/or trustworthiness. A "condition" in this realm includes such behaviors as irresponsibility, violence, self-harm, suicidality, paranoia, manipulative behavior, impulsivity, lying, deceit, exploitation, bizarre behaviors, pathological gambling (see the Guideline F: Financial Considerations section above), and/or failure to follow a treatment plan. Consider the following case.

Case 14.3. The Sergeant Who Cut Herself

The Army Sergeant had a history going back to her teenaged years of cutting herself with a razor blade when she became stressed. At no time did she consider suicide; rather, the cutting was a coping strategy that brought her stress relief. In light of this history, she was referred for a security clearance evaluation when she applied for a clearance in the context of a new job in the Army. Her evaluation revealed poor coping strategies, multiple attempts to replace the cutting behavior with healthier alternatives, and borderline personality traits but no diagnosis. When responding to the question "Does the person under investigation have a condition that could impair his or her judgment, reliability, or trustworthiness?," the psychologist responded with a "yes" and outlined the history of the cutting behavior and prognosis.

It is important for an interviewing psychologist to understand that most of the time when he or she identifies a "condition," this does not mean that the service member will not get a clearance. However, the requesting agency needs to have pertinent information, as it will be combined with other sources of information unknown to the psychologist in order to make a final determination. It is also important for the psychologist to know what "conditions" mitigate security concerns within the psychological conditions guideline. These include the following: that the condition is treatable, that the service member is currently actively participating in treatment and has a good prognosis, that the condition has been successfully treated, that the condition was temporary, and/or that there are no current problems. In the case presented above, the Sergeant went into treatment, was able to replace her cutting behavior with other coping strategies, and was granted a clearance.

It is important to note that government agencies encourage individuals to receive treatment in order to maintain optimal mental health. Consider this statement from the security clearance application (Standard Form 86; U.S. Office of Personnel Management, 2017):

> Mental health treatment and counseling, in and of itself, is not a reason to revoke or deny eligibility for access to classified information or for holding a sensitive position, suitability or fitness to obtain or retain Federal or contract employment, or eligibility for physical or logical access to federally controlled facilities or information systems. Seeking or receiving mental health care for personal wellness and recovery may contribute favorably to decisions about your eligibility.

It is also important to note that government agencies recognize that their personnel may experience trauma. Because of this, special instructions are provided to the following question on the security clearance application:

> Do you have a mental health or other health condition that substantially adversely affects your judgment, reliability, or trustworthiness even if you are not experiencing such symptoms today? (Note: If your judgment, reliability, or trustworthiness is not substantially adversely affected by a mental health or other condition, then you should answer "no" even if you have a mental health or other condition requiring treatment. For example, if you are in need of emotional or mental health counseling as a result of service as a first responder, service in a military combat environment, having been sexually assaulted or a victim of domestic violence, or marital issues, but your judgment, reliability, or trustworthiness is not substantially adversely affected, then answer "no."

Guideline J: Criminal Conduct

While criminal conduct will be thoroughly explored by the requesting agency, past offenses should be a part of the evaluation, as they are for any fitness-for-duty evaluation. Given that some conduct provides information regarding mental health (e.g., alcohol-related incidents) and personality functioning (e.g., antisocial personality disorder), questions about criminal offenses/behavior should be included in the security clearance evaluation.

Psychometric Assessment

Psychometric assessment is a critical tool in any evaluation in which impression management may be an issue. Given that individuals who are undergoing a security clearance evaluation are motivated to make a good impression, formal psychometric assessment provides important information about the psychological functioning of the service member. Specifically, a psychological test measuring potential psychopathology and maladaptive personality traits and includes validity measures is a key component of the evaluation. Face valid screening instruments are not considered useful in the conduct of a security clearance evaluation.

Record Review and Collateral Information

The psychologist should review the military medical record, any civilian mental health treatment records, all documentation provided by the requesting agency, and any other information/records deemed pertinent. Particularly when preservice mental health diagnoses and/or treatment are the issue, the mental health professional will need to review pertinent records or conduct a phone interview with the previous treating provider.

EXISTING OR PRIOR PATIENTS WITH SECURITY CLEARANCES

For those mental health providers who provide care to service members with clearances, there will be times when an investigator contacts them to ask the same four questions outlined above. Note that a treating provider is not expected to have the breadth of information gathered in the course of a formal security clearance evaluation, and the questions are answered based on what the psychologist already knows. When this occurs, the investigator will provide the medical disclosure form that has already been signed by the service member and in these cases the mental health provider does not need to seek additional releases of information for the information to be provided. With most concepts in the mental health field, there is some subjectivity in determining if someone has a "condition" of interest.[4] For example, an individual may be in treatment and have a formal diagnosis but not be considered to have a "condition" per the adjudicative guidelines. On the other hand, the individual may not have a diagnosis but have a "condition" per the guidelines (see also Case 14.3 above). Consider the following cases.

---

[4]The reader is directed to the adjudicative guidelines that provide behavioral definitions for each guideline for the most comprehensive and objective explanation of behaviors/concerns that constitute a condition (ODNI, 2017).

Case 14.4. The Major with Insomnia and a Clearance

The Marine Major was referred to the psychologist by his primary-care physician due to sleep difficulties, specifically to receive cognitive-behavioral therapy for insomnia (CBT-I). The psychologist provided this treatment, and in conjunction with some lifestyle changes, the Major's insomnia resolved. Ten months later when the Major's security clearance was up for renewal, the psychologist was interviewed by an investigator. The standard first question was posed: Does the person under investigation have a condition that could impair his or her judgment, reliability, or trustworthiness? The psychologist responded "no" to this question and the interview concluded.

Case 14.5. The Captain Who Tested Positive for Marijuana

The Air Force Captain tested positive for marijuana on a routine random drug screen. He was referred to the psychologist for a substance abuse evaluation upon which no diagnosis was given. His marijuana use was determined to be a one-time lapse in judgment. When asked by the investigator if the Captain had a condition that could impair his judgment, reliability, or trustworthiness, the psychologist answered "yes" and proceeded to answer the remaining questions as applicable. Any illegal drug use is considered a condition that could impair judgment, reliability, or trustworthiness given that substance use may result in psychological and cognitive impairment, and illegal substance use indicates that the individual is unable to follow basic regulations.

One final note about prior or existing patients: Psychologists should avoid conducting a formal security clearance evaluation on a known patient. Because the nature of the relationship with the service member is significantly different when conducting the security clearance evaluation than when serving as a care provider, this puts the psychologist in a problematic dual role (see Chapter 17, this volume) and can compromise the care of existing service member patients.

SECURITY CLEARANCE RECOMMENDATIONS WITHIN FITNESS-FOR-DUTY EVALUATIONS

While true security clearance evaluations are conducted at the request of the granting agency, and are forensic or operational in nature, clinical military psychologists will routinely interface with patients with clearances. Because mental health providers frequently see service members experiencing acute psychiatric crises or in the context of the diagnosis of a serious mental health condition, they end up having to consider clearances as they conduct fitness-for-duty evaluations on a regular basis. These may be as a result of voluntary self or medical referrals or as command-directed referrals (for a comprehensive discussion of fitness-for-duty evaluations, see Chapter 2, this volume). Either way, one of the critical responsibilities of these evaluations is an assessment of risk. Psychologists typically think of risk in the context of potential suicide or homicide; however, military psychologists also need to consider access to classified information and materiel. Depending on their specific job, service members may have routine access to a variety of classified programs and information, which if handled improperly could cause damage to national security. As a reminder, disclosure of confidential information can cause damage to national security; disclosure of secret information can cause serious damage; and disclosure of top secret information can cause grave damage (Executive Order No. 13526, 2010).

Assessing the risk of disclosing classified information is very similar to that of other areas of risk. Just as a psychologist is expected to provide recommendations regarding such areas as access to weapons and deployability on every fitness-for-duty evaluation, access to classified information should also be articulated for those with security clearances. Recall that key to concerns regarding mental health and security clearances are an individual's stability, judgment, reliability, and trustworthiness. Consider the following case.

Case 14.6. The Angry and Distraught Chief with a Top Secret Clearance

A Navy Chief Petty Officer (commonly referred to simply as Chief) presented for an emergent mental health evaluation following a referral from his primary-care physician due to concerns of potential suicide risk. His wife recently filed for divorce; he learned that she had been cheating on him with multiple men; she had emptied their bank account; and she had moved out of their apartment, taking their kids and dog with her.

He voiced thoughts of being better off dead to the primary-care physician, who walked him over to the mental health department. In the context of the evaluation, the Chief noted suicidal thoughts, but no current plan or intent. He presented angry, distraught, impulsive, in disbelief, agitated, and with urges and plans to go and confront his wife.

There was a lot for the provider to manage in this case; however, in the context of the security clearance, what should the psychologist do? Just like the psychologist will recommend that the command temporarily remove the Chief's access to weapons, the same principles are in play for his clearance. He is currently demonstrating poor judgment, emotionally is not himself, and the psychologist believes him to be impulsive. Recall that disclosure of information classified at the top secret level can cause grave damage to national security; thus, risk to others takes on an additional dimension. The psychologist in this case planned for aggressive outpatient

and command support until the crisis passed, and the Chief was thinking more rationally. The psychologist recommended to the command that the Chief not have current access to weapons or classified information, and it was arranged that one of his friends would come and pick him up and stay with him for emotional support and help guide his decision making in the crisis (e.g., rethink his decision to confront his wife at this time). The command provided the Chief with the time to address his home situation, and once the situation had stabilized, all of his privileges were restored.

CONCLUSION

Psychologists play an important role in the security clearance process. They have the ability to put together many facets of information, to look at an individual's past and current mental health status, and to provide critical information to the requesting agency. This makes the psychological evaluation an especially important tool in the agency's decision-making process and directly contributes to national security.

It is important to know that very few people lose their security clearances for mental health reasons alone. According to Shedler and Lang (2015), almost no one has a clearance denied or revoked exclusively due to mental health conditions. In fact, between 2006 and 2010, 0.002% of clearances were denied solely due to a mental health concern. Rather, personal conduct, specifically, alcohol-related incidents, criminal conduct, drug use, and significant financial problems are the most frequent causes of denial or loss of a security clearance (Fischer & Morgan, 2002). It is also important to note that the intelligence community is not motivated to deny or remove clearances, and that mental health services and employee assistance programs are encouraged in order to avoid significant problems and help people maintain both mental health and their clearance/career (Clavelle, 2009). Most mental health conditions of concern can be mitigated through treatment.

REFERENCES

Clavelle, P. R. (2009). Consulting to the intelligence community: An employee assistance program model. *Consulting Psychology Journal: Practice and Research, 61*(1), 14–24.

Executive Order No. 13526. (2010, January 5). Federal Register, Vol. 75, No. 2. Retrieved July 20, 2021, from *www.govinfo.gov/content/pkg/CFR-2010-title3-vol1/pdf/CFR-2010-title3-vol1-eo13526.pdf.*

Fischer, L. F., & Morgan, R. W. (2002). *Sources of information and issues leading to clearance revocations* (PERSEREC Technical Report 02-1). Retrieved July 7, 2021, from *https://apps.dtic.mil/sti/pdfs/ADA411037.pdf.*

Kennedy, C. H., Cook, J. H., Poole, D. R., Brunson, C. L., & Jones, D. E. (2005).
    Review of an overseas military gambling treatment program. *Military Medi-
    cine, 170*, 683–687.
Myers, C., & Trent, A. (2019). Operational psychology in insider threat. In M. A.
    Staal & S. C. Harvey (Eds.), *Operational psychology: A new field to sup-
    port national security and public safety* (pp. 157–184). Santa Barbara, CA:
    Praeger.
Office of the Director of National Intelligence. (2017). *Security Executive Agent
    Directive 4: National Security Adjudicative Guidelines.* Retrieved July 12,
    2021, from *www.dni.gov/files/NCSC/documents/Regulations/SEAD-4-Ad-
    judicative-Guidelines-U.pdf.*
Schendel, C., & Kennedy, C. H. (2020). Consultation within the military setting. In
    C. A. Falender & E. P. Shafranske (Eds.), *Consultation in health service psy-
    chology: Advancing professional practice—A competency-based approach*
    (pp. 301–318). Washington, DC: American Psychological Association.
Shedler, J., & Lang, E. L. (2015). *A relevant risk approach to mental health inqui-
    ries in Question 21 of the Questionnaire for National Security Positions (SF-
    86)* (PERSEREC Technical Report 15-01). Retrieved July 7, 2021, from *www.
    dhra.mil/Portals/52/Documents/perserec/TR_15–01_A_Relevant_Risk_
    Approach_to_Mental_Health_Inquiries_in_Question_21.pdf.*
U.S. Office of Personnel Management (2017, July). *Standard Form 86: Question-
    naire for National Security Positions.* Retrieved July 8, 2021, from *www.
    opm.gov/forms/pdf_fill/sf86.pdf.*
Young, J., Harvey, S., & Staal, M.A. (2011). Ethical considerations in the conduct
    of security clearance evaluations. In C. H. Kennedy & T. J. Williams (Eds.),
    *Ethical practice in operational psychology: Military and national intelligence
    applications* (pp. 51–68). Washington DC: American Psychological Associa-
    tion.

CHAPTER 15

Survival, Evasion, Resistance, and Escape Training

Preparing Military Members for the Demands of Captivity

Melissa D. Hiller Lauby and Charles A. Morgan III

In the ever-changing landscape of the battlefield, survival, evasion, resistance, and escape training (SERE) psychologists are being called on to ensure that members of the U.S. military are prepared to face emerging challenges and threats. A SERE psychologist in his or her many roles, as evaluator, educator, risk manager, researcher, and consultant, serves to assist U.S. servicemen and women in performing under stress, and when necessary, returning with honor. This chapter is intended to serve as a primer for those psychologists seeking to develop skills in SERE psychology.

HISTORY OF SURVIVAL SCHOOLS

Historically, those captured in battle or surrender have faced uncertain treatment at the hands of their enemies. During the 19th century, there were several efforts to ensure humane treatment for those captured in war, culminating in the Hague Convention in 1907 and the 1929 Geneva Convention on Prisoners of War. During World War II, there were several initiatives designed to increase military service member's chances of survival and escape from captivity. Among them was the predecessor of modern-day SERE training. The U.S. Army Air Force formed the 336th Bombardment Group and began training service men in basic skills for survival, evasion, and escape.

Following World War II, it was evident that the 1929 convention did not adequately provide protections for prisoners of war (POWs), resulting in the Geneva Convention of 1949, which provided more specific guidelines for the humane treatment of POWs. It was the Korean conflict, however, that dramatically changed the focus of the survival schools.

Although the Korean War has been referred to as the "forgotten war" (fought between World War II and the Vietnam War), this description marginalizes the physical and psychological injuries suffered by many POWs. Forty percent of the more than 7,000 POWs in Korea died in captivity. The only POW death rate higher was that for American POWs held by the Japanese during World War II. Additionally, following the end of the Korean War, 21 service members chose to remain in Korea. Many interrogation experts and consultants believe that this was directly related to false confessions, other forms of exploitation, and physical and psychological torture. Following these events, former POWs and senior military leaders began to take a long and serious look at how to better prepare our servicemen and women in survival training (Carlson, 2002) and particularly how to recognize and resist exploitation.

The experiences of American POWs held in Korea brought about two landmark changes to survival training. In 1955, the U.S. Military Code of Conduct was created and, one year later, President Dwight Eisenhower ordered the establishment of the 1956 SERE working group, a think tank composed of former POWs, military and intelligence experts, and clinical psychologists to study and recommend the best methodologies for training, particularly with regard to the exploitation prisoners may face at the hands of their captors. Because of the formidable task of enduring years of interrogation without revealing something other than name, rank, service number, and date of birth, other strategies were devised to help POWs manage interrogation without betraying their country and/or antagonizing their interrogators (Ruhl, 1978).

After the Vietnam POWs returned in 1972, a number of them aided their SERE schools by teaching students about their experiences with torture, lengthy interrogations, threats of execution, disease, physical injuries, communication with fellow POWs, and, most important, the means to keep hope alive. The most significant recommendation from the Vietnam veterans was to standardize training across the Services.

Over the years, several joint organizations were developed until ultimately the Joint Personnel Recovery Agency (JPRA) was established in 1999 under U.S. Joint Forces Command. The strategic purpose of this agency is to provide operational support and products to meet personnel recovery challenges; to provide training and education to prepare for, prevent, and respond to isolating events; to provide guidance and oversight in the standardization of training; to analyze personnel recovery capabilities and processes; and to ensure that relevant personnel recovery technologies are compatible, and interoperable with existing command and control architecture (Joint Personnel Recovery Agency [JPRA], n.d.).

In 2011, due to the disestablishment of U.S. Joint Forces Command, the Joint Chiefs of Staff was assigned as the executive agent for the JPRA. JPRA provides oversight for all SERE and Military Code of Conduct training. In addition to providing regular oversight inspections of each SERE schoolhouse, the JPRA hosts annual training forums for program directors, SERE psychologists, personnel recovery specialists, and planners to adjust and provide standardized guidance to all SERE schools and personnel recovery personnel. Viewed as integral training by all military service departments, SERE schools continue to develop and evolve to meet current challenges and ensure that all students are adequately trained to handle today's threats. JPRA has recently published new guidance on joint standards for SERE training in support of the U.S. Military Code of Conduct and on joint standards for SERE training, role-playing activities in an effort to ensure best practices and the safety of both students and staff in this high-risk training environment (JPRA, 2010a, 2010b).

Today, each of the service departments operates its own SERE schools under the accreditation of the JPRA. The Air Force was the first service to begin SERE training, beginning with evasion and escape training in 1943 and adding resistance training in 1953. The Air Force's survival school moved to its present location in Spokane, Washington, in 1966. The Navy SERE schools came online in 1962. Originally set up for desert survival in Coronado, California, and cold weather survival in Brunswick, Maine, they now offer standardized training. The Army established its program in 1963 at Fort Bragg, North Carolina. The Marine Corps initially developed a SERE school at Cherry Point, North Carolina, but ultimately chose to use the Navy schools, which are both now staffed with a detachment of Marines. Most recently, each of the special operations communities has established specialized schools to provide more in-depth training, focusing on the particular scenarios their personnel are most likely to experience.

OVERVIEW OF CURRENT SERE TRAINING

Given the changing landscape and increased risk for military personnel of isolation or capture, the DoD made SERE training more accessible for all service members. SERE Level A currently provides military personnel with an online orientation to survival and Code of Conduct principles. Recognizing that some servicemen and women may require more than the orientation, but not the full immersion experience, a Level B training was developed and implemented by each of the Services. Level B is composed of both academic and laboratory-based role-play scenarios, but does not include the full *in vivo* experience. Level C SERE training is the most intensive and is provided to those military personnel designated as at high risk of isolation, capture, kidnapping, or governmental detention (e.g., aviation personnel, snipers, members of Special Forces, and intelligence gatherers).

Level C SERE training is built around the fundamentals of stress inoculation training (Meichenbaum, 1985). The concept of *stress inoculation* (Meichenbaum, 1985) is akin to the concept of preventing illness through vaccination. Like a vaccine, stress inoculation occurs when training stress is high enough to activate the body's psychological and biological coping mechanisms but not so great as to overwhelm them. When stress inoculation occurs, an individual's performance is likely to improve when stressed again (Parker, 2004; Selye, 1983).

To achieve stress inoculation, training is delivered in three phases with increasing challenges and stressors. Students are first presented with didactic information in the classroom. After acquiring those concepts, students are then provided with opportunities to apply and develop the skills and concepts through classroom-based role-plays. Finally, students are provided with a full *in vivo* laboratory exercise to further refine and use their skills in an environment that is as realistic as possible.

All SERE schools prepare students for a variety of captivity contingencies, including peacetime/governmental detention, POW captivity, and various abduction and hostage scenarios. Given its sensitive nature and content, only an overview of the unclassified portion of the training may be provided here.

For basic survival, students are provided with academic lessons that review personal survival skills, navigation and evasion, as well as techniques to assist in successfully resisting interrogation and exploitation methods. Following academic lessons, students are provided with in-depth and practical experiences in the field, such as land navigation, as well as how to procure potable water, hunt and trap small animals, build shelters, and differentiate edible from poisonous plants. During this time, students are forced to deal with hunger, uncertainty, fatigue, and discouragement in an experiential manner rather than in an academic format. In the field component, students officially begin the live evasion portion of their training. Their primary task initially is to reach various navigation objectives several miles away by successfully moving through hostile territory, all while dealing with the discomforts associated with the aforementioned survival contingencies (temperatures, hunger, sleep deprivation, etc.). At a designated point in the training, the students are moved from the field to the resistance portion of the training.

During the resistance phase, students are captured by simulated hostile entities, where they are confronted with various captivity scenarios in which they must use their situational awareness, newly acquired resistance techniques, and the Code of Conduct to successfully survive captivity. Instructors work to make this experience as realistic as possible, instructing and assessing the students while fully "in role." Throughout this training period, students are provided with opportunities to defeat the various exploitation scenarios they may encounter if captured or detained. This is the most memorable, and ultimately the most physically and psychologically demanding, aspect of the training.

At the conclusion of the course, students are provided with a debrief and opportunity to discuss their performance and ask any questions that may have arisen. It is critical for students to understand the methods of exploitation they encountered as well as why and how they reacted in various situations so they can learn and grow. The ultimate goal is that students will walk away from the course with confidence that they are equipped with skills and their own personal fortitude to manage to survive if ever isolated or captured.

THE SERE PSYCHOLOGIST

Although there is a growing body of literature on the effects of extreme stress on performance, there has been little written about the varied roles of a SERE psychologist. In the past, SERE psychologists received their mandates from a variety of resources that included several U.S. DoD Directives (DoDD) and Instructions (DoDI) that articulated some of the roles and training requirements: DoDD 1300.7 (Department of Defense, 2000a); DoDD 2310.2; DoDI 2310.4 (Department of Defense, 2000b); and DoDI 1300.21 (DoD, 2001). In response to the need for a better articulated instruction, JPRA published the *Guidance on Qualification Criteria and Use of Department of Defense (DoD) Survival, Evasion, Resistance, and Escape (SERE) Psychologists in Support of the Code of Conduct* (2010c), as well as the *Guidance on Joint Standards for Survival Evasion, Resistance, Escape (SERE) Training Role Play Activities in Support of the Code of Conduct* (2010a). These documents articulated the qualifications needed to work in the SERE community as well as the roles and responsibilities of psychologists in both the schoolhouse and personnel recovery environment. Today, the DoD SERE Psychology Program is governed by the Chairman of the Joint Chiefs of Staff Manual 3500.11 (2013) and DoDI 3002.05 (2016).

There are currently two types of SERE qualifications for psychologists: SERE certification and resistance training (RT) qualification. A *SERE-certified psychologist* is a DoD psychologist who is certified by JPRA to assist JPRA, combatant commands, interagency partners, and military Services during the reintegration process. Certification requirements consist of an orientation course and a 1-year mentorship with a seasoned SERE psychologist focused on developing knowledge about the dynamics of captivity, isolation, and exploitation; how to promote resilience in returnees; and how to support reintegration. Additionally, the SERE-certified psychologist must participate regularly in reintegration exercises, complete continuing education in the field, and complete a Level C SERE course. An *RT-qualified SERE psychologist* is a DoD SERE-certified psychologist who is currently, or has been, assigned to a DoD SERE school or a high-risk unit and has obtained the necessary training and experience to oversee Code of Conduct high-risk training.

PRIMARY ROLES OF THE SERE PSYCHOLOGIST

The roles and functions of a SERE psychologist will depend on assignment, although they fall into five general categories: assessment and selection, safety observer, educator, consultant/researcher, and reintegration. According to JPRA 2010 guidelines, an RT-qualified SERE psychologist will be the commander's primary representative to ensure close supervision of training, including risk monitoring and assessment, training effectiveness and evaluation, assessment and selection, and ongoing evaluation of instructors. Additionally, the RT-qualified SERE psychologist will provide instructor training to reduce the risk to students and increase training effectiveness, provide interventions to students and staff as needed, and provide a debrief to SERE students at the completion of training. SERE-certified psychologists may also be called on to assist in the reintegration of isolated personnel (JPRA, 2010c).

Assessment and Selection

Assessment and selection (A&S) for high-reliability positions has increasingly been seen as a pillar of operational psychology (Picano, Williams, & Roland, 2006; Picano, Williams, Roland, & Long, 2011; Staal & Stephenson, 2006; Williams, Picano, Roland, & Banks, 2006; Weiss & Inwald, 2010; see Chapter 13, this volume) and is a foundational skill practiced by RT SERE psychologists in the schoolhouses. All SERE instructors, without exception, must undergo an intensive psychological evaluation prior to receiving orders as a SERE instructor. Like other challenging training programs, SERE is considered high risk by the DoD. This is the result of not only the physical challenges encountered by the students—including strenuous activity, procuring one's own food and water sources, and mitigating the effects of the environment and elements—but also the psychological challenges posed by isolation, mock captivity, and stress. DoD is highly cognizant of the potential consequences of exploitation at the hands of instructors. As demonstrated by the Stanford Prison Experiment (Haney, Banks, & Zimbardo, 1973), one of the most potentially dangerous roles of the SERE instructor is role-playing a captor, guard, or interrogator.

SERE psychologists approach A&S of instructors from a "select out"

perspective. That is, they utilize the information they have (i.e., psychological assessment data, record reviews, and interviews) to determine if the individual is suitable. When reviewing a candidate for selection, the psychologist will be examining both cognitive and personality factors. As with any A&S process, it is best practice for selection methods to include decision making based on a thorough job analysis. In general, the psychologist needs an understanding of the social, emotional, physical, personality, risk and stress tolerance, and cognitive characteristics that are indicators for success or considered risk factors to be weighed in determining suitability.

Historically, we know that this type of "prison" scenario can be high risk for all parties involved. In 1971, the U.S. Navy funded Phillip Zimbardo to examine the effects of perceived power in what is now known as the Stanford Prison Experiment (Haney et al., 1973). This study examined the behavior of 24 individuals who had been carefully evaluated and selected for emotional stability. They were randomly assigned to either a "guard" or "prisoner" group. The experiment was initially designed to last 2 weeks, but it was discontinued after 6 days because of increasing and arbitrary antisocial behavior in the role-playing environment. The subjects who were pretending to be guards became overly "negative, hostile, affrontive, and dehumanizing" (p. 80) in effect, ceasing to perceive the prisoners as research participants. The subjects pretending to be prisoners became overly compliant, docile, and conforming, and five of them had to be released prior to the premature end of the experiment because they developed "extreme emotional depression, crying, rage, and acute anxiety" (p. 81). To ensure safety for both instructors and students, SERE psychologists closely review known risk factors in the A&S process and are required to be present in all scenarios where students are held in captivity or exposed to training in exploitation methods.

The SERE instructor position requires an adaptable instructional style due to the need to provide instruction in the classroom utilizing more traditional teaching styles, through practical demonstration in the field, and while in role-play scenarios. Providing instruction in role is a cognitively challenging task, as the instructor is required to simultaneously role-play, provide instruction while in role, and assess the performance of the students. Therefore, psychologists closely review each candidate's relative cognitive strengths and weaknesses to best determine if he or she is suited to this duty.

A general profile of the SERE instructor indicates that the average individual is over 30 years of age (approximately 10 years older than the college students used in the prison study), has more than 15 years of military service, is married, has numerous personal awards, was his or her previous command's top performer, and has no legal, substance abuse, or disciplinary history. Psychologically, the SERE instructor has a high need for achievement, has a high frustration tolerance, enjoys being part of a group, and is able to tolerate the intense scrutiny of not only the evaluation process but, more important, the constant observation and oversight that occur throughout a tour at the SERE school. Two cases are provided to demonstrate an example of a disqualified sailor and a sailor deemed qualified for SERE instructor duty.

Case 15.1. The Sailor Who Was Disqualified from SERE Instructor Duty

A Petty Officer Second Class (PO2) presented voluntarily for an A&S evaluation to determine his suitability for SERE instructor assignment. The evaluation consisted of a brief cognitive screen: the Minnesota Multiphasic Personality Inventory-2 (MMPI-2), a semistructured interview that consists of a review of medical, mental health, developmental, social, family, military, and educational history, a collateral interview, as well as an in-depth discussion of motivation for assignment. The cognitive screening estimated the sailor to be in the high average range of intellectual functioning, and while the MMPI-2 did not indicate any clinical mental health concerns, it did indicate some concerns regarding impulsivity. During the interview, the service member's motivation for reporting to SERE instructor duty was his desire to do something different than his current job. A review of his medical records indicated a referral to anger management 5 years ago in the context of a hazing incident. A collateral interview with his supervisor revealed that he was perceived as having a quick temper. This service member was ultimately disqualified from SERE instructor duty due to the risks presented by his impulsivity observed in both psychological testing and via collateral information and questions regarding his judgment.

Case 15.2. The Army SGT Who Was Qualified for SERE Instructor Duty

The SGT presented for SERE instructor evaluation and completed the same evaluation process as described above. The service member's personality testing and interview did not indicate any clinical, personality, or social concerns. His cognitive testing estimated his intellectual functioning to fall in the average range. He exhibited a strong motivation to serve and train other service members, and had an impressive military history of small unit leadership. He was determined to be suitable for instructor duty and was accepted into the program.

Safety Observer

Perhaps the most important lesson from Zimbardo's Stanford Prison Experiment in relation to SERE training is the necessity of maintaining the physical and psychological health of participants through consistent monitoring of individuals and systematic evaluation of the process itself. SERE training necessarily incorporates certain levels of emotional and physical distress to maintain the integrity and efficacy of the training experience, essentially integrating many of the lessons learned from prior POW experiences. For example, captors (e.g., Germans and Japanese in World War II and North Koreans and Vietnamese during those respective conflicts) have generally utilized four tactics with captured personnel: isolation, deprivation, abuse, and interrogation (Sherwood, 1986). Isolation consists of not only physical separation from other prisoners but also a more general isolation strategy of breaking ties with family, country, and, most significantly, a former identity of oneself. Deprivation consists of withholding food, water, adequate clothing and shelter, sleep, access to constructive physical and cognitive activity, medical care, and adequate means of maintaining personal hygiene. Psychological abuse, such as threatening to harm or kill prisoners, and coercive physical abuse have been reported. Last, interrogations for the purpose of gathering military intelligence have been routinely performed, often utilizing combinations of the first three tactics.

Because these imprisonment strategies are brutal in and of themselves, and approximating them for learning purposes in training scenarios is a sophisticated task, the existence of stringent guidelines and protocols is basic for effective functioning. The just mentioned issues illuminate the need for in-depth training of staff in positions of power as well as in regimented safety procedures. The safety observer position was implemented to ensure that "captors and guards" do not cross the line and that "prisoners" do not become traumatized by their experience. Consequently, the role of safety observer is one of the key responsibilities of the SERE psychologist. When done correctly and consistently, the SERE psychologist can quickly be viewed as a trusted member of the team. When trusted, it is not uncommon for instructors to debrief difficult student encounters with the psychologist looking for feedback and guidance.

During SERE training, there are three to five personnel whose sole responsibility is serving as safety observers, ensuring the well-being of those participating in training. Although all SERE personnel at times act as safety observers, the psychologist's specific duty in this role is to monitor the instructors for cues that a "guard" or "captor" might be taking the role too seriously or too far. Other than the obvious scenario of a too aggressive instructor, the psychologist looks for subtle changes in instructors' typical mode of operating, which may indicate that they are having some difficulties. Some instructors might become more outspoken when they are typically quiet, become too gentle during an interrogation, exhibit real affect during or after an exercise, or even subtly or unconsciously target a specific student. Some of the more general indicators of behavioral drift include observed diffusion of responsibility, dehumanizing tendencies, or reliance on anonymity for decreased accountability. A key concept in training for instructors is "performing" the role versus "becoming" the role. The instructor must maintain the mind-set that he or she is an instructor, not an interrogator or guard, and that the purpose of the exercise is for the student to demonstrate resistance techniques.

In addition to monitoring in the training environment, instructors are also monitored outside of it. Many of the schoolhouses have created human factors boards or other types of mechanisms for routinely evaluating the health, welfare, and performance of their instructors. Accepting a job at SERE places a strain on even a healthy marital relationship, as much of the job cannot be discussed at home because of its classified nature. The combination of possibly bringing power roles home to spouses and children and being unable to discuss workday occurrences and stressors can be difficult on these military families. SERE personnel are taught how to monitor each other for warning signs, such as increases in irritability or alcohol consumption, decreased military bearing, or any shifts in behavior that might affect their ability to perform. The SERE psychologist formally and informally encourages instructors to decompress from the training environment through the use of healthy stress management techniques (such as physical exercise, relaxation strategies, and humor), and the SERE psychologist is one of many personnel who help ensure that SERE instructors are rotated from position to position. This not only helps to promote cross-training but also helps to move SERE instructors out of power roles for extended periods of time.

Although a main thrust of the safety observer's role is to closely monitor the instructors, the observers are ultimately there to maintain the integrity and realism of the training experience for the benefit of the students. Not unexpectedly, some students have strong maladaptive reactions to certain aspects of the training. Given the nature of the highly dedicated and trained SERE students (e.g., Special Forces members, aircrew and pilots, and intelligence operators), they are not always amenable to psychological intervention or performance direction. Although significant anxiety, irritability, and even hallucinations are considered normal, interventions may be initiated when they arise. Generally, this early intervention and assessment of psychological status are best delivered through subtle reminders by instructor staff that cue coping and performance skills. However, if a more formal intervention is required, a technician (e.g., corpsman, medic, psychological technician) or a psychologically minded senior instructor, under the supervision of the psychologist, can help to reduce stigma. Having a psychologist immediately intervene may create the perception that the SERE student is incapable of completing training or that his or her reaction is not normal (True & Benaway, 1992).

Perhaps most importantly, it should be pointed out that the psychologist does not provide data or guidance on the best ways to exploit students. This has been a reported misconception and critique of psychologists participating in SERE programs. At no time do psychologists provide specific student information to instructors to create a "more stressful or unique" training experience. This would constitute behavioral drift and mission creep on the part of the psychologist and be considered unethical.

Educator

The SERE psychologist provides multiple types of education for both staff and student trainees. All SERE personnel receive training in the dangers of behavioral drift and more specifically on role-playing situations in which individuals have power over others. The psychologist reviews in-depth information related to role immersion, the prison study findings, and the ethics involved in the mock imprisonment described earlier (Zimbardo, 1973). All personnel must exhibit a comprehensive understanding of the concepts raised by this research in order to work at SERE. In addition, the SERE psychologist teaches the safety observers what signs to look for, in both the instructors and the students, that would indicate a problem so appropriate intervention can be initiated, as well as principles of stress inoculation, reactions to stress and exploitation, common coping mechanisms, and principles of learning. The vast majority of SERE instructors care deeply about this mission, fully understanding that the training they offer may one day save a life. They are eager to continuously hone their instructional abilities.

In addition to regular training, the SERE psychologist also educates the trainees. In this role as educator, the operational psychologist explains the normal reactions to severe uncontrollable stress—including fear, anger, negative self-statements, crying, illusions, and hallucinations, dissociation, somatic complaints, and memory problems—and how long they are expected to last (Dobson & Marshal, 1997; Engle & Spencer, 1993; Mitchell, 1983; Sokol, 1989; Yerkes, 1993). This education has proven to be an integral part of the success of captured service members. A number of factors help individuals to be more resilient under stress (Morgan, Wang, Mason, et al., 2000a; Morgan, Wang, Southwick, et al., 2000b). From Korea and Vietnam POWs to the more recent EP-3 crew detained in China, service members reported that whereas their military training aided in the survival of a particular incident, it was the experiential nature of SERE training that facilitated their survival in captivity.

Research indicates that those individuals who functioned well in captivity possessed several characteristics, including a strong faith in their country, in each other, and in God. Those who focused on factors under their internal control, such as thinking about future plans (e.g., designing their dream house, down to the smallest detail) or developing a personal exercise program in their cell, were also much more successful (Ursano & Rundell, 1996). Successful former POWs had a tremendous sense of humor

(Henman, 2001), were older, had higher levels of education at the time of their imprisonment (Gold et al., 2000), and maintained an ability to reframe their situation even under the most dire circumstances. Research on former POWs from the Vietnam War has consistently demonstrated that this group is resilient (Coffee, 1990), and that SERE training provided experiential anchors and cues to help them effectively cope with the demands of captivity. An example of the ability to reframe events comes from the comments of a commanding officer who kept a piece of shrapnel on his desk and would explain to the curious: "That is a piece of shrapnel that flew over my head during the Vietnam War when I was serving as a corpsman. When I am having a bad day, I realize things could be a lot worse" (Captain A. Shimkus, personal communication, November 2003). Research at SERE indicates that individuals who view themselves as passive or vulnerable and who mentally disconnect from their environment under stress do not perform as well as those who remain grounded in the situation and who appraise it in an active manner (Taylor & Morgan, 2014). Teaching service members active, rather than passive, coping strategies is likely to enhance their stress tolerance.

Consultant and Researcher

Acquainted with the results of stress research (Meichenbaum, 1985), the U.S. military designs training to be physically and psychologically demanding and lifelike in stress intensity. Challenging and realistic training develops trainees' ability to perform on the battlefield, and exposure to realistic levels of stress is intended to inoculate them from the negative effects of operational stress. In the roles of consultant and researcher, the SERE psychologist explores a wide variety of research topics related to the effects that severe stress has on humans. SERE offers a unique opportunity to validate training parameters, establish predictors of superior performance, and develop new tools and techniques for the Global War on Terror. These topics have particular military relevance, and a brief synopsis of some of this research follows.

Validation of Training Parameters

Over the past two decades, civilian and military research teams have assessed the impact of acute stress on psychological, neurohormonal, and physiological parameters in students enrolled in U.S. and non-U.S. military survival school training (Taylor, Larsen, & Hiller Lauby, 2014a; Taylor et al., 2014b; Eid & Morgan, 2006; Dimoulis et al., 2007; Morgan, Wang, Mason, et al., 2000a; Morgan et al., 2001; Morgan et al., 2002; Morgan, Doran, Steffian, Hazlett, & Southwick, 2006; Morgan, Hazlett, Southwick, Rasmussen, & Lieberman, 2009; Morgan, Hazlett, et al., 2004a;

Taylor, Sausen, Mujica-Parodi, et al., 2007a; Taylor, Sausen, Potterat, et al., 2007b; Morgan, Southwick, et al., 2004b). This research has had the overarching goal of assessing the impact of realistic stress in healthy humans and to identify the factors that explain why and how people differ in their response to stress. By elucidating the factors that contribute to stress resilience, this research has led to better treatment strategies for individuals who suffer from trauma-related mental health problems and to better methods for recovery of cognitive functioning after exposure to high levels of stress (Morgan et al., 2009). The initial purpose of studies conducted at SERE was to assess whether or not SERE represented a venue in which valid studies of acute stress in humans could be conducted. Specifically, it was important to learn whether the stress experienced by participants was comparable to real-world stress (Morgan, Wang, Mason, et al., 2000a; Morgan, Wang, Southwick, et al., 2000b; Morgan et al., 2001; Morgan et al., 2002). Investigators examined the overall impact of each phase of SERE training (classroom, evasion, and detention) as well as several specific components. The results of these studies provided the following evidence:

1. SERE stress intensity is within a range of real-world stress and of a magnitude necessary for stress inoculation (Morgan, Wang, Mason, et al., 2000a; Morgan, Wang, Southwick, et al., 2000b; Morgan et al., 2001; Morgan et al., 2002).
2. Students who undergo SERE training recover normally and do not show negative psychological or neurobiological effects from having experienced this type of military training (i.e., students do not exhibit stress sensitization or increased psychological symptoms of dissociation 6 months after training; Morgan et al., 2001; Morgan et al., 2002; Morgan et al., 2006; Morgan, Hazlett, et al., 2004a; Morgan, Southwick, et al., 2004b).
3. Students' physiology and biological measures indicate a normal recovery from the various physical interrogation aspects of SERE training (Morgan et al., 2001; Morgan et al., 2002).

These findings are important in that they support the idea that the training stress experienced by students at SERE is at a level that will help, and not harm, their ability to cope with extreme stress in the future.

Establishment of Predictors of Superior Performance during Stress

The SERE research conducted to date has also provided clues as to why and how some students perform better under stress than others. More specifically, investigators have examined who and how some students remain mentally clear and experience fewer stress-induced cognitive deficits when stress increases. Researchers evaluated specific capacities such as resistance techniques, simple and complex problem-solving abilities during stress, and visual and verbal memory capacity (Morgan, Hazlett, et al., 2004a; Morgan, Southwick, et al., 2004b; Morgan et al., 2006; Morgan, Aikins, et al., 2007a; Morgan, Hazlett, et al., 2007b; Morgan, Southwick, Steffian, Hazlett, & Loftus, 2013; Morgan, Dule, & Rabinowitz, 2020). The results of this line of research indicate the following:

1. Specific psychological and biological differences at baseline (prior to stress exposure) predict objective performance (as assessed by cadre) during stress. Put briefly, students who have a vulnerable sense of self, higher baseline anxiety, and less capacity for regulating their sympathetic nervous system are more likely to have difficulties during stress. By contrast, those low in anxiety and high in neurobiological factors that modulate the stress response do well. (For a full review of the neurobiological and neuroanatomical elements of acute stress, see Eid & Morgan, 2006; McNeil & Morgan, 2010; Morgan, Wang, Southwick, et al., 2000b; Morgan et al., 2001; Morgan et al., 2002; Morgan et al., 2014).

2. Specific biological differences in the expression of stress hormones explain why some students are more focused, more clear-headed during stress, and show more accuracy in cognitive and memory tests both during and after stress. Although the reasons remain unclear, some students are protected from the negative impact of stress due to higher levels of dehydroepiandrosterone (a steroid hormone that can convert into estrogen and testosterone), whereas in others stress hardiness is mediated by neuropeptide Y (NPY). Both paths result in individuals who are more accurate in descriptions of what they encountered during stress (i.e., eyewitness memory). These studies are important in that they are directly related to aspects of the work performed by a SERE psychologist: namely debriefings of individuals who, in the course of their service, are captured or detained by the enemy. These studies highlight the complex nature, and fallibility, of human eyewitness memory under stress. SERE studies continue to help us develop specific interventions that may enhance operational abilities (Morgan et al., 2004b; Morgan, Aikins, et al., 2007a; Morgan, Hazlett, et al., 2007b; Morgan et al., 2013; Morgan et al., 2020; Taylor et al., 2007b; Taylor et al., 2008; Taylor et al., 2011; Taylor et al., 2012).

Sex Differences in Acute Stress Response

Over the years, most military stress research has been focused on males. The opening of infantry and combat ratings to females across all Services has highlighted the need to better understand the effects of stress and trauma on female service members. Taylor et al. (2014b) observed pronounced sex

differences in the psychological impact of and physiological response to mock captivity. When assessed following the most stressful and intense training scenarios, females scored higher on measures of posttraumatic stress for total impact, arousal, and intrusion. This is important as the literature has suggested females have higher risks of developing PTSD than their male counterparts (Mota et al., 2012; Breslau, 2009; Kesler, Sonnega, Bromet, Hughes, & Nelson, 1995; Oliff, Langeland, Draijer, & Gersons, 2007).

Physiological arousal is one of the cornerstone symptom clusters in PTSD. In an initial study of its kind, Taylor et al. (2014) reviewed sex differences in acute stress reactions during mock captivity. Females maintained lower systolic blood pressure and diastolic blood pressure throughout the course of evaluation, yet demonstrated greater elevation in residual systolic blood pressure. Additionally, while there was a nonsignificant trend in this study for females experiencing a higher heart rate under stress, modeling indicated that differences may be better accounted for by individual traits. This is congruent with existing literature that indicates that males may produce more of a vascular response under stress, while myocardial responses are more common in females (Lepore, Mata, Allen, & Evans, 1993; Steptoe, Fieldman, & Evans, 1996). Taken together with the findings of higher measures of posttraumatic stress, it may be suggested that stress-induced heart rate may partially mediate sex differences in the psychological impact of acute stress. This is certainly an area for continued research.

Specifically, reviewing sex differences in psychological impact and responses to stress, Schmeid et al. (2015) identified differences in coping strategy utilization and perceived psychological distress during and following a high-stress mock captivity environment. After controlling for education, female service members were significantly more likely to choose self-blame, denial, and positive reframing coping strategies. They also chose self-distraction and planning more often, but not to a significant degree more than their male counterparts. When these coping strategies were reviewed as mediators between sex and psychological distress, two specific strategies, behavioral disengagement and self-distraction, were directly tied to higher rates of psychological distress at a follow-up after completing training. Conversely, planning as a coping strategy was shown to not be related to follow-up distress. This is congruent with other studies that have shown the use of maladaptive coping strategies may increase the risk of developing PTSD following a traumatic event or situation (Nolen-Hoeksma, 2012).

Dimoulas et al. (2007) examined dissociation and somatic complaints in female SERE students and compared them with previous samples of male students that included special forces troops and general infantry soldiers. The research highlighted three points. First, both men and women who report previous trauma from which they thought they might die tend to experience greater levels of dissociation. Second, baseline measures of dissociation indicated that for the female participant, dissociation measures were most similar to those of the special forces comparison group and, as a sample, were lower than those of the general infantry students. One possible explanation for this is that women who self-select careers that require SERE training are likely a stress-hardy group, having already completed physically and mentally challenging training (i.e., flight school, officer candidate school) in their career pathways. Last, women with higher levels of dissociation tend to report more somatic complaints ($r = .76$, $p < .0001$) compared with their male counterparts ($r = .54$, $p < .02$). Unfortunately, this study was limited in that it was not able to determine whether this finding resulted from differences in the pathophysiology or homogeneity of this particular sample.

New Tools and Techniques for Professions Engaged in the Global War on Terror

In response to issues raised by the September 11, 2001, terrorist attacks on the United States, the Director of National Intelligence issued a report on what is currently known about interrogations: "Educing Information: Interrogation: Science and Art, Foundations for the Future" (Fein, Lehner, & Vossekuil, 2006). As noted in the report, there is little empirical evidence for many of the methods and techniques employed by law enforcement or government officials who conduct interrogations. A significant barrier to conducting research that could help determine whether specific questioning techniques or technologies (such as the polygraph) are effective is that most research laboratories cannot ethically expose research subjects to realistic stress comparable to that of a person being questioned in real-life circumstances. However, as noted by stress studies described previously, SERE training is a venue in which one can ethically examine the efficacy of some methods currently used by U.S. officials, such as the polygraph. Determining whether a traditional method loses efficacy when used on people who are experiencing significant stress would be helpful. Clarifying whether or not techniques that purportedly detect deception actually work under stressful conditions may provide empirical data that would inform law enforcement agencies and government officials about whether spending taxpayer money on these techniques, or believing the information gained by using such techniques, is valid.

Morgan and colleagues (2005) completed a study with SERE students that was designed to test the accuracy (sensitivity and specificity) of the traditional polygraph in detecting concealed knowledge. Analysis of the data indicated that traditional measures of the polygraph did no better than chance in detecting the guilty subjects. These findings are important and provide evidence that officials should *not* rely on such techniques to detect deception in people who are experiencing significant stress. This said, it is possible that new approaches, such as assessments for RSA norm (the respiration-driven speeding and slowing of the heart), can be used to accurately determine when a person is engaged in telling a deceptive story while under conditions of stress. While promising, these data need to be replicated in populations of SERE students who are not members of special operations units in order to assess whether the findings are likely to generalize to other members of the population.

Reintegration

A critical role for the SERE psychologist is the reintegration process. Verifying both the applicability and efficacy of SERE training to real-world situations can be a difficult task, given the significant hurdles or confounds of validation research of POW occurrences. However, one of the primary vehicles utilized by the DoD for assessment of individual performance and SERE training, in general, is the process of reintegration. DoDI 2310.4 (Department of Defense, 2000b), concerning personnel recovery, indicates that preserving the life and well-being of personnel who are placed in harm's way is one of the highest priorities. It states that "personnel recovery is a critical element in the DoD ability to fulfill its moral obligation to protect its personnel, prevent exploitation of U.S. personnel by adversaries, and reduce the potential of captured personnel being used as leverage against the United States" (p. 2).

In general, there are four basic types of personnel recovery. First and foremost, isolated personnel have an obligation to evade potential captors and, if captured or detained, to effect their own escape within the parameters of the Military Code of Conduct and the Geneva Conventions. In essence, service members are expected to attempt to facilitate their own recovery. The term *isolated* is used here to describe personnel who are supporting a military mission and are temporarily separated from their units in an environment requiring them to survive and evade capture or to resist and escape if captured. The second form of personnel recovery is characterized as conventional combat search and rescue (CSAR), whereby trained military forces on land or sea recover the isolated individual. An example would be the recovery of a downed pilot, in danger of being captured but not yet detained. The third form of recovery, typically a far more fluid and dangerous proposition, is described as an unconventional assisted recovery. In this situation, special forces personnel might be inserted into the equation to contact, authenticate, and extract detained U.S. personnel. In essence, the CSAR mission becomes an armed recovery from enemy forces, with the goal of returning detainees to U.S. control. Certainly, this can be fraught with danger to both the detainees and recovery forces, and will have important implications in the repatriation process debriefings. The fourth method of personnel recovery involves a negotiated release, typically with diplomatic initiatives between governments. Of course, these four methods are general descriptions and contain a number of variants and convergences as the situation dictates.

Once isolated or detained personnel are recovered and returned to U.S. control, the work of reintegration begins. Reintegration can be thought of as an established process that bridges two entirely different contexts: the readjustment from captivity back into life as a U.S. citizen and/or service member. The reintegration of recovered DoD personnel is an extraordinarily important process for the well-being of the individual and for safeguarding U.S. government interests. The SERE psychologist must assist the returnee as well as help the reintegration team understand and meet the needs of the returnee within the context of the broader DoD and interagency community requirements. Through the process of reintegration, the returnee will achieve medical and psychological stabilization, regain their ability to predict and reestablish control over themselves and their environments, and reengage in a healthy lifestyle to include their social and family connections as well as work and other aspects of their lives. Additionally, throughout the reintegration process, the DoD will seek to gather intelligence and valuable lessons learned toward strategic and operational planning. Last, the interagency will seek to gather intelligence and evidence that may be used to prosecute criminals and protect U.S. citizens abroad. Despite these many needs, DoDI 2310.4 (Department of Defense, 2000b) guides the reintegration process and explicitly states, "The well-being and legal rights of the individual returnee shall be the overriding factors when planning and executing repatriation operations. Except in extreme circumstances of military necessity, they must take priority over all political, military, or other considerations" (p. 3). Subsequently, the operational aspects of each stage of the reintegration process will be carried out in accordance with thoughtful consideration of the hardships endured and the physiological, psychological, and spiritual needs of the returnee. Other inclusive aims involve the recovery of personal dignity and pride that may have been affected by captivity and the restoration of confidence in one's person and country.

The primary aim of the reintegration process is to restore the health of the recovered personnel through a protocol of psychological decompression, which is specifically designed to minimize the impact of unrealistic expectations on the service member's recovery and provide an individually tailored plan for transition from isolation/captivity back to full duty. Throughout the decompression process, the overlaying assumption is that the recovered personnel are emotionally healthy and resilient and are having normal reactions to abnormal events.

Because of the nature of exploitation during isolation and captivity, personnel very quickly lose their ability to predict and control their environments. One of the early tasks throughout the decompression process is to slowly allow the returnee to begin to regain his or her sense of control and predictability. This can be accomplished through initially providing a highly structured environment that becomes more flexible over time, allowing the returnee to make choices when able, and creating action plans for upcoming events and challenges.

As the returnee moves through the reintegration process and begins telling his or her story, reactions and emotions to the event that service member has experienced should be accepted and normalized within the context of isolation. It is important that the returnee be allowed to repeatedly tell his or her story in a manner that feels natural so he or she can more fully understand the event that occurred and contribute to the mission by providing critical and time-sensitive information.

Last, it is important that decompression include periods of downtime and time alone. In some cases, returnees may be in a hurry to get back to life, catch up on things they have missed, particularly when it comes to their families. Unfortunately, this can quickly become overwhelming to the returnee; thus, downtime is critical to the process. It is during these down periods where returnees can begin to process their emotional reactions, practice individual coping skills, and be provided with physical rest and recovery time.

Reintegration is accomplished over a series of three phases depending on the needs of the returnee, the DoD, and the interagency community. The reintegration team is typically composed of a SERE-certified psychologist, a medical officer, a carefully selected key unit member, a chaplain, a public affairs officer (PAO), and a legal officer. While the SERE psychologist does not serve as the reintegration team leader, he or she plays an important role in helping to manage the reintegration team's expectations and perceptions, setting the pace for reintegration and decompression activities, and facilitating the various formal debriefing activities. A new psychologist will typically be assigned at each phase of reintegration. This allows for the theaters to maintain SERE capability while the returnee moves through the process.

Phase I begins when recovered personnel are returned to U.S. control and lasts anywhere from 24 to 48 hours. Phase I typically takes place within the same theater of operations and is intended to allow for safe and efficient reintegration. Proximity allows for greater flexibility in assessing the returnee's needs as well as potentially returning the service member to duty with his or her assigned unit when appropriate. The main priorities for Phase I reintegration are to quickly provide medical and psychological assessment and stabilization, conduct debriefing to gain time-sensitive intelligence, and make return-to-duty determinations.

The reintegration team will make a return-to-duty determination based on a number of factors that may include the medical and psychological health of the service member, the needs of the DoD and interagency community, as well as the complexity of the isolating or captivity event.

The decision to return to duty from this secure area is consistent with the BICEPS concept of combat stress control: *Brevity* of treatment, *Immediacy* of the response, *Centrality* of the treatment area, *Expectancy* of recuperation, *Proximity* of treatment near the incident location, and *Simplicity* of the interventions. Since the returnees are considered to not be in need of psychological services, the focus can be directed at transitioning them back to duty unless their condition suggests otherwise. They would still complete critical operational and/or intelligence debriefings for immediate dissemination but then would return to their primary duty.

If the returnees have experienced a prolonged period of evasion from or detention by hostile forces, then the Phase I secure area will probably be a short transition point en route to a Phase II location, which is typically a major regional medical center near that theater of operation. General duties of the SERE psychologist during this phase may include (1) initial and ongoing psychological assessment to address the needs and psychological status of the returnees, which will subsequently direct future interventions and debriefing operations; (2) education of the returnees (and their chain of command) about what they may expect in the near future; and (3) the moderation of their activities and public or familial exposure to aid in decompression and transition. These factors will continue to be revisited and adjusted as needed while the SERE psychologist accompanies the returnee to the Phase II location.

In general, most returnees continue on to Phase II of the reintegration. Phase II typically takes place in a military medical treatment facility or other secure location outside of the area of responsibility (AOR) over the course of 4–5 days. It is during this phase that the service member will receive a more thorough medical assessment, begin the psychological decompression protocol, make initial family contact, and begin to participate in more formal debriefings. These might include operational or intelligence debriefs, SERE training debriefs, or psychological debriefs to aid in decompression. They are carried out separately to avoid convergence of details or facts and are generally moderated by a SERE psychologist in accordance with the psychological condition of the returnees. The SERE psychologist monitors for situations that detract from the returnees' readjustment and will advocate for protocols that maximize the accuracy of recalled information. Each of these debriefs is part of the larger decompression effort formulated to allow returnees maximum reintegration success in their military and civilian lives.

Operational and intelligence debriefs are oriented toward the returnee's mission. Military members, in general, are routinely asked to complete postmission debriefs with superiors, often focusing on successes and failures, lessons learned, intelligence gleaned from the enemy or given away (if contact was made), or changes in standard operating procedures should the situation warrant it. These military debriefs are carried out in a professional manner, are behaviorally or factually focused, and are tactical or strategic in nature. Operational and/or intelligence debriefers in a repatriation context try to mirror routine, typical debriefs. There is an important decompression element as well, since returnees are able to obtain relevant feedback from authorities who can answer nagging concerns or questions they may have about their own performance. In this manner, returnees are allowed conceptually to "complete the mission." The relevant information from these debriefs is immediately disseminated to the appropriate commanders for tactical purposes.

Psychological debriefing primarily provides decompression for the returnees through a guided process of "telling their story." This process can be particularly helpful when there is more than one returnee, as experiences are shared and each recipient receives a fuller understanding of the situation and everyone's experiences. It is important to note that based on data from over 1,400 SERE participants, we know that human eyewitness memory for experiences when under stress is highly fallible and subject to change (Morgan et al., 2004a; Morgan et al., 2007b; Morgan et al., 2013; Morgan et al., 2020). A person's level of confidence is not related to eyewitness accuracy. These data should underscore the need for accurately documenting memories about experiences during debriefings. Human memory for traumatic events is malleable and frequently changes over time (Southwick, Morgan, Niclaou, & Charney, 1997). If the information that is acquired in a SERE debrief is retained in a high-fidelity manner, it permits over time a comparison to other objective data that may become available. It is important for SERE psychologists who are involved in debriefings to remember that what they document may be useful in both forensic and intelligence settings. The SERE psychologist should also be aware when concerns exist that the returnee may have legal issues related to his or her isolation or captivity. In those cases, the psychologist should take care.

Furthermore, since returnees are not necessarily considered psychologically impaired as a result of their experiences, much effort is expended to educate and normalize their psychological reactions to the situations they encountered. Returnees generally find comfort in understanding their past and/or current reactions as "normal human responses to abnormal events" and the knowledge that these reactions will improve over time. Some of the typical psychological reactions to release from captivity are sleep disruption (nightmares, insomnia, or hypersomnia); changes in concentration (memory deficits or disorientation); mood fluctuations (irritability, hostility, depression, guilt, anxiety, and euphoria); and reevaluation of life goals and conviction. The extent of these symptoms largely depends on the preexisting traits of the individual, the level of sleep and sensory deprivation or isolation experienced, the type of duress and coercive attempts endured, and possibly the duration of captivity. Much of the psychological decompression occurring in Phase II involves the SERE psychologist's ability to (1) educate and normalize the returnees' reactions to the events they experienced and (2) clarify the context in which their actions occurred, with the goal of providing meaning and connectedness to their actions.

A reciprocal benefit of SERE debriefs is the ability to provide feedback to the SERE training institutions in a research and development continuum. In other words, clarifying difficulties encountered with personnel recovery, learning about the enemy's interrogation methods or aims of exploitation, or assessing the treatment of captives is directly applicable to the validation efforts of the current training methodologies and course of instruction. It is important in this educative process that returnees be able to ask direct questions and receive direct feedback about their own performance. Since military members are held to the standards of the Military Code of Conduct, it is often part of their psychological decompression to know that they have comported themselves well and "returned with honor."

In Phase II, reintegration with the returnee's family also begins. Generally, the initial contact with family is by telephone, as personal visitation in Phase II has been found to be problematic in the past. Although this principle would seem to be counterintuitive in some ways, experience has shown that the returnees' immediate integration with their families can be conflictive with their own long-term psychological decompression needs as well as with the general efforts of a repatriation operation. For instance, there may have been significant shifts in family roles during detention, or family issues may have already existed, making it difficult for the returnees to receive assistance in decompressing while engaged in familiar needs. Accordingly, a PAO and legal officer are also assigned to the returnee to assist with any information or interview requests, as well as any relevant legal concerns caused by the detention. Again, with the returnee's needs foremost, the SERE psychologist will work closely with the PAO to jointly decide on the appropriate level of media exposure. A key unit member also aids the decompression process by providing familiarity to predetention life, liaison assistance between the returnee and the unit, and assistance with other administrative or logistical concerns.

A service member may be returned to duty following Phase II reintegration. As with Phase I, there are a number of variables that will determine whether a service member returns to duty or continues on to Phase III reintegration. Factors may include the need for further psychological or medical assessment or treatment, further debriefing requirements, or national security or command interests.

If required, Phase III is a more Service-specific phase of reintegration that occurs in the continental United States. It also typically serves as the first opportunity for the returnees to be physically reunited with their families, unit members, and friends. The objectives for Phase III reintegration

include completing any remaining debriefing activities, continuing any needed medical treatment, and developing the skills and action plans to successfully reintegrate into family, social, and work life. Family reunification is handled in a structured and tiered approach. While the initial desire may be to immediately immerse with one's family and loved ones, that has at times proven to be detrimental. Family reunification is best managed in a structured approach, over the course of several days, increasing in frequency and decreasing in structure over time. If significant changes occurred in the family structure because of the returnee's absence, a period of transition or adaptation may be indicated. It is highly beneficial for the SERE psychologist to provide coaching in preparation for family reunification (both for the family as well as the returnee), help establish healthy expectations, and create action plans for the reunification process. Furthermore, if family members wish to address their own needs or concerns related to the returnee's absence, it can be provided by contact with the military unit or through JPRA and SERE psychologists.

Despite the probable desire to be immediately sheltered by family, loved ones, or friends, it is equally important for returnees to maintain contact with their military unit or captivity peers upon returning home, particularly for those who had been held in group captivity and were reintegrated together. Generally, there may have been some unique experiences and psychological reactions that are best worked through with the same reintegrated peers or with guides familiar with the psychology of captivity. Continued affiliation with groups that have experienced traumatic or difficult events together has proven helpful in the past.

As returnees begin to venture into the public eye, action planning regarding media exposure and communication will be important. With constant access to 24/7 news, social media, and other communication modalities, it is important for returnees to think through and plan for managing the media and public commentaries available on many social media sites. Media may present an inaccurate depiction of the circumstances or event, paint the returnee in a negative or conversely a too positive light, or second-guess the actions of the returnee. This is particularly true for social media. Early exposure without an appropriate action plan may distort the returnee's image of themselves and impact his or her ability to feel as if he or she has returned with honor and remains connected to communities. This can greatly affect the recovery process.

For the returnee's aftercare, medical needs will continue to be attended to as necessary, along with follow-up by the affiliated SERE psychologist for any ongoing psychological needs. By protocol, the SERE psychologist will continue to remain available and provide aftercare as indicated throughout the following year. Also, all detainees and former POWs are eligible for annual screenings and continued medical and psychological services through the Robert E. Mitchell Center for Repatriated POW Studies Center in Pensacola, Florida (Moore, 2010).

DOD SUPPORT FOR POST-ISOLATION SUPPORT ACTIVITIES

Occasionally, DoD SERE psychologists will be requested to act in a supporting role for Post-Isolation Support Activities (PISA). PISA is an activity that is similar to the reintegration process, with the purpose of providing services and support for private citizens who have been isolated or in captivity. While similar in structure and goals, PISA is a service offered, not mandated, unlike reintegration for military members, with the express purpose of ensuring the welfare of returnees. In PISA operations, DoD SERE psychologists may be requested for support to the mission; however, the interagency community is the agency responsible. In these circumstances, it is important for the SERE psychologists to be in constant contact and consultation with the SERE representative for the appropriate agency (i.e., the Federal Bureau of Investigations).

SUMMARY

SERE training aids and equips service members to cope with the unthinkable demands of captivity. Although SERE training may induce temporary psychological changes and demands while one is being held captive by a simulated enemy for several days, the psychological and physical effects of truly being held prisoner can result in permanent damage. One of the key functions of SERE training, and the experiential learning and preparation therein, is to give service members the tools and confidence needed to mitigate problematic future effects of the demands of captivity.

The SERE psychologist plays a vital role in this training environment as an evaluator, safety observer, educator, researcher, and consultant. When service members are recovered, the SERE psychologist functions as a consultant and clinician during the reintegration process. The SERE environment is a laboratory of realistic stress, and the research that has been conducted provides a greater understanding of how to enhance performance under severe stress, improve a student's ability to learn during exposure to stress and about the ways to recover from stress exposure. The research from SERE also assists the SERE psychologist in understanding the ways high stress affects human memory and which aspects of memory are more, or less, vulnerable to alteration. The SERE psychologist is in a unique position to help nonpsychology professionals involved in forensic or intelligence investigations understand the science of human memory so as to better appreciate information acquired in post stress debriefings.

REFERENCES

Breslau, N. (2009). The epidemiology of trauma, PTSD, and other posttrauma disorders. *Trauma, Violence & Abuse, 10*, 198–210.

Carlson, L. (2002). *Remembered prisoners of a forgotten war: An oral history of the Korean War POWs*. New York: St. Martin's Press.

Chairman of the Joint Chiefs of Staff Manual. (2013). Department of Defense (DoD) *Survival, evasion, resistance, and escape psychology program* (CJCMS 3500.11). Washington, DC: U.S. Department of Defense.

Coffee, G. (1990). *Beyond survival: Building on the hard times*. New York: Putnam.

Department of Defense. (2000a, December 8). *Training and education to support the code of conduct (CoC)* (Department of Defense Directive 2310.2). Washington, DC: Author.

Department of Defense. (2000b, November 21). *Repatriation of prisoners of war (POW) hostages, peacetime government detainees and other missing or isolated personnel*. (Department of Defense Directive 2310.4). Washington, DC: Author.

Department of Defense. (2001, January 8). *Code of conduct training and education* (Department of Defense Directive 1300.21). Washington, DC: Author.

Department of Defense. (2016). *Personnel recover (PR) education and training* (Department of Defense Instruction 3002.05). Washington, DC: Author.

Dimoulas, E., Steffian, L., Steffian, G., Doran, A. P., Rasmusson, A. M., & Morgan, C. A. (2007). Dissociation during intense military stress is related to subsequent somatic symptoms in women. *Psychiatry, 4*, 66–73.

Dobson, M., & Marshall, R. (1997). Surviving the war zone: Preventing psychiatric casualties. *Military Medicine, 162*, 283–287.

Eid, J., & Morgan, C. A. (2006). Dissociation, hardiness and performance in military cadets participating in survival training. *Military Medicine, 158*, 533–537.

Engle, C., & Spencer, S. (1993). Revitalizing division mental health in garrison: A post Desert Storm perspective. *Military Medicine, 158*, 533–537

Fein, R. A., Lehner, P., & Vossekuil, B. (2006). *Educing information. Interrogation: Science and art. Foundations for the future*. Bethesda, MD: National Intelligence University. Retrieved October 16, 2011, from *www.fas.org/irp/dni/educing.pdf*.

Gold, P. B., Engdahl, B. E., Eberly, R. E., Blake, R. J., Page, W. F., & Frueh, B. C. (2000). Trauma exposure, resilience, social support, and PTSD construct validity among former prisoners of war. *Social Psychiatry and Psychiatric Epidemiology, 36*, 36–42.

Haney, C., Banks, C., & Zimbardo, P. (1973). Interpersonal dynamics in a simulated prison. *International Journal of Criminology and Penology, 1*, 69–97.

Joint Personnel Recovery Agency. (n.d.). JPRA Strategic Goals. Available at *www.jpra.mil/links/About/StrategicGoals.html#*.

Joint Personal Recovery Agency. (2010a). *Guidance on joint standards for survival evasion, resistance, escape (SERE) training role play activities in support of the Code of Conduct*. Spokane, WA: Author.

Joint Personal Recovery Agency. (2010b). *Guidance of joint standards for survival, evasion, resistance, escape (SERE) training in support of the Code of Conduct.* Spokane, WA: Author.

Joint Personal Recovery Agency. (2010c). *Guidance on qualification criteria and use of Department of Defense (DoD) survival evasion, resistance, and escape (SERE) psychologists in support of Code of Conduct.* Spokane, WA: Author.

Kesler, R. C., Sonnega, A., Bromet, E., Hughes, M., & Nelson, C. B. (1995). Post-traumatic stress disorder in the National Comorbidity Survey. *Archives of General Psychiatry, 52,* 1048–1060.

Lepore, S. J., Mata, K. A., Allen, B. A. & Evans, G. W. (1993). Social support lowers cardiovascular reactivity to an acute stressor. *Psychosomatic Medicine, 55,* 518–524.

McNeil, J. A., & Morgan, C. A. (2010). Cognition and decision making in extreme environments. In C. H. Kennedy & J. L. Moore (Eds.), *Military neuropsychology* (pp. 361–382). New York: Springer.

Meichenbaum, D. (1985). *Stress inoculation training.* New York: Pergamon Press.

Mitchell, J. (1983). When disaster strikes: The critical incident stress debriefing process. *Journal of Emergency Medical Services, 8,* 36–39.

Moore, J. L. (2010). The neuropsychological functioning of prisoners of war following repatriation. In C. H. Kennedy & J. L. Moore (Eds.), *Military neuropsychology* (pp. 267–295). New York: Springer.

Morgan, C. A., Aikins, D., Steffian, G., Coric, V., & Southwick, S. M. (2007a). Relation between cardiac vagal tone and performance in male military personnel exposed to high stress: Three prospective studies. *Psychophysiology, 44,* 120–127.

Morgan, C. A., Doran, A., Steffian, G., Hazlett, G., & Southwick, S. M. (2006). Stress induced deficits in working memory and visuo-constructive abilities in special operations soldiers. *Biological Psychiatry, 60,* 722–729.

Morgan, C. A., Dule, J., & Rabinowitz, Y. (2020). Impact of interrogation stress on compliance and suggestibility in U.S. military special operations personnel. *Ethics Medicine and Public Health, 14,* 100499.

Morgan, C. A., Hazlett, G., Baronoski, M., Doran, A., Southwick, S. M., & Loftus, E. (2007b). Accuracy of eyewitness identification is significantly associated with performance on a standardized test of recognition. *International Journal of Law and Psychiatry, 30,* 213–223.

Morgan, C. A., Hazlett, G., Doran, A., Garrett, S., Hoyt, G., Thomas, P., et al. (2004a). Accuracy of eyewitness memory for persons encountered during exposure to highly intense stress. *International Journal of the Law and Psychiatry, 27*(3), 265–279.

Morgan, C. A., Hazlett, G., Southwick, S. M., Rasmusson, A., & Lieberman, H. (2009). Effect of carbohydrate administration on recovery from stress induced deficits in cognitive function: A double blind, placebo controlled study of soldiers exposed to survival school stress. *Military Medicine, 174,* 132–138.

Morgan, C. A., Hazlett, G. A., & Steffian, G. (2005, June). *Efficacy of the polygraph and RSA in detecting deception in Special Operations Forces* (Scientific Report). Fort Leavenworth, KS: Joint Institute of Concepts and Requirements Division.

Morgan, C. A., Rasmusson, A., Wang, S., Hoyt, G., Hauger, R., & Hazlett, G. (2002). Neuropeptide-Y, cortisol, and subjective distress in humans exposed to acute stress: Replication and extension of previous report. *Biological Psychiatry, 52,* 136–142.

Morgan, C. A., Southwick, S., Hazlett, G., Rasmusson, A., Hoyt, G., Zimolo, Z., et al. (2004b). Relationships among plasma dehydroepiandrosterone in humans exposed to acute stress. *Archives of General Psychiatry, 61,* 819–825.

Morgan, C. A, Southwick, S. M., Steffian, G., Hazlett, G. A., & Loftus, E. F. (2013, January–February). Misinformation can influence memory for recently experienced, highly stressful events. *International Journal of Law & Psychiatry, 36*(1), 11–17.

Morgan, C. A., Wang, S., Hazlett, G., Rassmusson, A., Anderson, G., & Charney, D. S. (2001). Relationships among cortisol, catecholamines, neuropeptide Y and human performance during uncontrollable stress. *Psychosomatic Medicine, 63,* 412–442.

Morgan, C. A., Wang, S., Mason, J., Southwick, S., Fox, P., Hazlett, G., et al. (2000a). Hormone profiles of humans experiencing military survival training. *Biological Psychiatry, 47,* 891–901.

Morgan, C. A., Wang, S., Southwick, S. M., Rasmusson, A., Hazlett, G., Hauger, R. L., et al. (2000b). Plasma neuropeptide-Y concentrations in humans exposed to military survival training. *Biological Psychiatry, 47,* 902–909.

Mota, N. P, Medved, M., Wang, J., Asmundson, G. J. G., Whitney, D., & Sareen, J. (2012). Stress and mental disorders in female military personnel: Comparisons between the sexes in a male dominated profession. *Journal of Psychiatric Research, 46,* 159–167.

Nolen-Hoeksma, S. (2012). Emotional regulation and psychopathology: The role of gender. *Annual Review of Clinical Psychology, 8,* 161–187.

Oliff, M., Langeland, W., Draijer, N., & Gersons, B. P. R. (2007). Gender differences in posttraumatic stress disorder. *Psychological Bulletin, 133,* 183–204.

Parker K. P., Buckmaster, C. L., Schatzberg A. F., & Lyons, D. M. (2004). Prospective investigation of stress inoculation in young monkeys. *Archives of General Psychiatry, 61*(9), 933–941.

Picano, J. J., Williams, T. J., & Roland, R. R. (2006). Assessment and selection of high-risk operational personnel. In C. H. Kennedy & E. A. Zilmer (Eds.), *Military psychology: Clinical and operational applications* (pp. 353–370). New York: Guilford Press.

Picano, J. J., Williams, T. J., Roland, R. R., & Long, C. (2011). Operational psychologists in support of assessment and selection: Ethical considerations. In C. H. Kennedy & T. J. Williams (Eds.), *Ethical practice in operational psychology: Military and national intelligence applications* (pp. 29–49). Washington DC: American Psychological Association.

Ruhl, R. (1978, May). The Code of Conduct. *Airman,* 63–66. Retrieved from *www.au.af.mil/au/awc/awcgate/au-24/ruhl.pdf.*

Selye, H. (1983). The stress concept: Past, present, and future. In C. L. Cooper (Ed.), *Stress research: Issues for the eighties* (pp. 1–20). New York: John Wiley & Sons.

Sherwood, E. (1986). The power relationship between captor and captive. *Psychiatric Annals, 16,* 653–655.

Sokol, R. (1989). Early mental health intervention in combat situations: The *USS Stark. Military Medicine, 154,* 407–409.

Southwick, S. M., Morgan, C. A., Nicolaou, A. L., & Charney, D. S. (1997). Consistency of memory for combat-related traumatic events in veterans of Operation Desert Storm. *American Journal of Psychiatry, 154,* 173–177.

Staal, M. A., & Stephenson, J. A. (2006). Operational psychology: An emerging sub-discipline. *Military Psychology, 18,* 269–282.

Steptoe, A., Fieldman, G., & Evans, O. (1996). Risk and responsivity to mental stress: The influence of age, gender and risk factors. *Journal of Cardiovascular Risk, 3*(1), 83–93.

Taylor, M. K., Larsen, G. E., & Hiller Lauby, M. D. (2014a). Genetic variants in serotonin and corticosteroid systems modulate neuroendocrine and cardiovascular responses to intense stress. *Behavioral Brain Research, 270,* 1–7.

Taylor, M. K., Laurent, H. K., Larsen, G. E., Rauh, M. J., Hiller Lauby, M. D., & Granger, D. A. (2014b). Salivary nerve growth factor response to intense stress: Effect of sex and body mass index. *Psychoneuroendocrinology, 43,* 90–94.

Taylor, M. K., Markham, A. E., Reis, J. P., Padilla, G. A., Potterat, E. G., Drummond, S. P., et al. (2008). Physical fitness influences stress reactions to extreme military training. *Military Medicine, 173,* 738–742.

Taylor, M., & Morgan, C. A. (2014). Spontaneous and deliberate dissociative states in military personnel: Relationships to objective performance under stress. *Military Medicine, 179*(9), 955–958.

Taylor, M. K., Padilla, G. A., Stanfill, K. E., Markham, A. E., Khostravi, J. Y., Dial Ward, M. E., et al. (2012). Effects of dehydroepiandrosterone supplementation during stressful military training: A randomized, controlled, double-blind field study. *Stress, 15*(1), 85–96.

Taylor, M. K., Sausen, K. P., Mujica-Parodi, L. R., Potterat, E. G., Yanaqi, M. A., & Kim, H. (2007a). Neurophysiologic methods to measure stress during survival, evasion, resistance, and escape training. *Aviation Space Environmental Medicine, 78,* 224–230.

Taylor, M. K., Sausen, K. P., Potterat, E. G., Mujica-Parodi, L. R., Reis, A. E., Markham, A. E., et al. (2007b). Stressful military training: Endocrine reactivity, performance, and psychological impact. *Aviation Space Environmental Medicine, 78,* 1143–1149.

Taylor, M. K., Stanfill, K. E., Padilla, G. A., Markham, A. E., Ward, M. D., Koehler, M. M., et al. (2011). Effect of psychological skills training during military survival school: A randomized, controlled field study. *Military Medicine, 176*(12), 1362–1368.

Tennant, C., Fairley, M. J., Dent, O. F., Suway, M., & Broe, G. A. (1997). Declining prevalence of psychiatric disorder in older former prisoners of war. *Journal of Nervous and Mental Disease, 185,* 686–689.

True, B., & Benaway, M. (1992). Treatment of stress reaction prior to combat using the "BICEPS" model. *Military Medicine, 157,* 380–381.

Ursano, R. J., & Rundell, J. R. (1996). The prisoner of war. In R. J. Ursano & A. Norwood (Eds.), *Emotional aftermath of the Persian Gulf War: Veterans, families, communities, and nations* (pp. 443–476). Washington, DC: American Psychiatric Press.

Weiss, P. A., & Inwald, R. (2010). A brief history of personality assessment in police psychology. In P. A. Weiss (Ed.), *Personality assessment in police psychology: A 21st century perspective* (pp. 5–28). Springfield, IL: Charles C Thomas.

Williams, T. J., Picano, J. J., Roland, R. R., & Banks, L. M. (2006). Introduction to operational psychology. In C. H. Kennedy & E. A. Zillmer (Eds.), *Military psychology: Clinical and operational applications* (pp. 193–214). New York: Guilford Press.

Yerkes, S. (1993). The "un-comfort-able" making sense of adaptation in a war zone. *Military Medicine, 58,* 421–423.

Zimbardo, P. G. (1971). *The power and pathology of imprisonment.* Congressional Record (Serial No. 15, 1971-10-25). Hearings before Subcommittee No. 3 of the United States House Committee on the Judiciary, Ninety-Second Congress, First Session on Corrections, Part II, Prisons, Prison Reform and Prisoner's Rights: California. Washington, DC: U.S. Government Printing Office.

Zimbardo, P. G. (1973). On ethics of intervention in human psychological research: With special reference to the Stanford Prison Experiment. *Cognition, 2,* 243–256.

Crisis Negotiations in a Military Context

Michael J. Craw and Russell E. Palarea

Those interested in the field of crisis negotiation have a wide selection of resources available to develop this important trade craft. There are comprehensive books written by consulting psychologists (e.g., McMains & Mullins, 2015), research articles with conceptual models published in peer-reviewed journals (e.g., Taylor, 2004; Taylor & Donald, 2009; Taylor & Thomas, 2008), and books written by experienced crisis negotiators (e.g., Noesner, 2018; Strentz, 2013, 2018). For consulting psychologists, there are resources on applying the Ethical Principles and Code of Conduct of the American Psychological Association (2002/2017), hereafter referred to as the Ethics Code; to crisis negotiations (e.g., Craw & Catanese, 2020; Gelles & Palarea, 2011). This chapter reviews the psychological principles of crisis negotiations (CN) with emphasis placed on negotiating with members of the military. Familiarity with military culture and rank structure is paramount in these situations. Leveraging positive images of the individual's military service will be discussed. Contemporary issues such as a suggested reformulation of Stockholm syndrome and recommendations for research to empirically validate CN techniques will be covered. The current effort is intended to provide practical guidance regarding a wide range of available psychological conceptualizations, techniques, and strategies.

DEVELOPING AND IMPLEMENTING
CN STRATEGIES WITH AVAILABLE EVIDENCE

The field of CN has a rich history of utilizing concepts from psychology to provide structure to communicate with subjects during crisis situations,

including hostage taking, barricaded subjects, and potential suicide. Early adaptations of psychological theories were derived primarily from clinical psychology and the mental health field to explain subjects' behavior. Later work emphasized the use of behavioral profiles, recommendations for negotiating with specific diagnoses, and sensitivity to context (e.g., spontaneous vs. anticipated vs. deliberate incidents; McMains & Mullins, 2015; Strentz, 2018). Taylor (2002) and Wells, Taylor, and Giebels (2013) outlined the importance of moving toward an empirically derived foundation for describing communication behavior within the negotiation context, including first impressions, rapport building, communication skills, understanding motivations, and application of persuasion strategies. This chapter will focus on psychological strategies that emphasize communication behavior with the subject as the crisis unfolds.

TEAM STRUCTURE AND GENERAL ASSUMPTIONS

The command and control structure of a negotiation may vary depending on jurisdiction, with teams having separation between tactical and negotiation elements or integration with one high-ranking commander in charge of both elements, often referred to as the incident commander. The composition of the negotiation team may vary slightly, but typically has a designated primary negotiator who dialogues with the subject and a secondary negotiator who coaches the negotiator and provides support. Sometimes the secondary negotiator and primary negotiator switch roles if the dialogue is not having the desired effect and it's believed that the secondary negotiator may be a better match for the situation. Many agencies also have a pool of officers with specialized language skills trained in negotiations to fill a vital need when the subject speaks a different language than English. The psychologist acts in a consultant role, monitoring the negotiations and suggesting various strategies to improve communication and rapport. The psychologist's role will be further delineated later in this chapter. Investigators or detectives support the negotiation by providing intelligence, including mental health and criminal background. They also endeavor to locate family members or other collaterals who can provide additional information to aid in negotiations.

Several assumptions can be made upon the outset of a crisis situation based on the universals of human nature and how people respond to a crisis. The utility, and even necessity, of assumptions is that they allow for a starting point based on the limited information available to the negotiation team.

1. Crisis situations are typically emotionally driven events. Rather than bargaining for substantive demands, most situations negotiators encounter are emotionally driven, and crisis management is a reasonable approach to

begin working the problem. If the incident is driven by preplanned events or deliberate hostage taking, rather than spontaneous emotions, the team can adjust its approach accordingly.

2. The use of a host of verbal de-escalation skills, especially active listening, helps to decrease emotionality and increase rationality in the subject. The emotional areas of the brain have a privileged position in brain physiology because of their survival value in split-second reactions involving fight or flight, and can short-circuit the thinking parts of the brain, resulting in irrational thinking and an inability to problem-solve (Pinizzotto, Davis, & Miller, 2004). Not only do the problem-solving areas of the brain shut down when in crisis, but negative emotions increase, and the subject may further believe he or she is losing control. This increases the likelihood that the subject will perceive others as threatening (Boyatzis & McKee, 2005). Therefore, it is important to initially avoid problem solving with the subject and, instead, focus on using verbal de-escalation strategies and building rapport.

3. Human behavior is malleable, and even the most challenging circumstances can be transformed into a peaceful resolution with the use of sound negotiation strategies. Experienced incident commanders may echo this sentiment by reminding their teams that the outcome can never be predicted, and negotiation teams may reflect on many peaceful resolutions in circumstances where it seemed unlikely.

4. There is a science and structure to getting people to cooperate through persuasion principles that are universal across cultures. Social psychology, which is the study of how people behave in context (Ross & Nisbett, 2011), offers many useful strategies the negotiator can combine with active listening skills to de-escalate emotions and help move subjects toward a peaceful resolution. Cialdini's (2004) six psychological strategies (reciprocity, commitment, social proof, liking, authority, and scarcity) are important tools for negotiators to integrate into their dialogue. See McMains and Mullins (2015) for a discussion of persuasion principles in CNs.

5. The passage of time can cause high-intensity emotions to de-escalate and allow for the return of rational thought. Emotionally driven crises often de-escalate naturally through the passage of time. Negotiation is an excellent strategy to facilitate the passage of time and the return of rational thought in the subject (Noesner, 2018).

We now turn to specific psychological conceptualizations that apply to CNs with case examples. The chosen models follow contemporary trends that emphasize the dynamic and context between how the subject and negotiator relate to each other.

CYLINDER MODEL

The cylinder model (Taylor, 2002) is an empirically derived conceptualization of CNs developed through an analysis of nine hostage situation transcripts. The model defines three levels of subject behavior organized as a cylinder: avoidant, competitive (distributive), and cooperative. The analysis identified that subjects' communications often occur at the level of these three orientations. The goal of the CN is to move the subject up the cylinder to higher levels of integration and cooperation. Within each cylinder level, there are three themes of communication or motivation: identity, instrumental, and relational. Subjects may talk about themselves (identity), what they want or demand (instrumental), or the interaction between them and the negotiator (relational). By identifying the subject's level of cooperation and matching with his or her theme of communication, the negotiator may notice increased congruous dialogue and de-escalation of emotions as the subject moves up the cylinder to greater levels of cooperation. The model helps identify when the subject and negotiator are out of sync so that the negotiator can adjust the dialogue. This framework provides an enhanced ability to anticipate the subject's behavior and determine the progression through the negotiations, as illustrated in the following case.

Case 16.1. The Veteran with Substance-Induced Psychosis in Hollywood

A native of New York and Army veteran moved to Hollywood with the unrealistic belief that he would become a famous actor. He returned home from his job as a waiter, began to use methamphetamine, and entered a state of psychosis. He assaulted his roommate with a knife during an argument and barricaded himself in his apartment. His roommate escaped and called the police. Initially, the CN dialogue lasted for a few seconds and centered around antagonistic behavior (competitive) as he yelled and used profanity toward the negotiator (relational). He demanded that the police vacate the area (instrumental), and he spoke of his anger toward a society that had thwarted his success in show business (identity). He remained at the level of competitive/antagonistic behavior in the cylinder model for several hours. During a natural break from dialogue, the tactics team reported that he threw a framed picture out of the second-story dwelling, and it was brought to the negotiations team. It was a photo of the subject at the age of 10 standing next to his father, who was in full dress uniform at a police graduation ceremony (these facts were confirmed by collateral information from his mother), and the picture was covered in blood. The negotiation team reasoned that the subject had negative attitudes toward male authority figures, and it was suggested that dialogue about his father and his police background be avoided. His mother also indicated that he wanted to become a police officer but was rejected from several agencies so he joined the Army instead, hoping to achieve his father's approval as a man in uniform. His experience in the Army was negative, and he was disciplined several times for conflicts with authority, making mention of his military service unlikely to improve rapport. To move the subject toward greater levels of cooperation and circumvent negative attitudes about men in authority, a female negotiator was brought in. The passage of time helped de-escalate his emotions, and the effects of the stimulant narcotics began to wear off. His demeanor changed dramatically when he heard a female voice on the phone, and meaningful dialogue began to take place at the level of cooperative/relational communication and behavior. The intensity of his emotions also decreased, resulting in a more rational subject accepting his fate of being arrested when the SWAT team made entry. Even though he refused to surrender, negotiations set the stage for a tactical intervention with lowered risk for a use of force.

OBSERVING RAPPORT-BASED INTERPERSONAL TECHNIQUES AND MOTIVATIONAL INTERVIEWING

Similar to the cylinder model's (Taylor, 2015) development from studying transcripts of negotiated resolutions, observing rapport-based interpersonal techniques (ORBITS) was borne out of field validation studies of interviews with high-value detainees in counterterrorism investigations (Alison et al., 2013). The researchers devised the ORBITS system after analyzing over 1,000 hours of video footage of terrorism suspects in an interrogation setting to determine communication strategies that resulted in actionable intelligence and greater cooperation. The researchers were particularly interested in how the interviewers developed rapport and used different skills and techniques in response to the suspect's behavior. They defined adaptive and maladaptive communication behaviors, and observed that adaptive interviewer behaviors resulted in more cooperation and a greater yield of information from the interview.

The ORBITS model is based on motivational interviewing (MI; Miller & Rollnick, 2013), which was developed in the field of psychotherapy and has gained prominence in law enforcement settings for de-escalation of subjects with mental illness. It involves five interrelated concepts that are imbued into the communication:

- *Autonomy* involves providing the subject with choice for his or her own self-determination and decision making.
- *Acceptance* involves accepting the views and beliefs of the subject without judgment.
- *Adaptation* allows flexibility to changing circumstances throughout the interaction.

- *Evocation* is used to draw out the subject's beliefs or feelings without passing judgments.
- *Empathy* is used to demonstrate sensitivity and respect for the subject's perspective without necessarily agreeing with his or her views. In this way, empathy is expressed as compassion, as the negotiator seeks clarification and understanding of the subject's point of view, while expressing concern for his or her well-being.

MI is more than a communication approach; it is a way of being with people when dialogue is embued with the above qualities. It is recommended that negotiators explore these concepts in MI as part of an overall development plan. Within this backdrop of communication, ORBITS describes a range of positive or negative interactions between the negotiator and subject, with suggestions for adaptive responses to counter the subject's maladaptive verbalizations. For instance, if the subject is pleading, the negotiator responds with kindness. Aggressiveness and verbal attacks are met with the negotiator being direct, frank, and forthright. Should the subject react with rigidity, the negotiator responds by being humble and seeking guidance. Any weakness or submissiveness on the subject's part is met with the negotiator being firm and setting the agenda. Table 16.1 displays the maladaptive responses with corresponding suggested adaptive responses. Once the negotiator notices the subject has moved to adaptive responses, the negotiator is advised to do the same as he or she selects dialogue. The ORBITS model encourages versatility from the list of adaptive responses as the negotiator wordsmiths the dialogue and responds to the subject. The adaptive list provides a starting place for countering the subject's maladaptive communications, and it is suggested that the negotiator respond with adaptive responses generally opposite the subject's response on the maladaptive list, although any adaptive verbalizations may prove effective.

The following negotiation with a military veteran provides an example of applying the ORBITS model.

Case 16.2. Negotiation with a Subject Threatening Suicide

The negotiation team responded to the scene of a subject named Tom, who was a 68-year-old male Vietnam veteran threatening suicide with a handgun. Tom was communicating from the demanding and rigid theme of maladaptive responses by forcefully asking the primary negotiator a series of personal questions. The primary negotiator was responding with weakness and submissiveness by dutifully answering the questions in a shy and timid fashion. Thus, both the subject and negotiator were communicating from a maladaptive theme. The primary negotiator did not notice when Tom mentioned his military service in Vietnam. The CN supervisor recommended a switch in negotiators. The secondary negotiator took

TABLE 16.1. ORBITS Model

Maladaptive response	Adaptive response
Passive and resentful	Confident and assertive
Weak and submissive	In charge and sets the agenda
Uncertain and hesitant	Supportive and conversational
Overfamiliar and desperate	Social and warm
Parental and patronizing	Respectful and trusting
Demanding and rigid	Humble and seeking guidance
Argumentative and competitive	Patient and pensive
Attacking and punishing	Frank and forthright

Note. Adapted from Alison et al. (2013).

over and approached Tom's demanding and domineering tone with a humbling and seeking guidance framework: "Help me understand what's happened today" and "I'm trying to get a better sense of how you are feeling." Dialogue then focused on Tom's underemployment as an airport shuttle driver, disenfranchisement by his own children, and his divorce. The focus soon shifted to his service in the military. A turning point came when the negotiator asked Tom about the unit to which he was assigned. Tom quickly recited his unit designation with pride. Extensive dialogue took place in the supportive/conversational theme. The negotiator actively listened to Tom's description of his military service, how denigrated he felt by society upon his return home due to unpopular sentiment surrounding the Vietnam conflict, and the challenges he faced in finding employment. When Tom switched back to maladaptive communications and went on a profanity-laced tirade (attacking and punishing), the negotiator responded by being social and warm, acknowledging his emotions and setting an appropriate boundary for courteous dialogue (frank and forthright). Tom began to cry, and the depth and intimacy of the dialogue reflected the strong rapport the negotiator established, setting the stage for an eventual negotiated resolution.

This case illustrates a number of important considerations when negotiating with current service members or veterans.

• Be on guard for the presence of unlocked and accessible firearms in the household of veterans and consider that veterans who become the subject of negotiations are likely to possess firearms and may maintain unsafe firearm practices (Simonetti, Azrael, Rowhani-Rahbar, & Miller, 2018).

• Facilitate discussion about their individual experiences in the military given the wide range of situations veterans may have encountered while in the military. Veterans will be on guard with regard to whether they can trust the negotiator with their most private thoughts and perceptions. They may be particularly untrusting of those who make assumptions or hold stereotypes about veterans.

• Develop relevant knowledge of various ranks, insignia, and terminology related to military service. If the negotiator is unfamiliar with military rank structure and culture, acknowledge this fact and allow the subject to instruct him or her. Express a willingness and curiosity to learn about the subject's experiences and perceptions of the military.

NEGOTIATING WITH CURRENT AND FORMER MILITARY MEMBERS: LEVERAGING POSITIVE IMAGE IN THE MIDST OF A CRISIS OR CRIMINAL BEHAVIOR

Case 16.3. Full-Dress Uniform on a Bridge

Rob had been separated from the Army after only 60 days because of a drug possession charge. Many years later, he scaled a tall bridge and waited for a police response. He was in crisis because the drug charge was preventing him from receiving certain benefits that he believed he was entitled to, and his efforts to get his record expunged had been thwarted. He exhibited instrumental needs/demands in terms of securing benefits after clearing his criminal record and expressive needs related to his perception of unfair treatment. The negotiation dialogue revolved around his anger at the Veterans Administration (VA) and what he saw as endless bureaucracy and red tape. A negotiated resolution was achieved by providing Rob with the opportunity to vent his emotions with a caring negotiator and by securing assurances from VA representatives (who were summoned to the scene) that his case would be reexamined. Months later, Rob experienced similar grievances and repeated his trip to the top of the bridge, but not before spending the last of his funds on a full dress Army uniform. Rob took great pride in his short time with the military, and the strategy of invoking the power of this positive identity was critical in the negotiations. By dialoguing about the positive aspects of his service, however brief, it undermined his low opinion of himself. The negotiator avoided being conflated with bureaucratic institutions by taking on a relaxed, almost glib demeanor. He introduced himself by first name to Rob instead of using a law enforcement title. The negotiator sensed that Rob would be amenable to surrender, and the dialogue transitioned to a plan to recover Rob from the bridge with additional assurances from VA representatives that they would consider his appeal, although it was unlikely that he qualified for benefits.

This case highlights the importance of utilizing the persuasion principle of *consistency* when negotiating with present or former military members. The consistency principle reflects that people value being perceived by others as consistent in their beliefs and actions. Consistency takes two forms: the rationalization trap and the image protection trap. While its name might imply coercion, a rationalization trap is simply used by the negotiator to gently point out to a subject how his current behavior is inconsistent with his stated or implied values. The created dissonance then provides an opportunity to suggest how the subject can bring his behavior in line with his values and beliefs. Cognitive dissonance and the ambivalence it generates pave the way for attitude change and behavior change. An image protection trap is used similarly to prop up a person's self-esteem by talking about positive aspects of his character and values. Let's examine an example illustrating the use of the consistency principle.

Case 16.4. The Reservist in a Custody Dispute

A member of the Army Reserves graduated from the police academy, but was terminated during his probationary period due to unsatisfactory performance. Several years later, he refused to return his 4-year-old son to his ex-wife after visitation. The SWAT team made a stealth entry due to concerns about the child's safety after failed attempts to establish dialogue. Upon entry, one of the tactical officers, who was also cross-trained as a negotiator, noticed the police academy diploma prominently framed above the fireplace as the team searched for the subject and his son. They found the father and son asleep in an upstairs bedroom unharmed, but the SWAT team's presence quickly roused the father from sleep and he took a fighting stance. The SWAT officer remembered the diploma in the living room and said, "We don't want to hurt you, you're one of us." The message evoked feelings of positive identity in the subject, and the SWAT officers instantly became colleagues instead of a perceived threat. He submitted to arrest without incident.

A natural extension to building the suspect's positive identity is instilling a sense of meaning and purpose (for a review, see Barnes, Banks, & Albanese, 2011). Persuasive messages to choose a peaceful course of action are powerful hooks when they are imbued with meaning and purpose. In the military, there is a well-developed sense of purpose that can be evoked during negotiations in the subject, regardless of his or her length of service, record, or discharge status. Negotiation teams are encouraged to familiarize themselves with the various rank structures in the different branches of the military, receive training from veterans groups about current issues facing veterans, and maintain contacts with the VA for resources and consultation.

ROLES OF THE CONSULTING MENTAL HEALTH PROFESSIONAL

The various roles of the mental health professional who consults with the negotiation team include pre-incident, intra-incident, and post-incident duties. Psychologists play a major role prior to a negotiation. They provide training for negotiators on a wide range of topics—including active listening skills, persuasion techniques, crisis intervention, interpersonal relationships, psychiatric disorders and pharmacological treatment, assessment of personality types, threat assessment, and aggression potential—as well as participate in training exercises (Fuselier, 1981; Galyean, Wherry, & Young, 2009).

The psychologist has several functions as a consultant to a negotiation team during incidents (Fuselier, 1988). As an on-scene participant-observer, the psychologist monitors negotiations, translating relevant information and behavior of the subject, with an emphasis on the assessment of potential violence. Also, the psychologist manages the stress level of the negotiator and liaisons with collateral sources and other professionals to support the ongoing assessment of the subject in crisis. The psychologist must help negotiators in not only assessment, but also management of the different behaviors that are presented during a negotiation. The differing patterns of behavior and clinical syndromes presented in negotiation scenarios call for a variety of approaches in managing the subject. Given the complexity of CN situations, there is a high risk that events will agitate the subject. The psychologist assists the negotiator in moving beyond any misperceptions or problems and helps to prevent escalation of the incident.

Because all behavior occurs within a context, the psychologist is in a position to assess the critical interface between the mental state of the subject and the situation that is unfolding. The key to initial assessment in a negotiation scenario is to evaluate the motivation for the subject to engage in negotiation, and it is critical to understand the events that led to a barricaded situation and interaction with law enforcement. An assessment of the context allows the psychologist to evaluate more clearly the motivation of the subject. For example, is the situation based on a terrorist group's attempt to promote a political or religious cause and gain publicity? Are the subjects going to use violence as the punctuation to their communication? Is the situation the result of a botched robbery, with the subject motivated to negotiate an escape? Is the subject suicidal and barricaded, with or without hostages, getting over a failed relationship, and experiencing a sense of helplessness? Is the subject delusional or hallucinating? Are hallucinations the result of drugs or mental illness?

Assessing the situation also includes evaluating whether the subject has engaged in predatory or affective violence (Meloy, 1992). In cases of predatory violence, the subject demonstrates minimal levels of arousal, does not demonstrate emotion, acts in a purposeful and planned manner, and demonstrates behavioral responses that are not time-limited. Generally, these subjects demonstrate a level of heightened awareness, as is often the case in criminal escapes, botched robberies, or terrorist acts. When the subject demonstrates indicators consistent with affective violence, the goal is threat reduction (Van Hasselt et al., 2005). These individuals show an intense level of arousal and considerable emotion in the form of anger and fear; they are often reactive, and there is a heightened but diffuse level of awareness. This phenomenon is generally observed in domestic violence situations, with the serving of warrants, and with individuals who are either under the influence of a substance or mentally ill.

In any context in which a negotiation is initiated and an assessment pursued, it is critical to evaluate the subject's motivation for negotiation. For example, an individual who has been interrupted during a homicide–suicide may have little interest in negotiating if he or she has already made a decision on the eventual outcome. The approach will be more solution-oriented, geared toward buying time and offering alternatives. In situations in which the subjects are reactive and emotional, the preferred strategy is to create some sense of containment, using time to allow them to utilize their available resources and reduce the tendency to act impulsively.

The art and science of psychological consultation in CNs have evolved over the years. The concept of psychological profiles has become increasingly outdated and of little use to negotiators. Traditional psychiatric diagnosis is also of limited relevance. Rather, demonstrated critical variables include behavioral indicators or behavioral constellations and their associated personality styles, which are assessed by accounting for the contexts in which they occur.

Psychological consultants to the negotiator engage in ongoing, context-specific behavioral assessment, which generates inferences and hypotheses they want to corroborate. However, most critically, psychologists assess the motivation behind each communication and try to determine throughout the negotiation whether the subject is *making* or *posing* a threat (Fein & Vossekuil, 1998, 1999). As consultants, psychologists are interested in what a person says and does, giving insight into whether the negotiation process is increasing or decreasing the potential for violence or peaceful resolution.

Turner and Gelles (2003) discuss several variables that help assess a communication for violence potential: the degree to which the communication is organized, fixated on a theme, or blaming; whether it is focused on a specific person or target; and whether an action plan or time imperative is articulated. Today, as a result of considerable work in the area of targeted violence (Fein & Vossekuil, 1998, 1999), psychologists can help assess the potential for violence in the behavior and communication of CN situations. Also, with current developments in indirect assessment, psychologists contribute significantly to the analysis of gathered intelligence through interviews with family members, assessing the subject's mental status, recognizing potential mental illness, and utilizing data about the subject's actions and patterns of behavior. However, given ethical dilemmas regarding the boundaries between a clinical health care provider and operational psychology consultant, consultations with other mental health professionals should be approached with caution (Gelles & Palarea, 2011; see below as well as Chapter 17, this volume, for more on operational psychology ethics).

Psychologists function as an adjunct resource to the team, offering expertise in understanding behavior (Bahn & Louden, 1999), and helping to translate behavior for the on-scene commander and the negotiator. As a mental health professional, the psychologist thinks and interprets behavior differently than a tactical commander, who serves as a strategic decision maker. Because CN is a law enforcement function, psychologists *do not and should not* function as a negotiator. It is uncommon for psychologists to know about the process of negotiations, the resources of law enforcement, or the public safety responsibility of law enforcement (McMains & Mullins, 2001). Using a psychologist as a negotiator may also escalate a situation by implying that an individual is mentally ill or by dredging up previous negative experiences with the mental health system (Hatcher, Mohandie, Turner, & Gelles, 1998). Psychologists function as consultants, and their expertise is used by the negotiation team to plan its strategy. One difficulty for psychologists is that, after hours and possibly days of negotiations, the final resolution may require tactical operations to capture or kill the subject (Fuselier, 1981). This may also cause serious injury and/or the death of the hostages, law enforcement officers, and bystanders.

In addition to focusing on the subject, monitoring the stress of the negotiators is a key role of the psychologist consultant. Crisis negotiators are highly trained, have superior verbal skills, and are able to think quickly and perform effectively under tremendous stress. But even these superior performers experience a high level of stress both during and after negotiations. The negotiators are under significant pressure to successfully conclude negotiations and prevent harm to innocent people. Although time is a great ally for the negotiators, increasing the chances of a positive resolution, the more time that passes, the more impatient the tactical arm of the crisis response team becomes. This creates added pressure for the negotiators, who must remain collected and rational. Psychologists should monitor the negotiators and provide feedback. If they believe a negotiator is losing objectivity, they can recommend bringing in a new negotiator. The internal and external pressures on negotiators ebb and flow throughout the process, and psychologists are a great asset in monitoring these stressors. To the extent possible, they can also monitor and promote the well-being of hostages (Giebels, Noelanders, & Vervaeke, 2005).

Following an incident, psychologists provide stress management education, particularly when incidents have an adverse outcome, as well as team debriefings and counseling to team members. Unsuccessful negotiations that result in death and injury are a significant cause of stress for the hostage negotiator. One example occurred in September 2004 in Beslan, Russia, where Chechen terrorists were holding children and teachers hostage. After authorities stormed the school, more than 300 victims were killed. When there are adverse outcomes like this, negotiators commonly feel guilty, angry, and depressed (Bohl, 1992). Although initially these feelings are considered normal, a psychologist consultant can help restructure the perception of the event, showing the negotiator and the team how to use the experience to learn and move forward. When negotiators fail to manage symptoms appropriately after a poor outcome, long-term problems may occur, such as mood disturbance, occupational or marital problems, and substance abuse. Negotiators are also at risk of developing posttraumatic stress disorder (Bohl, 1992). A psychologist's expertise is invaluable when helping negotiators in this capacity.

ETHICAL ISSUES IN CNS

CNs present numerous ethical dilemmas to the psychologist consultant and have received attention in the literature (Gelles & Palarea, 2011; Rowe, Gelles, & Palarea, 2006), including a recent update from Craw and Catanese (2020). Gelles and Palarea (2011) reviewed the various roles psychologists provide in CNs and identified typical ethical dilemmas that arise from these roles. They noted that ethical conflicts naturally arise between the needs of the law enforcement agency (the client), the needs of any persons taken hostage (society), and the needs of the subject in crisis. In order to anticipate and proactively address these role conflicts and mixed agency issues, the consulting psychologist is advised to identify the different roles in the consultation process, to draw boundaries between these roles, and to not violate these boundaries (see also Kennedy, 2012). For example, the psychologist should remain in the objective role as consultant to the negotiation process and not serve as the actual negotiator or as the on-scene strategic decision maker. The psychologist needs to also be mindful of keeping his or her operational and clinical roles separate, and must not provide clinical mental health services to the negotiation team when functioning as an operational member of the same team. Instead, a separate clinical psychologist should be brought in to provide mental health support and debrief the negotiation team members, including the operational psychologist serving on the team.

Additionally, Gelles and Palarea (2011) conducted an analysis of the Ethics Code on specific applications to CNs, indirect assessment issues, training and competency issues, and other considerations in consulting with law enforcement. One common argument against psychologists serving on negotiation teams is that it violates the "do no harm" principle (Principle A & Ethical Standard 3.04), as the psychologist may participate in a negotiation that ultimately ends with a tactical intervention in which the subject is killed by the police (Call, 2008). However, they point out that the purpose of the psychological consultation is to preserve life and thus avoid harm. Furthermore, they argue that the psychologist's role is to assist the negotiation team with gaining insight into the subject's mental health, motivations, and risk for violence in order to ensure the safety of the subject in crisis, any hostages taken, the police, and bystanders, and to assist with bringing the situation to a peaceful resolution.

Craw and Catanese (2020) provided further clarification and refinement regarding application of the Ethics Code in CN operations, specifically the concern related to being perceived as a participant to the tactical action (McCutcheon, 2017). Previous writings advised that the consultation ends when tactical action begins (Gelles & Palarea, 2011), a recommendation not easily implemented in fluid situations. The nature of critical incidents and organization or placement of tactical versus negotiation cadres may create an inability to know if and when tactical action might occur, leaving the psychologist unable to end the consultation. Knapp, Younggren, VandeCreek, Harris, and Martin (2013) advise psychologists to guard against absolutist thinking because such recommendations have no other purpose than to increase the consultant's legal protection. Such false risk management strategies deny the psychologist the opportunity to think through ethical issues to arrive at the best decision.

Craw and Catanese (2020) suggest that consulting psychologists define their consultation during SWAT call-outs along a continuum of engagement and disengagement. That is, the psychological consultant decides on his or her level of participation, based on ethical considerations, and perhaps disengages, but remains present, when circumstances arise that may conflict with ethical principles. Craw and Catanese (2020) discuss areas not previously addressed in the literature that may create potential ethical dilemmas and signal potential disengagement, such as involving third-party intermediaries. They argue the most common reason to consider less participation or disengagement is when the situation violates the aspirational principle of beneficence.

Other key elements of the Ethics Code addressed by Gelles and Palarea

(2011) include identifying and avoiding multiple relationships (Ethical Standard 3.05), establishing and maintaining competence (Ethical Standards 2.01 and 2.03), and conducting an indirect assessment of the subject in crisis (Ethical Standard 9.01).

Finally, Gelles and Palarea (2011) provided the following guidelines in order to more clearly define roles and boundaries in psychological consultation for CNs:

- *Identify the client, the psychologist's role, and the roles of other team members.* The client is the law enforcement organization, not the subject, hostages, or other involved parties. The psychologist's role is to consult with the law enforcement team as they conduct the negotiation.

- *Remain in the role of an expert psychologist consultant.* The psychologist should remain in the objective role as subject matter expert consultant and should never become the negotiator.

- *Remain autonomous in consultation and free from external influence and pressure.* The psychologist should be mindful of not letting the high-energy environment, the scene commander's agenda, or the political agendas of senior leadership influence the consultation.

- *Identify the boundaries of the psychologist's role.* The psychologist only serves as a consultant and never as the on-site strategic decision maker. The psychologist consults with the negotiator and scene commander on the negotiation process, but never makes operational decisions, such as shifting from negotiation to tactical resolution.

- *Appreciate the uniqueness of each crisis situation.* The psychologist gives careful thought and consideration to each negotiation and subject in crisis, understands the limitations of models and templates, and keeps his or her biases and prejudices in check.

- *Clearly delineate the boundaries between operational consultants and health care providers.* The psychologist must keep the clinical health care provider and operational consultation roles separate. Before entering into an operational consultation role, the psychologist must first receive appropriate training and supervision.

- *Establish and maintain professional competence.* Psychologists conducting consultation on this mission should receive CN training and supervision, join their local CN association and conduct liaison with other CN professionals, and establish a network of psychologists consulting on this mission in order to discuss and resolve ethical dilemmas.

NEGOTIATOR DEVELOPMENT

Leaders in military and police organizations may be tempted to enlist psychologists to perform preselection psychological assessments (Corey, 2007) for negotiator assignments with the idea that selection is paramount for the specialized skills of CN. There are a number of problems associated with performing psychological assessments on incumbent employees, including potentially negative consequence if their tests reveal they are not suitable. Existing psychological instruments may also not be valid and reliable for such purposes. Instead of formal psychological selection, it is suggested that CN training programs employ various opportunities for team members to introspect about their life experiences, personality, and character strengths that may relate to how subjects perceive them.

One way to enhance negotiator development is to complete a branding matrix (Shepherd, 2005), a tool borrowed from marketing and product placement. Create a personal branding statement based on the information gleaned from the following questions: (1) How does the subject see him- or herself? (2) How does the subject see us? (3) How do we see the subject? (4) How do we need the subject to see us?

By responding to the above questions, the negotiator is in a position to craft first impressions, anticipate personal questions, and predict subject reactions. The horns and halos effect describes our human tendency to make an immediate judgment regarding whether we like or dislike someone upon meeting that individual (Nisbett & Wilson, 1977). This global and automatic evaluation occurs without sufficient evidence to make such judgments. We also tend to trust our first impressions even when presented later with contradictory information. In the negotiation context, the metaphor of horns and halos illustrates why branding is so important. The negotiator needs to project a positive, nonthreatening tone at the outset of the dialogue, with an emphasis on first impressions.

The branding matrix can be completed for the negotiator, the negotiation team, or even the entire SWAT team and police department. For instance, the narratives, stories, and Hollywood portrayals that subjects hold toward SWAT teams is a horns effect; they assume the SWAT team is likely to use lethal force against them. The negotiator can anticipate this assumption and change the suspect's perception to a halo effect by creating the suggestion of a peaceful resolution and sharing that uses of force are rare.

THE IMPACT OF HOSTAGE BEHAVIOR ON INCIDENT OUTCOMES: MOVING BEYOND STOCKHOLM SYNDROME

When first described, Stockholm syndrome (named for a bank robbery in Stockholm, Sweden in which hostages formed a bond with their hostage takers) was an urgent attempt to explain what law enforcement saw as con-founding—the development of positive feelings in hostages toward hostage takers and concomitant feelings of hostility toward the police, presumably in an effort to survive the encounter. Even though the term appears in the negotiation literature, no rigorous research or definitions are associated with Stockholm syndrome. It may best be thought of as a legacy term accounted for by modern conceptualizations of trauma. The key to developing such reactions is prolonged and extreme exposure to traumatic stress, as seen in human/sex trafficking, intimate partner abuse, incest, prisoners of war, or cult membership. With prolonged confinement and traumatic abuse, a hostage may develop paradoxical reciprocal positive feelings toward their captors to enhance their coping and survival (Cantor & Price, 2007). These survival strategies are manifestations that take more time to develop than is typical in a hostage-taking incident (J. Leipsic, personal communica-tion, 2017). It is important for negotiation teams to think broadly about an array of behaviors in hostages that may impact the incident and label such behavior in an effort to understand what is occurring. Behavioral manifes-tations include survival attachment, trauma response, or misinterpretation of arousal cues for positive feelings toward the captor (Catanese & Pultz, 2019). Some examples illustrate a host of hostage behaviors that can occur.

Case 16.5. The Hostages Who Took Care of the Hostage Taker

A car-jacking subject took three members of a family hostage while fleeing custody. He forced his way into their home as the mother was entering the front door with groceries. Colloquially known as the "look who's come to dinner" caper, the grandmother said to the mother in Spanish, "Let's be nice to him" and proceeded to cook the subject dinner. As the negotia-tion team waited for them to finish dinner to re-engage in a dialogue, they reflected on what appeared to be Stokholm syndrome. The true nature of the hostages' influence turned out to be very different and wasn't revealed until interviews and debriefings occurred afterward. Prolonged negotia-tions revolved around the suspect's focus on the amount of time he would likely serve in prison for his crimes and other issues related to his past criminal history. They negotiated the release of the mother, which left the grandmother and teenage daughter still inside the location. There were tense periods of time without dialogue, and unknown to the negotiation team, the daughter was trying to convince a now suicidal subject to not shoot himself. He agreed but didn't promise to not attempt other meth-ods of suicide. He then drank a mixture of orange juice and bathroom cleaner. The daughter could have self-evacuated, but instead continued to tend to his needs. When he vomited, the elderly grandmother cleaned his vomitus, comforted him, and upon release, gave him the leather scapu-lar necklace she had received at Holy Communion many decades earlier.

When interviewed in prison, the subject still wore the scapular necklace and described how he was overwhelmed by the dispositional kindness shown by the family, which led to his eventual surrender. The hostages, motivated by their own humanity rather than trauma or fear, also showed no evidence of hostility toward law enforcement. The hostages' actions toward their captor proved to be a substantial factor in the outcome.

Case 16.6. The Hostage Who Got Drunk in Order to Cope

A police pursuit terminated at a convenience store. The two suspects took the cashier hostage and threatened to cut off his fingers with pruning shears unless the police retreated. The hostage, in an attempt to dull his experience, began to imbibe heavily. By the time the SWAT team performed a dynamic entry, the hostage was unable to assist in his own rescue, having consumed a 12-pack of beer. He had no positive feelings toward the suspects or hostility toward the police and reacted to the suspects' threats of violence with passive resignation.

Case 16.7. The Physician Who Kept Her Cool

A paranoid subject persisted in a delusional belief that doctors at a local hospital had performed medical experiments on him by injecting acid into his bloodstream. He walked into the hospital with a plan of vengeance, stating, "I'm going to shoot whitecoats." He murdered several physicians before taking a physician and a clerk hostage in a back office. Negotiations led to an agreed hostage release in which the hostages would exit first, followed by the suspect. Neither hostage developed any positive feelings toward the suspect, nor did they manifest hostility toward the police. The physician remained calm and participated in dialogue with the negotiators when the subject allowed communication, while the clerk was terrified and unable to speak. At the moment of hostage release, the physician decided that it was too risky to turn her back on the suspect, so she influenced the subject to exit at the same time. This led to last-second adjustments by the tactical team, who expected to only receive the hostages. The physician continues to send chocolates annually to the SWAT team on the anniversary of the incident to express her gratitude to law enforcement.

INSIGHTS FROM SUBJECTS REGARDING NEGOTIATIONS

Some agencies have conducted interviews with subjects who were involved in negotiations to learn more about what they found effective and what wasn't helpful. The most fruitful interviews were conducted in prison well after the incident and following criminal proceedings. These interviews are time intensive, but can glean meaningful information with regard to the suspect's perception of the negotiations process, as compared to the short debriefs from the back of a squad car following the incident. While no systematic research has been conducted on these interviews, the senior author interviewed a former SWAT commander (M. Albanese, personal communication, February 2020) who conducted these interviews and reviewed a number of interview videos. Three themes emerged that benefit negotiators: (1) Suspects perceive rapport and trust with the negotiator as paramount. (2) It was important to the subject that no deception be attempted by the negotiator, resulting in the perception of the negotiator as honest, direct, and frank. (3) Suspects often reported they felt as if the negotiator treated them better than other officers with whom they had interacted in the past. These qualitative findings suggest negotiators should master active listening skills and motivational interviewing, two powerful techniques from the psychotherapy field that are useful for developing rapport (see the previous sections). Emerging evidence from the field of investigative interviewing indicates rapport-based strategies achieve positive results; the field of CN would benefit from utilizing the same research methodology.

FUTURE DIRECTIONS FOR RESEARCH: THE EVIDENCE BASE FOR NEGOTIATIONS

With the collaboration of the Federal Bureau of Investigation, Defense Intelligence Agency, and Central Intelligence Agency, the High Value Detainee Interrogation Group (HIG) was formed in 2009, to transition American law enforcement toward evidence-based and noncoercive interrogation methods (White House Press Briefing, August 24, 2009). The model of field-validating interrogation methods and establishing an empirical base for certain techniques can also be applied to negotiations (Brimbal, Kleinman, Oleszkiewicz, & Meissner, 2019; Brimbal, Meissner, Kleinman, & Phillips, 2019; Meissner, Surmon-Böhr, Oleszkiewicz, & Alison, 2017). The research methodology involves coding and statistically analyzing transcripts to identify fidelity to certain tradecraft and techniques with measured outcomes. In validating rapport-based interrogation techniques, the desired outcome is not a confession, but rather development of new information that can be used to further an investigation. Similarly, in negotiations, the outcome variables may include continued dialogue, evidence of rapport, and higher levels of cooperation as described in the cylinder model (Taylor, 2002). Such research methodology would advance the field of CNs by establishing empirical support for techniques that lead to meaningful dialogue and successful resolution.

CONCLUSION

In closing, psychologists and other mental health professionals provide valuable consultation to CN teams. Across the nation, law enforcement agencies have integrated mental health consultants as a vital part of the negotiation team. The community expectation for de-escalation, negotiation, and nonlethal means of resolving crises has never been more intense, whether the jurisdiction is in a military context or municipal, state, federal, or tribal setting. This leads to the need for law enforcement and mental health professionals to be well trained and prepared to engage in dialogue that is geared toward increasing the chances of a peaceful resolution for a wide variety of crisis scenarios.

REFERENCES

Alison, L. J., Alison, E., Noone, G., Elntib, S., & Christiansen, P. (2013). Why tough tactics fail and rapport gets results: Observing Rapport-Based Interpersonal Techniques (ORBIT) to generate useful information from terrorists. *Psychology, Public Policy, and Law, 19*(4), 411–431.

American Psychological Association. (2002/2017). *Ethical principles of psychologists and code of conduct* (amended June 1, 2010, and January 1, 2017). Retrieved from *www.apa.org/ethics/code.*

Bahn, C., & Louden, R. J. (1999). Hostage negotiation as a team enterprise. *Group, 23,* 77–85.

Barnes, D. M., Banks, C. K., & Albanese, M. (2011). Meaning-making: The search for meaning in dangerous contexts. In P. J. Sweeney, M. D. Matthews, & P. B. Lester (Eds.), *Leadership in dangerous situations: A handbook for the Armed Forces, emergency services, and first responders* (pp. 139–159). Annapolis, MD: Naval Institute Press.

Bohl, N. K. (1992). Hostage negotiator stress. *FBI Law Enforcement Bulletin, 61,* 24–26.

Boyatzis, R., & McKee, A. (2005). *Resonant leadership: Renewing yourself and connecting with others through mindfulness, hope, and compassion.* Boston: Harvard Business Press.

Brimbal, L., Kleinman, S. M., Oleszkiewicz, S., & Meissner, C. A. (2019). Developing rapport and trust in the interrogative context: An empirically-supported and ethical alternative to customary interrogation practices. In S. J. Barela, M. J. Fallon, G. Gaggioli, & J. D. Ohlin (Eds.), *Interrogation and torture: Integrating efficacy with law and morality* (pp. 141–171). Oxford: Oxford University Press.

Brimbal, L., Meissner, C. A., Kleinman, S. M., & Phillips, E. (2019). *Validating a conceptual framework for resistance in investigative interviewing.* Paper presented at the American Psychology-Law Society Annual Meeting, New Orleans, LA.

Call, J. A. (2008). Psychological consultation in hostage/barricade crisis negotiations. In H. Hall (Ed.), *Forensic psychology and neuropsychology for criminal and civil cases* (pp. 263–288). Boca Raton, FL: CRC Press.

Cantor, C., & Price, J. (2007). Traumatic entrapment, appeasement and complex post-traumatic stress disorder: Evolutionary perspectives of hostage reactions, domestic abuse and the Stockholm syndrome. *Australian & New Zealand Journal of Psychiatry, 41*(5), 377–384.

Catanese, S. A., & Pultz, J. (2019). *Stockholm syndrome: Implications for crisis negotiation teams.* Paper presented at California Hostage Negotiators Association (CAHN) quarterly training, Anaheim, CA.

Cialdini, R. B. (2004). The science of persuasion. *Scientific American Mind, 284,* 76–84.

Corey, D. (2007). Analysis of the ADA as it pertains to medical examinations of police officers applying for special assignments. *AELE Monthly Law Journal, 7,* 501–513.

Craw, M. J., & Catanese, S. A. (2020). Identifying points of engagement versus disengagement when consulting during crisis negotiations: A flexible model for applying the ethics code. *Journal of Police and Criminal Psychology, 35,* 92–97.

Fein, R. A., & Vossekuil, B. (1998). *Protective intelligence and threat assessment investigations* (NCJ Publication No. 170612). Washington, DC: U.S. Department of Justice.

Fein, R. A., & Vossekuil, B. (1999). Assassination in the United States: An operational study of recent assassins, attackers, and near-lethal approachers. *Journal of Forensic Sciences, 44,* 321–333.

Fuselier, G. D. (1981). A practical overview of hostage negotiations, Part 2. *FBI Law Enforcement Bulletin, 50,* 10–15.

Fuselier, G. D. (1988). Hostage negotiation consultant: Emerging role for the clinical psychologist. *Professional Psychology: Research and Practice, 10,* 175–179.

Galyean, K. D., Wherry, J. N., & Young, A. T. (2009). Valuation of services offered by mental health professionals in SWAT team members: A study of the Lubbock, Texas SWAT team. *Journal of Police and Criminal Psychology, 24*(1), 51–58.

Gelles, M., & Palarea, R. (2011). Ethics in crisis negotiation: A law enforcement and public safety perspective. In C. Kennedy & T. Williams (Eds.), *Ethical practice in operational psychology: Military and national intelligence applications* (pp. 107–125). Washington, DC: American Psychological Association.

Giebels, E., Noelanders, S., & Vervaeke, G. (2005). The hostage experience: Implications for negotiation strategies. *Clinical Psychology and Psychotherapy, 12,* 241–253.

Hatcher, C., Mohandie, K., Turner, J., & Gelles, M. (1998). The role of the psychologist in crisis/hostage negotiations. *Behavioral Sciences and the Law, 16,* 455–472.

Kennedy, C. H. (2012). Institutional ethical conflicts with illustrations from police and military psychology. In S. Knapp & L. Vandecreek (Eds.), *APA handbook of ethics in psychology: Vol. 1. Moral foundations and common themes* (pp. 123–144). Washington, DC: American Psychological Association.

Knapp, S., Younggren, J. N., VandeCreek, L., Harris, E., & Martin, J. N. (2013). *Assessing and managing risk in psychological practice: An individualized approach.* Rockville, MD: The Trust.

McCutcheon, J. L. (2017). Emerging ethical issues in police and public safety psychology: Reflections on mandatory vs. aspirational ethics. In C. Mitchell & E. Dorian (Eds.), *Police psychology and its growing impact on modern law enforcement* (pp. 314–334). Hershey, PA: Information Science Reference.

McMains, M. J., & Mullins, W. (2001). *Crisis negotiations: Managing critical incidents and hostage situations in law enforcement and corrections* (2nd ed.). Cincinnati, OH: Anderson.

McMains, M. J., & Mullins, W. C. (2015). *Crisis negotiations managing critical incidents and hostage situations in law enforcement and corrections.* London: Routledge.

Meissner, C. A., Surmon-Böhr, F., Oleszkiewicz, S., & Alison, L. J. (2017). Developing an evidence-based perspective on interrogation: A review of the U.S. government's high-value detainee interrogation group research program. *Psychology, Public Policy, and Law, 23*(4), 438–457.

Meloy, J. R. (1992). *Violent attachments.* Northvale, NJ: Jason Aronson.

Miller, W. R., & Rollnick, S. (2013). *Motivational interviewing: Helping people change.* New York: Guilford Press.

Nisbett, R. E., & Wilson, T. D. (1977). The halo effect: Evidence for unconscious alteration of judgments. *Journal of Personality and Social Psychology, 35*(4), 250–256.

Noesner, G. (2018). *Stalling for time: My life as an FBI hostage negotiator.* New York: Random House.

Pinizzotto, A., Davis, E. F., & Miller, C. E. (2004). Intuitive policing: Emotional/rational decision making in law enforcement. *PsycEXTRA Dataset.*

Ross, L., & Nisbett, R. E. (2011). *The person and the situation: Perspectives of social psychology.* London: Pinter & Martin.

Rowe, K. L., Gelles, M. G., & Palarea, R. E. (2006). Crisis and hostage negotiations. In C. H. Kennedy & E. A. Zillmer (Eds.), *Military psychology: Clinical and operational applications* (pp. 310–331). New York: Guilford Press.

Shepherd, I. D. H. (2005). From cattle and Coke to Charlie: Meeting the challenge of self marketing and personal branding. *Journal of Marketing Management, 21*(5–6), 589–606.

Simonetti, J. A., Azrael, D., Rowhani-Rahbar, A., & Miller, M. (2018). Firearm storage practices among veterans. *American Journal of Preventative Medicine, 55*(4), 445–454.

Strentz, T. (2013). *Hostage/crisis negotiations: Lessons learned from the bad, the mad, and the sad.* Springfield, IL: Charles C. Thomas.

Strentz, T. (2018). *Psychological aspects of crisis negotiation.* New York: Routledge.

Taylor, P. J. (2002). A cylindrical model of communication behavior in crisis negotiations. *Human Communication Research, 28,* 7–48.

Taylor, P. J., & Donald, I. (2004). The structure of communication behavior in simulated and actual crisis negotiations. *Human Communication Research, 30,* 443–478.

Taylor, P. J., & Thomas, S. (2008). Linguistic style matching and negotiation outcome. *Negotiation and Conflict Management Research, 1,* 263–281.

Turner, J. T., & Gelles, M. G. (2003). *Threat assessment: A risk management approach*. Binghamton, NY: Haworth.

Van Hasselt, V. B., Flood, J. J., Romano, S. J., Vecchi, G. M., de Fabrique, N., & Dalfonzo, V. A. (2005). Hostage-taking in the context of domestic violence: Some case examples. *Journal of Family Violence, 20,* 21–27.

Wells, S., Taylor, P. J., & Giebels, E. (n.d.). Crisis negotiation: From suicide to terrorism intervention. *Handbook of Research on Negotiation,* 473–496.

Ethical Dilemmas in Clinical, Operational, Expeditionary, and Combat Environments

Carrie H. Kennedy

Military psychology ethics has received significant visibility in recent years, with unprecedented use of psychologists during the war. Psychologists used psychometric expertise in assessing blast concussion in the combat zone, increased consultation roles, and continued to expand other evolving skill sets (e.g., prescription privileges, telehealth, embedded psychology, assessment and treatment of military stress reactions). In an organization in which consultation activities and clinical decisions can have dire consequences, military psychologists routinely address a number of difficult ethical issues. While every area of psychological practice contends with potentially conflicting loyalties, guidance, and regulations, military psychology faces a high degree of ethical dilemmas, with the added dynamics and potentially conflicting interactions of the American Psychological Association's *Ethical Principles of Psychologists and Code of Conduct* (2017; hereafter referred to as the Ethics Code), APA policy, military instructions, and military laws (i.e., Uniformed Code of Military Justice; see also Johnson, Grasso, & Maslowski, 2010; Coyne, 2019). Given the complexity of some of these interactions, the sometimes ambiguous wording of ethics codes in general, and the impossibility of ethics codes to cover every potential situation, simply following the Ethics Code is insufficient for ethical decision making (Kitchener & Kitchener, 2012).

This chapter focuses on the four environments in which military psychologists practice—traditional military treatment facilities, operational commands, noncombat expeditionary environments, and the combat zone—and highlights the most prominent ethical dilemmas experienced in each locale. Finally, recommendations for prevention and mitigation of conflicts are presented.

TRADITIONAL MILITARY TREATMENT FACILITIES

Traditional military treatment facilities (MTFs) include both military and veterans' hospitals and clinics and encompass all aspects of mental health care, including primary-care behavioral health services, mental health outpatient assessment and treatment, addictions services, and inpatient treatment. Military providers in MTFs enjoy routine access to resources most clinical psychologists take for granted: electronic medical records, soundproofed offices, support staff, office equipment, and generally predictable schedules and patient caseloads, to name a few. Ethical conflicts tend to be those normally associated with traditional mental health care with the added dynamics of military practice.

The practice of clinical psychology in MTFs dates back to World War II, when many psychologists transitioned from primarily research and psychometric assessment to the provision of mental health care. This occurred largely because of the overwhelming mental health needs of World War II veterans and insufficient numbers of psychiatrists (see Chapter 1, this volume; see also Kennedy, Boake, & Moore, 2010). Consequently, a robust analysis of ethical dilemmas in the military comes from practice in traditional military treatment environments given the eight decades that military psychologists have been able to identify and examine these challenges. These primary ethical dilemmas include multiple/dual relationships and roles (Johnson, 2008; McCauley, Hughes, & Liebling-Kalifani, 2008; Barnett, 2013), competence (Johnson, 2008; Dobmeyer, 2013), informed consent, cultural/multicultural competence (Kennedy, Jones, & Arita, 2007; Reger, Etherage, Reger, & Gahm, 2008; Kennedy, 2020), confidentiality (Johnson, 2008; McCauley et al., 2008; Hoyt, 2013), and mixed/dual agency (e.g., Stone, 2008; Kennedy & Johnson, 2009; Johnson, 2013).

Multiple/Dual Relationships and Roles

In the day-to-day role of any active-duty military psychologist, dual roles and relationships are unavoidable. The psychologist is a military officer with inherent regulations and expectations given his or her rank, in addition to the fact that the psychologist is a member of the command and community with collateral duties, community involvement, friendships, and so on. In a large stateside MTF, these relationships are fairly easy to mitigate given significant options for referral (e.g., other military providers within the MTF and civilian referrals outside of the MTF). However, akin to rural

environments, multiple relationships are particularly common in solo and remote billets, and these can be harder to manage. It is not uncommon for a psychologist to have to enter into a clinical relationship with a subordinate, a senior officer, a roommate, or even a friend (Staal & King, 2000; Johnson, 2011). Standard 3.05, Multiple Relationships, states:

> (a) A multiple relationship occurs when a psychologist is in a professional role with a person and (1) at the same time is in another role with the same person, (2) at the same time is in a relationship with a person closely associated with or related to the person with whom the psychologist has the professional relationship, or (3) promises to enter into another relationship in the future with the person or a person closely associated with or related to the person.
>
> A psychologist refrains from entering into a multiple relationship if the multiple relationship could reasonably be expected to impair the psychologist's objectivity, competence, or effectiveness in performing his or her functions as a psychologist, or otherwise risks exploitation or harm to the person with whom the professional relationship exists.
>
> Multiple relationships that would not reasonably be expected to cause impairment or risk exploitation or harm are not unethical.
>
> (b) If a psychologist finds that, due to unforeseen factors, a potentially harmful multiple relationship has arisen, the psychologist takes reasonable steps to resolve it with due regard for the best interests of the affected person and maximal compliance with the Ethics Code.

Not all multiple relationships are contraindicated. It is important for the military psychologist to be able to objectively determine whether a dual-role/multiple relationship could be potentially harmful prior to entering into the relationship (Sommers-Flanagan, 2012). Treating a member of the command who does not work in your department, for example, and then serving on the military ball committee with that same person are not likely to qualify as potentially harmful. It is important, however, that thorough informed consent be done with every military patient, since these dual relationships arise frequently and unexpectedly and are not always so benign. Let's examine a case in which there is a clear, problematic, yet unavoidable dual relationship.

Case 17.1. The Psychologist with a Dual Relationship Problem

The psychologist was a junior officer in an overseas location. One afternoon, she received a phone call from the Commanding Officer (CO) of the hospital (also the psychologist's CO), who noted that he was command-directing another high-ranking officer in the chain of command (also one of the psychologist's superiors) for emergent mental health evaluation. The other officer's wife reported to the CO that her husband had an uncontrollable gambling habit, had lost their life savings, was now $200,000 in debt, and was voicing suicidal statements.

The psychologist knew that she should not see this officer as a patient. He was in her chain of command, which put him in a position that was not conducive to effective mental health care. The psychologist was also in a vulnerable position as he wielded power over her fitness reports and career. Although there were two other available psychologists as well as a psychiatrist, they were also in the same chain of command and thus the dual relationship was an issue for all of them. Given the specific overseas location and the lack of civilian referral options, they were unable to refer to a local provider. Given concerns about suicidality, they were unable to request a provider be flown in to do the assessment or request a telehealth appointment as neither of these options was available urgently.

Consequently, the psychologist had to do the evaluation. She mitigated this as much as possible through informed consent and openly addressing the dual relationship problem at the beginning of the assessment. Ultimately, she facilitated referral to a program in the United States, where the officer received residential treatment for his severe gambling problem.

This type of multiple relationship should obviously be avoided whenever possible and when not possible be mitigated by informed consent and other strategies. While the psychologist believed there was no option but to do the assessment, the officer's treatment needs were more ethically and effectively addressed by specialists who were not a part of his command. Unfortunately, these kinds of dual roles and relationships are not uncommon, and most seasoned military psychologists have a story similar to this one.

Competence

Competence is a particularly complicated issue in the military because there are a wide variety of jobs that psychologists may be assigned (e.g., embedded in primary care, inpatient treatment, infantry unit, aviation command, operational billet, aircraft carrier, submarine command, etc.). Although professional competence is clearly a matter for junior psychologists, this concern is not solely the domain of the new military psychologist. It is common for active-duty psychologists to hold disparately different jobs throughout their career, requiring new training for each position. As an example, one midcareer officer in the Navy has been assigned to an HIV clinic, an alcohol and drug rehab, an aviation command, a detainee mental health clinic, a combat zone hospital, in a counterintelligence position, and then back to leading a clinic in an MTF. This wide variety of experiences is not unusual for a military psychologist; however, "the range of professional competence within psychology is sufficiently broad that expertise in one area does not necessarily readily translate into another" (Nagy, 2012,

p. 170). Consequently, military psychology competence is a constantly moving target. Standard 2.01, Boundaries of Competence, states:

> (a) Psychologists provide services, teach, and conduct research with populations and in areas only within the boundaries of their competence, based on their education, training, supervised experience, consultation, study, or professional experience.
> (c) Psychologists planning to provide services, teach, or conduct research involving populations, areas, techniques, or technologies new to them undertake relevant education, training, supervised experience, consultation, or study.
> (d) When psychologists are asked to provide services to individuals for whom appropriate mental health services are not available and for which psychologists have not obtained the competence necessary, psychologists with closely related prior training or experience may provide such services in order to ensure that services are not denied if they make a reasonable effort to obtain the competence required by using relevant research, training, consultation, or study.

In addition to the routine reassignment of active-duty clinical psychologists, new demands have provided increasing challenges to competency. Within traditional MTFs, two of these ways are the dramatically increased utilization of telehealth in light of COVID-19 (Pierce, Perrin, Tyler, McKee, & Watson, 2021) and the rapidly evolving science supporting different treatments for a variety of mental health disorders, but especially posttraumatic stress disorder (PTSD). Note that these are simply two examples of evolving strategies in traditional military mental health care. Psychologists working with military members and in the clinical psychology field in general face advances and changes to treatment provision on a regular basis.

With the increased need for military mental health care, the decreased stigma associated with seeing mental health care providers (Kennedy, 2020), and the need for physical distancing related to COVID-19, in addition to coincident advances in technology, telehealth has become a more viable option for both active-duty and veteran service members. Studies of the efficacy and implementation of telehealth as a mainstream option for treatment are growing (see, e.g., Gros, Yoder, Tuerk, Lozano, & Acierno, 2011; Tuerk, Yoder, Ruggiero, Gros, & Arcieno, 2010; Glassman et al., 2019; Glynn, Chen, Dawson, Gelman, & Zeliadt, 2021). Although telehealth may prove to be a great option for some service members, providing better access to treatment, ethical dilemmas ultimately arise. Specific concerns related to the various modalities of telehealth are risks to privacy and confidentiality, technological competence required by the provider, assessment of client appropriateness for telehealth, empirical base of various assessment and treatment techniques delivered via telehealth, and availability and accessibility of emergency resources when needed (Ragusea, 2012; Chenneville & Schwartz-Mette, 2020).

A second area of rapid change is the rate of publications on mental health treatments, expanding the evidence base to a degree that an individual provider cannot keep up with the science in order to provide state-of-the-art care. This has been no more true than in the case of PTSD. An APA PsycNet search revealed 2,397 journal articles and 21 testing instruments published in 2019 alone. The Department of Veterans Affairs (VA) and Department of Defense (DoD) counter this glut of information through the use of clinical practice guidelines (CPGs), systematic reviews that are revised approximately every 5 years and clearly define scientifically backed effective treatments (VA & DoD, 2017). It is up to individual providers to maintain their knowledge and competence regarding any disorder they are treating or treatment they are using, and the CPGs enable providers to do so.

While maintaining competency in a wide array of jobs with a diverse population (see the later "Cultural/Multicultural Competency" section) is a challenging task, the military provides the opportunity for a wide range of competency development. This is achieved through formal internships, fellowships and other training programs, mentorship programs, continuing education, supervision, and the encouragement of individual professional development, such as board certification by providing monetary bonuses to diplomates.

With regard to postdoctoral fellowship, between the three services, formal training is provided in clinical psychopharmacology (i.e., prescribing psychology; see Laskow & Grill, 2003, for an overview of the DoD Psychopharmacology Demonstration Project), neuropsychology, child psychology, forensic psychology, operational psychology, and health psychology. Fellowship training is approached differently between the three services, with some fellows training in military sites (e.g., Army neuropsychology postdoctoral fellows) and others in civilian sites (e.g., Navy child psychology postdoctoral fellows).

Informed Consent

Informed consent is an integral part of all mental health evaluation and care, and it is essential for service members and other individuals whom the military psychologist will evaluate or treat. In addition to more traditional information included in informed consent, the military provider must also discuss military-specific privacy and confidentiality issues (see the later discussion of confidentiality) related to military service or status of the individual in question (e.g., command-directed evaluation, special-duty evaluation) as well as all of the potential outcomes inherent in contact with military mental health providers (e.g., fitness-for-duty issues, potential loss-of-flight status). Standard 3.10, Informed Consent, states:

(a) When psychologists conduct research or provide assessment, therapy, counseling, or consulting services in person or via electronic transmission or other forms of communication, they obtain the informed consent of the individual or individuals using language that is reasonably understandable to that person or persons except when conducting such activities without consent is mandated by law or governmental regulation or as otherwise provided in this Ethics Code.

(b) For persons who are legally incapable of giving informed consent, psychologists nevertheless (1) provide an appropriate explanation, (2) seek the individual's assent, (3) consider such persons' preferences and best interests, and (4) obtain appropriate permission from a legally authorized person, if such substitute consent is permitted or required by law. When consent by a legally authorized person is not permitted or required by law, psychologists take reasonable steps to protect the individual's rights and welfare.

(c) When psychological services are court ordered or otherwise mandated, psychologists inform the individual of the nature of the anticipated services, including whether the services are court ordered or mandated and any limits of confidentiality, before proceeding.

(d) Psychologists appropriately document written or oral consent, permission, and assent.

Informed consent should be thoroughly discussed in any first session with a military patient prior to any disclosures by that individual. Only in the case of a command-directed evaluation may a service member undergo involuntary military mental health evaluation (see Chapter 2, this volume, for a discussion of command-directed and emergent evaluations), so it is important that the service member understand the potential career repercussions of any disclosure and have the option of not revealing information. Informed consent, particularly as it relates to confidentiality, the provision of information to the service member's command, and fitness for duty should be revisited in each session.

Cultural/Multicultural Competency

Although professional competence is paramount for military psychologists, cultural and multicultural competence must be equally considered. In the military, cultural competence generally refers to the ability to evaluate, treat, and make informed decisions for both service member patients and the organization in the context of rank, Military Occupational Specialty (MOS)/rate, officer/enlisted, branch of service, mission, military instructions, and military laws. Multicultural competence, on the other hand, refers to the ability to evaluate, treat, and make informed decisions regarding a diverse array of individuals with differing backgrounds. Age, gender, race/ethnicity, religion, disability, socioeconomic status, sexual orientation and so on all play key roles in the psychological assessment and treatment of military members. One needs not only to establish competency to work within the military with different groups but also to address any issues of individual bias and prejudice toward these same groups (Nagy, 2012).

To further explore the notion of cultural competence in military psychology, it is necessary to examine the various ways in which both civilians and active-duty psychologists come to be in the military or working in a military setting. Civilian military psychologists may have years of military experience (i.e., veterans) but in many cases may have none. In recent years, given increased demands for military mental health care, an unprecedented number of civilian psychologists have been hired by MTFs. Individuals without some type of prior military experience (e.g., prior active duty, the Reserves or National Guard) are especially at risk of decision-making mistakes because of a general lack of familiarity and understanding of the military culture (Johnson & Kennedy, 2010). Some of these errors can impact rapport, for instance, failing to use the individual's correct rank or calling a Marine a soldier, and some can be dire, such as not understanding an individual's MOS/rate and returning him or her to duty when this is contraindicated. (For an in-depth look at military cultural competence in the context of clinical evaluation and treatment, see Kennedy, 2020.)

Additionally, some multicultural issues interact significantly with military cultural competence. For example, in 2018, women made up 16.2% of enlisted ranks and 18% of officer ranks across the military (DoD, Office of the Deputy Assistant Secretary of Defense for Military Community and Family Policy, 2018). It is only recently that women have been able to fill many jobs in the military, previously denied to them due to gender. In 2015, the combat exclusion on women's military service was lifted, and the Services are slowly integrating women into these roles. However, women face unique challenges in serving, not due to these new roles, but in the male-dominated military in general. Understanding the history of women in the military (Kennedy & Malone, 2009), their day-to-day reality, and the unique medical and mental health needs of women in general is critical to the effective provision of mental health care. Other minority populations have similar challenges and a history of exclusion from military service (e.g., lesbian, gay, and bisexual individuals; Johnson, Rosenstein, Buhrke, & Haldeman, 2015). Consequently, providers must be familiar with the history, day-to-day challenges, current military instructions, and any ongoing issues related to cultural minorities and military service (e.g., transgender policy; Dunlap et al., 2021).

With regard to multicultural competency, in 2018, 31% of the active-duty force identified themselves as a racial minority (32.7% of enlisted personnel and 23.5% of officers), with 17.1% Black or African American, 4.5% Asian, 4.2% Other, 3% multiracial, 1.1% American Indian or Alaska Native, and 1.1% Native Hawaiian or other Pacific Islander. Additionally, 16.1% endorsed Hispanic or Latino ethnicity (DoD, Office of the Deputy Assistant Secretary of Defense for Military Community and Family Policy,

2018). Furthermore, approximately 40,000 immigrants are currently serving in the U.S. military, and the military enlists about 5,000 noncitizens every year (National Immigration Forum, 2017).

Standard 2.01, Boundaries of Competence, states:

> (b) Where scientific or professional knowledge in the discipline of psychology establishes that an understanding of factors associated with age, gender, gender identity, race, ethnicity, culture, national origin, religion, sexual orientation, disability, language, or socioeconomic status is essential for effective implementation of their services or research, psychologists have or obtain the training, experience, consultation, or supervision necessary to ensure the competence of their services, or they make appropriate referrals, except as provided in Standard 2.02, Providing Services in Emergencies.

Multicultural competence is of principle importance for the military psychologist. Not only does one work with the various ethnic, racial, and religious groups from within the United States, one works with U.S. service members from foreign countries (a person does not need to be a U.S. citizen to enlist in the U.S. military), with foreign nationals, and with wartime detainees (Toye & Smith, 2011; Kennedy, Malone, & Franks, 2009; Kennedy & Johnson, 2009; Kennedy, 2011).

Confidentiality

Confidentiality is a continuous challenge for the military psychologist. Given the dual-role challenge (see the prior discussion) and the mixed-agency challenge (see the following section), knowing when something needs to be reported and to whom while maintaining the best interests of service members can be complicated. Standard 4.01, Maintaining Confidentiality, states:

> Psychologists have a primary obligation and take reasonable precautions to protect confidential information obtained through or stored in any medium, recognizing that the extent and limits of confidentiality may be regulated by law or established by institutional rules or professional or scientific relationship.

Service members understand that when they see military medical providers, some of their information is not private. Their attendance at annual physical health assessments, whether or not they are up-to-date on immunizations, and the state of their dental readiness, for example, are all tracked by the command to ensure a state of continuous mission readiness and deployability. However, mental health evaluation and treatment are differentiated from this kind of routine medical maintenance. A lot of service members fall into categories in which there are strict requirements and procedures for disclosure (e.g., service members with access to classified information, service members in special operations or other high-risk special duties, service members displaying symptoms that they are not fit for duty, etc.). On the other hand, service members who have been sexually assaulted and are seeking mental health care are protected from military disclosures (see Chapter 8, this volume). Cultural competence is key to knowing when, to whom, and what must be disclosed (Hoyt, 2013). It is notable that there is a military command exception within the Health Insurance Portability and Accountability Act (HIPAA), located in Title 45 Part 164.512 of the Code of Federal Regulations. Essentially, a health care provider, be that person civilian or military, may "use and disclose the protected health information of individuals who are Armed Forces personnel for activities deemed necessary by appropriate military command authorities to assure the proper execution of the military mission." Thus, as an example, if a service member is deemed not fit for duty, this may be disclosed without the consent of the service member.

However, in an attempt to decrease mental health stigma and increase help-seeking, in August 2011, the military implemented an unprecedented instruction regarding confidentiality and mental health care. Department of Instruction (DoDI) 6490.08 states, "[T]he DoD shall foster a culture of support in the provision of mental health care and voluntarily sought substance abuse education to military personnel in order to dispel the stigma" (2011, p. 2). The instruction further states that "healthcare providers shall follow a presumption that they are not to notify a Service member's commander when the Service member obtains mental health care or substance abuse education services" (p. 2). This is negated when one of the following notification standards is met: harm to self, harm to others, harm to mission, special personnel, inpatient care, acute medical conditions interfering with duty, substance abuse treatment program, and command-directed evaluation. In these cases, however, the mental health provider is directed to "provide the minimum amount of information to the commander concerned as required to satisfy the purpose of the disclosure" (p. 2). This means that most service members who are considered fit for full duty may seek help from a military mental health provider in full confidence for a wide variety of problems (e.g., postdeployment adjustment, relationship problems, non-duty-limiting mental health concerns).

It should always be remembered, however, that often the command may be better able to help solve problems and reduce mental health symptoms than the mental health provider, even in instances where no disclosure needs to be made to the command. When you consider that the command has full control over such major life variables as living arrangements, leave, and deployments, and also has the power to intervene when individuals are having pay problems or severe personal or family problems, at times it is better for the command to know that a service member is having difficulty. This allows the command to better support the service member. Consequently, in the military, psychologists should be careful about defaulting

to a view that strict confidentiality is always best and be prepared to have conversations with military patients regarding bringing their command onboard. As an example, Schendel and Kennedy (2020) present the descriptive case of a sailor in treatment for insomnia. After comprehensive evaluation, it was determined that the cause of the sleeping problem was the sailor had a roommate on an opposite shift. Getting permission to speak to the command or encouraging the sailor to request a change in room or roommate was the cure for the sailor's chronic sleep problems. This might seem simplistic, but remember that the military culture is one where you are responsible for your own problems and good service members learn to "embrace the suck." Consequently, not all personnel default to informing their chain of command when they are having difficulties.

Finally, similar to rural communities, it is important for military psychologists to address with their military patients what their expectation is when seeing them in public. It is common knowledge among military psychologists that once they have been at the same duty station for just a few months, they inevitably run into patients at the commissary, exchange, gas station, and so on. Some military patients do not want to acknowledge their care provider so as to preserve confidentiality, while others want to say hello. It is recommended that this be addressed in the first session, especially in remote and overseas bases.

Mixed Agency

Mixed agency is present in every professional interaction that a military psychologist has with an active-duty patient. This is also true at times in VA settings, given that many Reserves personnel deploy or are activated multiple times (Stone, 2008). With every clinical decision made, the psychologist has a simultaneous responsibility to the service member patient, the military/organization, and society at large. The most common clinical psychological mixed-agency dilemma occurs in the context of returning a service member to duty. For example, when making a decision regarding the aeromedical qualifications of a military aviator, one must consider the aviator-patient (e.g., best interests of the patient), the military (e.g., can the aviator currently meet mission requirements?), and society (e.g., is the aviator safe in the air; is there a threat to others?). There are a variety of ethical standards pertaining to mixed agency, the three most pertinent of which are as follows:

- 1.02, Conflicts Between Ethics and Law, Regulations, or Other Governing Legal Authority, which states:

    If psychologists' ethical responsibilities conflict with law, regulations, or other governing legal authority, psychologists clarify the nature of the conflict, make known their commitment to the Ethics Code, and take reasonable steps to resolve the conflict consistent with the General Principles and Ethical Standards of the Ethics Code. Under no circumstances may this standard be used to justify or defend violating human rights.

- 1.03, Conflicts Between Ethics and Organizational Demands, which states:

If the demands of an organization with which psychologists are affiliated or for whom they are working are in conflict with this Ethics Code, psychologists clarify the nature of the conflict, make known their commitment to the Ethics Code, and take reasonable steps to resolve the conflict consistent with the General Principles and Ethical Standards of the Ethics Code. Under no circumstances may this standard be used to justify or defend violating human rights.

- 3.11, Psychological Services Delivered to or through Organizations, which states:

(a) Psychologists delivering services to or through organizations provide information beforehand to clients and when appropriate those directly affected by the services about (1) the nature and objectives of the services, (2) the intended recipients, (3) which of the individuals are clients, (4) the relationship the psychologist will have with each person and the organization, (5) the probable uses of services provided and information obtained, (6) who will have access to the information, and (7) limits of confidentiality. As soon as feasible, they provide information about the results and conclusions of such services to appropriate persons.

(b) If psychologists will be precluded by law or by organizational roles from providing such information to particular individuals or groups, they so inform those individuals or groups at the outset of the service.

Johnson and Wilson (1993) and Johnson (1995) reviewed three strategies military psychologists have used in the past to attempt to manage the mixed-agency dilemma: the military manual approach, the stealth approach, and the best-interest approach. To review, the military manual approach attempts to manage ethical conflicts by using literal applications of military rules. This approach is considered potentially harmful, tending to prevent the identification of ethical conflicts. The stealth approach is the other extreme, covering up issues that may impact the military and other military members by attempting to work solely in the context of the individual. While psychologists using this approach may believe they are working ethically in the best interests of the individual, this approach also has the potential to cause significant problems for the service member (e.g., occupational difficulty, life-threatening mistakes on the job). The best-interest approach, on the other hand, takes both the individual's and the military's needs into consideration and applies both the Ethics Code and military regulations. This approach involves the most creative problem solving and knowledge of pertinent ethical standards, military regulations, and laws but tends to demonstrate the best outcomes (see Kennedy & Johnson, 2009). This approach is advocated throughout this chapter as the only ethical approach of the three noted to manage the mixed-agency conflict.

While fitness for duty is the most frequently encountered mixed-agency dilemma for the clinical military psychologist, a second mixed-agency dilemma unique to the current war is that of mental health care for detainees. This war marked the first time that detained enemy combatants have been provided with mental health care during their incarceration. In this case, the mixed-agency triad consists of the detainee patient, the military/other government organizations involved, and society. However, the mental health care of detainees took an unusual turn. Some have criticized that this care is provided by military mental health providers, as opposed to providers from an independent agency (Aggarwal, 2009). In 2008, members of APA voted to make it a violation of APA policy for military psychologists to work in wartime detention facilities except to treat service members (APA, 2008). Consequently, any military psychologist providing mental health care to detainees in a wartime detention facility is in violation of APA policy. However, APA policy does not affect the APA Ethics Code and is not enforceable, so psychologists may be in violation of policy while not committing an ethical violation (see Kennedy, 2012). To make this matter more difficult for military psychologists is that no other medical specialty, to include psychiatry, implemented any similar policy. This confusing situation, and consequent decision, are then left to individual psychologists as to whether or not to deploy to a wartime detention facility and, if they do, to whom they will provide services.

OPERATIONAL ENVIRONMENTS

Operational psychology is "the application of the science and profession of psychology to the operational activities of law enforcement, national intelligence organizations, and national defense activities" (Kennedy & Williams, 2011b, p. 4). Operational psychological activities do not typically involve clinical responsibilities and include such activities as assessment and selection of personnel for high-risk jobs (e.g., special operations forces, embassy security guards, aviation personnel; Picano, Williams, Roland, & Long, 2011; see also Chapter 13, this volume), security clearance evaluations (Young, Harvey, & Staal, 2011; see also Chapter 14, this volume), support for repatriated U.S. prisoners of war (see Chapter 15, this volume), counterintelligence and counterterrorism activities (Kennedy, Borum, & Fein, 2011), consultation to interrogation (Dunivin, Banks,

Staal, & Stephenson, 2011; Department of Defense, 2019), and crisis negotiation (Gelles & Palarea, 2011; Greene & Banks, 2009; Kennedy & Williams, 2011a; Kennedy & Zillmer, 2006; Shumate & Borum, 2006; see
also Chapter 16, this volume).

Operational psychological activities are not as well established and
studied as military psychology's clinical activities, although some of these
functions (e.g., assessment and selection) predate clinical military psychology (see Chapter 1, this volume). Some of these less traditional applications
of psychology have come under significant scrutiny, particularly as they
pertain to the role of consultation to interrogation. This singular issue has
resulted in strong emotions and great debate (see Abeles, 2010; Galvin,
2008). Some psychologists believe that members of their profession should
not perform this role, that psychologists who participated were involved
in the engineering of torture, and that the APA was complicit in these
activities (e.g., see Soldz, 2008). Others believe that military psychologists
are in a good position to influence policy, research, and practice (e.g., see
Fein, Lehner, & Vossekuil, 2006) by focusing on issues such as memory
distortion, effective questioning strategies, and the detection of deception
(Loftus, 2011), thereby making a positive impact on current war efforts,
increasing ethical and effective intelligence gathering (Brandon, Arthur,
Ray, Meissner, Kleinman, Russano, & Wells, 2019), and preventing atroci-
ties such as those that occurred at Abu Ghraib (Greene & Banks, 2009;
Staal & Stephenson, 2006; Staal, 2019).

This singular disagreement within the field of psychology/APA brought
the ethics of operational psychology as a whole under significant examination. Kennedy and Williams (2011b) identify four primary ethical dilemmas in these environments, namely mixed agency, competence, multiple
relationships, and informed consent. Note that there is considerable overlap
of ethical dilemmas within each of the four practice environments. The
reader is directed to the Traditional Military Treatment Facilities section
for applicable ethical standards when indicated.

Mixed Agency

Mixed agency (also called dual agency, divided loyalty, and dual loyalty;
see prior discussion for the pertinent ethical standards) occurs when a psychologist has a responsibility to two or more simultaneous entities. Within
clinical venues, this dilemma usually involves a service member, the military, and society at large. In operational psychological environments, this
typically comes in the form of a responsibility to an individual, a government or military agency, and to society at large (Kennedy, 2012). Using
crisis negotiations as an example (see also Chapter 16, this volume), the
psychologist has a simultaneous responsibility to the law enforcement/
military/government agency (i.e., the primary client), society at large (e.g.,

hostages, bystanders), and the individual in question (i.e., barricaded individual or hostage taker). It is notable that the psychologist in crisis negotiations will not have face-to-face interactions with the hostage taker and the hostage taker will not know that there is a psychologist consulting, yet the purpose of the consultant psychologist is to optimize the chances of a peaceful surrender and minimize/prevent loss of life. Gelles and Palarea (2011) recommend that in order to ethically manage the mixed-agency and other dilemmas inherent in crisis negotiation consultation, the psychologist must identify the client, remain in the role of expert consultant (see also Mullins & McMains, 2011), remain autonomous in consultation and free from external influence, identify boundaries and delineate the boundaries between operational consultant and healthcare provider, appreciate the uniqueness of each crisis situation, and establish and maintain professional competence. Craw and Catanese (2020) emphasize the fluidity of these incidents and the need for a flexible model of ethical decision making in order to be able to address these volatile situations as they evolve and change.

Competence

Operational psychology has grown into a subdiscipline of psychology; however, it is still in the early stages as it pertains to the development of a formal training curriculum and professional standards for competency. Standard 2.01, Boundaries of Competence, states (for other pertinent standards related to competency, see the prior MTF discussion above):

> (e) In those emerging areas in which generally recognized standards for preparatory training do not yet exist, psychologists nevertheless take reasonable steps to ensure the competence of their work and to protect clients/patients, students, supervisees, research participants, organizational clients, and others from harm.

Like the prior advances made by military psychologists during various conflicts, the evolution of the practice of operational psychology is growing on a grand scale. Fostered and predated by the work of psychologists in law enforcement, operational psychology has become a force for national security. As with the development of clinical internships following WWII as a result of the relative newness of the field of clinical psychology (see Chapter 1, this volume), the expansion of operational roles for psychologists requires the same considerations for formal education and training. The military has implemented postdoctoral fellowship training in the Navy and the Army has developed a number of formal courses (e.g., Operational Psychology, Assessment and Selection), which are used by operational psychology trainees in all Services; conferences specific to operational psychologists are held annually (e.g., National Security Psychology Symposium; survival, evasion, resistance, and escape [SERE] psychology conference); and formalized mentorship opportunities and professional networks have been established. Military psychologists may also seek board certification in Police and Public Safety—as operational psychology functions mirror those in traditional law enforcement. This provides for the highest formal standard of professional competency awarded to psychologists in any subspecialty.

Multiple Relationships

Multiple relationships occur in operational psychology environs as they do in traditional MTFs, although the circumstances differ significantly. An important difference between operational psychologists and those military psychologists treating service members within MTFs is that operational psychologists typically do not perform clinical duties primarily. However, in any small, embedded, and/or deployed command, the military psychologist is at risk of having to manage the emergent mental health situation of a coworker or of being approached by a coworker for services. In an operational position, this may be a guard, police officer, or Special Forces personnel. This is the most frequently occurring multiple relationship dilemma in the operational psychology environment. It should be mitigated whenever possible through referrals; however, when this is not possible because of an emergency or lack of referral options, thorough informed consent (see prior Traditional Military Treatment Facilities section and Informed Consent section next) is the primary way in which to mitigate the conflict until a more appropriate referral option can be obtained.

Informed Consent

Much of the work of operational psychologists differs dramatically from the work of traditional military clinical psychologists with regard to the individual in question. When working with a service member-patient, informed consent is a standard process that includes the individual (see prior discussion for pertinent standards). In some cases, informed consent is standard for operational psychologists as well, such as in cases of security clearance evaluations or assessment and selection procedures. In these instances, the individual is readily identifiable and involved in the process of obtaining/reviewing appropriateness for a security clearance or undergoing evaluation to obtain/maintain a special duty. However, in many cases, the psychologist will have no direct contact with the individual in question when performing operational psychological responsibilities (e.g., hostage negotiation consultation, interrogation consultation, counterterrorism consultation), and informed consent will be unable to be obtained for a variety of reasons. In all cases however, the psychologist maintains a duty to identifiable individuals even in cases where informed consent cannot reasonably be obtained and the individual does not know of the presence of the consulting psychologist (Koocher, 2009).

NON-COMBAT-ZONE EXPEDITIONARY ENVIRONMENTS

Expeditionary environments are those in which the psychologist is embedded within a military unit and provides the gamut of mental healthcare (i.e., prevention, early intervention, outpatient care, and at times inpatient treatment) to the members of that unit as well as consultation to its leadership. Examples include Operational Stress Control & Readiness (OSCAR) providers who provide clinical assessment, care, and consultation for U.S. Marine ground units (Hoyt, 2006; Vaughn, Farmer, Breslau, & Burnette, 2015), and Navy shipboard psychologists who are responsible for the crew of an aircraft carrier and the accompanying battle group (Wood, Koffman, & Arita, 2003; Berg, 2019). Expeditionary environments and embedded practice may or may not include duty within a combat zone. This section focuses on those noncombat roles and locations.

Embedded, or integrated, providers become well known to the leadership of a specific unit and to the service members within that unit. Routine interactions and a "one of us" conceptualization serve to establish a comfort level with the provider, who is seen as an approachable and credible resource. This credibility and acceptance, in turn, serve to reduce stigma and increase receptiveness on the part of both individual service members and leadership to interventions and recommendations (Hoyt, 2006). In addition, the embedded psychologist provides continuity of care. This can be a significant problem for service members receiving care at a traditional MTF who require a course of psychotherapy. Not only do service member-patients deploy frequently but so do their MTF providers. Consequently, a traditional mental healthcare model can result in significant inconsistency and disruption of care (Ralph & Sammons, 2006). Embedded mental health is able to provide continuity of care since the providers are always with the unit wherever it might be. This embedded or expeditionary care is believed to be a powerful means to prevent problems, provide informed early interventions, facilitate better care when serious problems develop, and preserve the military's resources. For example, the billeting of a psychologist on each aircraft carrier has reduced the number of medical evacuations from Navy ships (Wood et al., 2003). However, with these significant advantages come increased ethical challenges. Johnson, Ralph, and Johnson (2005) describe dual agency and multiple roles as the most significant ethical challenges in these embedded environments.

Dual Agency and Multiple Roles

Dual or mixed agency and multiple roles are significant conflicts in all areas of military practice (see prior discussion on MTF and operational environments for the pertinent ethical standards and additional information). Although dual/mixed agency has already been described in depth and is highly similar to the dual agency found in traditional MTFs, multiple roles in expeditionary environments are the most magnified of any area of military psychology practice. This is because the psychologist is always a member of the same command hierarchy, is dedicated to provide care to the members of his or her same unit, is managing the same stressors as the unit, and often does so in austere locations where there may be no referral options or relief of any kind.

As potentially the sole mental health care provider, especially when deployed, the psychologist will find him- or herself in a position of multiple roles on a regular basis. Most of the time these roles are benign or manageable; however, at times they can be significantly problematic. Johnson et al. (2010), for example, describe a case of a carrier psychologist who has to perform a security clearance evaluation for a known patient, which resulted in the patient not receiving a clearance and consequently a better job. This secondary role placed the therapeutic alliance with that patient in serious jeopardy and compromised the service member's sole source of mental health care.

Johnson et al. (2005) provide considerable analysis of multiple relationships in expeditionary environments. These authors note several ways in which psychology practice is unique for the expeditionary psychologist.

1. The psychologist has multiple roles with every service member-patient, given that the psychologist is always an officer.
2. The psychologist has no choice as to whether or not to engage in a clinical relationship with someone. Because there are no other choices available, the psychologist cannot choose to begin a therapeutic relationship, transfer care, or even terminate treatment at times.
3. The psychologist may find him- or herself in a position of having to shift psychology roles with the same individual in order to make fitness-for-duty decisions, perform a forensic evaluation, or conduct a security clearance evaluation.
4. The psychologist represents a decision maker with authority in some matters. "Embedded military psychologists frequently influence the client's life thoroughly, and salient go/no-go decisions by the psychologist commonly impact whether a client will achieve promotions or even remain on active duty" (p. 75).
5. The psychologist will have ongoing personal contact with patients. Within an embedded unit, encountering patients, for example, in

their work space, in the gym, or at command functions is a normal matter of course.

6. The psychologist will inevitably end up providing services to friends, coworkers, and even superiors.

Although it is believed that expeditionary/embedded psychology significantly reduces adverse outcomes and the need for medical evacuation, and increases service member's willingness and probability of seeking care, these are significant challenges that must be carefully and thoughtfully managed by the provider.

COMBAT ZONE

Duty in a combat zone brings all of the ethical hazards of expeditionary psychological practice (for embedded providers) as well as traditional practice in an MTF (for providers assigned to combat stress units or combat hospitals), but in a physically more dangerous and emotionally charged environment where resources may be extremely limited. Challenges develop beyond dual agency and multiple roles, as military psychologists are at increased risk of being asked to do something they are not trained to do as well as policy and nonmedical decision makers effecting clinical care. The dilemmas of dual agency, multiple roles, potential unlawful orders, professional competency, multicultural competency, and personal problems are heightened issues in the combat zone.

Dual Agency and Multiple Roles

Dual agency and multiple roles take on a new dimension in the combat zone, because without the dual roles psychologists can have a very difficult time treating service members and managing ethical dilemmas. In other words, psychologists must not only be skilled clinicians but also competent military officers. An understanding of the military hierarchy, the weapons, vehicles and other equipment used in the current conflict, military strategy, and military objectives in pertinent areas is not normally equated with skills needed by psychologists. However, understanding exactly what one's patients are being expected to do, where they may be returning to, and what operations are ongoing as well as the ability to interface effectively with the command are keys to clinical decision making and effective implementation of mental health interventions in a war zone. A competent military officer will make informed decisions regarding return to duty and will be able to effectively negotiate plans with the command, which are in the best interest of both the service member and the unit. Simply being an excellent clinician in the combat zone is insufficient to provide care for service members (see prior discussions of MTF and cultural competence).

Unlawful Orders

Occasionally, a psychologist in a combat zone may be ordered to do something either unlawful or inherently unethical. When this occurs, it is typically in the context of a superior officer (usually not an officer in the medical field) not understanding what he or she has asked the psychologist to do and thus are "a result of the senior officer not having adequate information about psychology practice, regulations or the Ethics Code, as opposed to nefarious purposes or disregard for the law by the senior officer" (Kennedy, 2012, p. 134). Brief education on psychology/medical ethics and brainstorming to effectively troubleshoot the problem usually resolve any problems related to unlawful orders. In rare cases, however, this may become an issue. Kennedy (2009) presents a case of a junior psychologist, without prescriptive authority, being ordered by a senior medical officer to prescribe medication in the combat zone in the absence of a psychiatrist. The danger is that the junior psychologist will obey the order, even though it is not lawful. Recommendations for mitigation of unlawful orders if education and alternate problem solving are ineffective are to consult with senior members of the military psychology community and the local military lawyer.

Competence

Just because someone is an excellent clinician in garrison does not mean that he or she is going to enjoy the same efficacy in the combat zone. Treating combat trauma in a war zone requires competencies very infrequently used in a traditional mental health clinic. Everything changes in the combat zone to include diagnoses (e.g., combat stress reaction; combat exhaustion), risk mitigation, and treatment options. Each war also brings unique competency challenges for military psychologists. A modern example of an ethical dilemma is the situation involving blast concussion. Psychologists were assigned the task of using neurocognitive assessment measures in theater, yet few had received formal training in neuropsychology, neurocognitive testing, or concussive/neurological injuries. Further complicating the issue was that at the height of the war there was little published on acute blast concussion and little empirically validated basis for the use of neuropsychological testing instruments in theater (Bush & Cuesta, 2010). Standard 9.07, Assessment by Unqualified Persons, states:

> Psychologists do not promote the use of psychological assessment techniques by unqualified persons, except when such use is conducted for training purposes with appropriate supervision.

(For additional ethical standards relevant to competence, see prior Traditional Military Treatment Facilities section.) Issues regarding the Automated

Neuropsychological Assessment Metrics (ANAM) and the requirement for neuropsychological evaluation in theater for those with multiple concussions (DoD, 2010) provided significant pressure to generalists to practice neuropsychology without appropriate training. Take the following example.

Case 17.2. The Artillery Marine with a Blast Concussion

The Marine SGT was an 0811 (Field Artillery Canoneer, pronounced Oh-8-eleven). He was on a convoy when his MRAP (Mine Resistant Ambush Protected vehicle, pronounced Em-rap) hit an IED (Improvised Explosive Device). He experienced a blast concussion without loss of consciousness, but with significant confusion, approximately 10 minutes of posttraumatic amnesia, balance problems, tinnitus, severe headache, dizziness and nausea. Symptoms resolved over the course of 37 days; his ANAM scores were consistent with his pre-deployment baseline scores; and he passed exertional testing (physical exercise designed to trigger return of concussion symptoms when the concussion is not fully resolved). The issue now is, can he return to duty?

Only in the context of intersecting abilities in both cultural and professional competence can you determine the answer. The Marine's job is that he leads the crew of a Howitzer, a large weapon that fires 100-pound projectiles up to 25 miles. If he were returned to duty, there is a high likelihood that the repeated sub-concussive impacts from the weapon would cause him further problems. This is a good example of the need for both cultural (must understand the service member's job) and professional competence (must understand the dynamics of concussion as opposed to just being able to administer the cognitive testing) when making a return to duty decision of a service member.

Multicultural Competency

Another issue that arises in the combat zone is that of providing mental health services to the local population (see Tobin, 2005) or to friendly forces from other nations. Some issues arise in that different cultures define mental health and stress differently; something in one culture may be normal, where in another culture that same thing may conceived as abnormal; the vocabulary to describe mental health concepts may be very different. Additionally, even when an assessment may be able to be competently conducted, there may be no avenues to follow up or obtain treatment, particularly in war torn countries. Take the following example.

Case 17.3. The Local Soldier Who Could Get No Treatment

The patient was a member of the Afghan National Army (ANA) who was brought to a U.S. combat hospital after jumping from a guard tower after receiving some bad news. He was physically unharmed but had voiced suicidal intent prior to jumping. The U.S. military psychologist was the only mental health provider available. To make matters more complicated, the combat hospital is only for acute admissions; there were no ANA mental health resources in that region, as well as no civilian mental health resources. The psychologist was faced with a situation in which he possessed minimal cultural competency to evaluate the individual and lacked any referral option at all.

The psychologist worked with the individual and the ANA leadership to support him as best as possible and had the medical asset attached to his unit agree to follow up. These kinds of situations are not uncommon in war zones and they can result in distress to the psychologist.

Personal Problems

In addition to the ethical challenges and logistical hurdles of managing patients outside of a traditional clinic or hospital, military psychologists are at risk of developing personal problems secondary to their own deployment stress and potentially traumatic incidents (Johnson et al., 2011). While there are no empirical studies addressing the psychological health of military mental health providers, the reality is that no one is impervious to the stressors of the combat zone, and the frequency and at times unpredictability of deployments takes a toll on military mental health providers (Johnson, 2008). Routine combat zone stressors for medical personnel can include fairly continuous exposure to the seriously wounded, dying, and dead; environmental stressors (e.g., sleep deprivation, extreme temperatures, wearing of heavy and restrictive personal protective equipment); taking indirect fire (i.e., rockets and mortars) or being fired at directly; and "nearly constant vicarious exposure to trauma through the stories of traumatized clients" (Johnson & Kennedy, 2010, p. 299). This is in addition to any of the "normal" challenges encountered in trying to manage any unexpected problems on the homefront from a war zone. Maintaining one's own mental health is a significant challenge. Standard 2.06, Personal Problems and Conflicts, states:

> (a) Psychologists refrain from initiating an activity when they know or should know that there is a substantial likelihood that their personal problems will prevent them from performing their work-related activities in a competent manner.
> (b) When psychologists become aware of personal problems that may interfere with their performing work-related duties adequately, they take appropriate measures, such as obtaining professional consultation or assistance, and determine whether they should limit, suspend, or terminate their work-related duties.

While there are multiple conceptualizations of the stressors associated with secondary trauma, compassion fatigue, and burnout (for a review, see Linnerooth, Mrdjenovich, & Moore, 2011; Maltzman, 2011), there has been no empirical study of the experience of military mental health providers in the combat zone as it relates to potentially traumatic experiences, no follow-up beyond the routine postdeployment health assessments, and no exit assessments as to whether or not this is a factor in some military psychologists' decisions to leave the military. There also is little in the way of guidance in recognizing a detriment in professional competence and then acting upon it. Johnson et al. (2011) recommend the development of a "comprehensive program for both supporting and monitoring the health and competence of deployed military psychologists, both in theater and following their return" (p. 97).

PREVENTING, MITIGATING, AND MINIMIZING RISK

While there are a multitude of ethical dilemmas that may arise in any work setting, there are also many strategies available to individual military psychologists, both active duty and civilian, that can assist significantly.

- *Know the Ethics Code, relevant state, federal and military laws, and relevant military instructions.* The practice of psychology is governed by law, and complying with the Ethics Code is often a requirement of state licensure. Understanding the requirements of the law as it relates to the field and general practice of psychology is a minimum prerequisite for psychologists (Behnke & Jones, 2012). Beyond the basic understanding of the regulation of psychology and in order to practice military psychology in an informed manner, one must be able to also apply relevant military laws and instructions (Johnson et al., 2010) and understand how these organizational regulations interact with the Ethics Code and APA policy (Kennedy, 2012).

- *Build a network of mentors, peers, and other pertinent professionals.* Military psychologists are expected to perform a wide variety of jobs, and requests for them to engage in unique duties or consultative roles occur daily. In order to manage these requests, it is essential that military psychologists have an existing network of professionals to consult (Johnson et al., 2005; Schank, Helbok, Haldeman, & Gallardo, 2010). At a minimum, it is recommended that each military psychologist have one to two senior mentors, have several peer consulting relationships, be in contact with an individual who had their job in the past, and have a good working relationship with a military lawyer (i.e., judge advocate general).

- *Take advantage of every training opportunity.* The military provides a vast amount of training, and the military psychologist should take advantage of any opportunities, even if they do not seem particularly relevant to current duties. Formal trainings such as rifle/pistol qualification, SERE training, Assessment and Selection Course, Field Medical Service Officer school, and aeromedical officer training increase cultural competency and provide essential skills for future use.

- *Adopt a personal ethical decision-making model.* There are a number of ethical decision-making models (e.g., Barnett & Johnson, 2008), some of which are military specific (e.g., Staal & King, 2000). Psychologists are urged to evaluate and adopt a decision-making model in order to systematically and objectively evaluate ethical dilemmas as they arise (Johnson et al., 2010; McCutcheon, 2011).

- *Always work toward a best interest solution.* Considering the needs of both the individual and the military can be challenging, but there is usually a course of action that will benefit both parties (Johnson & Wilson, 1993; Johnson, 1995; Johnson et al., 2010). Cultural competence is key to being able to do this well.

- *Obtain appropriate informed consent.* In situations where informed consent can be obtained, military psychologists should discuss the realities of military instructions and laws on confidentiality, where and how records are kept, what the psychologist can reasonably do for the service member-patient, other treatment options, and how the various types of treatment/intervention may impact a current military career and/or future military career goals (Johnson, 1995; Johnson et al., 2005; Schank et al., 2010).

- *Become culturally savvy.* When just beginning to work in the military environment or with military personnel, one must make a concerted effort to understand military rank structure, military jargon and acronyms, military law, and the cultural differences between the Services. Military psychologists should coordinate visits to the various commands that they serve, learn their mission, and understand the environments in which their patients/clients operate.

- *Become multiculturally savvy.* The military psychologist should seek out both multicultural-specific continuing education and a diverse array of social events; travel to different areas and experience other cultures; explore and be open to one's own beliefs and personal biases (see Kennedy et al., 2007). Prior to duty station transfer or deployment, military psychologists should study the culture into which they are going and seek cultural opportunities once they arrive.

• *Within embedded and remote billets, the military psychologist should assume that everyone is a future patient.* Experienced military psychologists have reported how they can end up in a professional relationship with just about anyone in the command. Psychologists can prepare for this by remaining as neutral as possible on controversial issues, avoiding significant self-disclosure, and building a strong support system that is not a part of the command (see Johnson et al., 2005).

• *In remote and solo environments, have a backup plan should you have to provide an evaluation to someone that creates a potentially harmful situation for that person.* If this occurs, it will most likely be someone in your direct chain of command. These plans often include an agreement to send the military member elsewhere for evaluation (possibly to another Service's base or to another country altogether) or, if the situation warrants it, to request an additional psychologist to travel to the command to perform the evaluation.

• *Within embedded and operational billets, educate the military chain of command.* With some of the newer roles for psychologists, not all commands and commanders understand both the breadth of services as well as the limitations of services that embedded/expeditionary and operational psychologists can provide. An upfront educational session for the chain of command and other pertinent members of the command can gain the psychologist significant support to keep the psychologist working within appropriate boundaries and avoiding ethical dilemmas.

• *Be prepared to say no, but have an alternate suggestion.* In the rare case where you may be asked to do something unlawful or something that you are not competent to do, be prepared to refuse the request and propose alternative options. Leaders rarely ask for something without a legitimate reason. A culturally competent psychologist can almost always propose an alternate course which meets the needs of the leader without compromising the psychologist or a service member patient. Preparation includes understanding the Ethics Code, your professional responsibilities, and being able to articulate the specific problem with the request. However, in that rare instance where an alternate course of action cannot be agreed upon, know who in your chain of command or the military psychology community you can consult and depend on for top cover.

• *Be active in your profession.* Join pertinent organizations in order to network and remain current on practice issues and advances.

• *Rely on clinical practice guidelines and the accompanying clinical support tools in order to maintain clinical professional competency.* The

VA and DoD provide clinical practice guidelines (CPGs) for PTSD, Major Depressive Disorder, Substance Use Disorders, suicide risk, and Insomnia. Additionally, VA and DoD collaborate to make clinical support tools which accompany each CPG to distill the vast amount of scientific literature into useable information for clinicians. The website to download these free materials is the Department of Veterans Affairs site (*www.healthquality. va.gov/guidelines/MH*).

- *Take care of yourself.* Our own mental health definitely impacts our abilities to provide care for others and make good decisions on the job. Military psychologists need to understand how a variety of life and job circumstances affect them (e.g., stressors, mood, medical issues, medication side effects, exposure to combat trauma, and secondary traumatization) and take action to make routine healthy lifestyle choices (Nagy, 2012; Johnson, Bertschinger, Snell & Wilson, 2014) and create a network of support through other military psychologists and mentors (Johnson et al., 2011).

CONCLUSIONS

The job of military mental health providers continues to be a dynamic one, with service in every aspect of the military mission. With each new challenge comes accompanying ethical dilemmas and the need to develop new competencies. Applying the expertise provided within this volume, getting formal education and training in aspects of the military mental health mission and the military, staying tied into professional organizations for networking and skill development and maintenance, and maintaining a vast mentorship and support network are key to managing the ethical challenges that arise.

REFERENCES

Abeles, N. (2010). Ethics and the interrogation of prisoners: An update. *Ethics and Behavior, 20,* 243–249.

Aggarwal, N. K. (2009). Allowing independent forensic evaluations for Guantanamo detainees. *Journal of the American Academy of Psychiatry and the Law, 37,* 533–537.

American Psychological Association. (2008). *Report of the APA Presidential Advisory Group on the implementation of the petition resolution.* Retrieved March 6, 2011, from *www.apa.org/ethics/advisory-group-final.pdf.*

American Psychological Association. (2017). *Ethical principles of psychologists and code of conduct, 2010 and 2016 amendments.* Retrieved September 9, 2020, from *https://www.apa.org/ethics/code.*

Barnett, J. E. (2013). Multiple relationships in the military setting. In B. A. Moore

& J. E. Barnett (Eds.), *Military psychologists' desk reference* (pp. 103–107). New York: Oxford University Press.

Barnett, J. E., & Johnson, W. B. (2008). *Ethics desk reference for psychologists.* Washington, DC: American Psychological Association.

Behnke, S. H., & Jones, S. E. (2012). Ethics and ethics codes for psychologists. In S. J. Knapp, M. C. Gottlieb, M. M. Handelsman, & L. D. VandeCreek (Eds.), *APA handbook of ethics in psychology: Vol. 2. Practice, teaching, and research* (pp. 43–74). Washington, DC: American Psychological Association.

Berg, A. (2019). Diary of an aircraft carrier psychologist. *Psychological Services, 16*(4), 647–650.

Bush, S. S., & Cuesta, G. M. (2010). Ethical issues in military neuropsychology. In C. H. Kennedy & J. L. Moore (Eds.), *Military neuropsychology* (pp. 29–55). New York: Springer.

Brandon, S. E., Arthur, J. C., Ray, D. G., Meissner, C. A., Kleinman, S. M., Russano, M. B., et al. (2019). The high-value detainee interrogation group (HIG). In M. A. Staal & S. C. Harvey (Eds.), *Operational psychology: A new field to support national security and public safety* (pp. 263–285). Santa Barbara, CA: Praeger.

Chenneville, T., & Schwartz-Mette, R. (2020). Ethical considerations for psychologists in the time of COVID-19. *American Psychologist, 75*(5), 644–654.

Coyne, K. (2019). The forensic psychologist in the military justice system. In C. T. Stein & J. N. Younggren (Eds.), *Forensic psychology in military courts* (pp. 13–38). Washington, DC: American Psychological Association.

Craw, M. J., & Catanese, S. A. (2020). Identifying points of engagement versus disengagement when consulting during crisis negotiations: A flexible model for applying the ethics code. *Journal of Police and Criminal Psychology, 35,* 92–97.

Department of Defense. (2010, June). *Directive type memorandum 09–033 policy guidance for management of concussion/mild traumatic brain injury in the deployed setting.* Washington, DC: Author.

Department of Defense. (2011, August). *Command notification requirements to dispel stigma in providing mental health care to service members* (Department of Defense Instruction 6490.08). Washington, DC: Author.

Department of Defense. (2019, September). *Behavioral science support (BSS) for detainee operations and intelligence interrogations* (Department of Defense Instruction 2310.09). Washington, DC: Author.

Department of Defense, Office of the Deputy Assistant Secretary of Defense for Military Community and Family Policy. (2018). *2018 Demographics: Profile of the military community.* Washington, DC: Author. Retrieved September 10, 2020, from *https://download.militaryonesource.mil/12038/MOS/Reports/2018-demographics-report.pdf.*

Department of Veterans Affairs & Department of Defense. (2017). *VA/DoD Clinical Practice Guideline for the management of posttraumatic stress disorder and acute stress disorder.* Retrieved September 9, 2020, from *www.healthquality.va.gov/guidelines/MH/ptsd/VADoDPTSDCPGFinal.pdf.*

Dobmeyer, A. C. (2013). Primary care behavioral health: Ethical issues in military settings. *Families, Systems, & Health, 31*(1), 60–68.

Dunivin, D., Banks, L. M., Staal, M. A., & Stephenson, J. A. (2011). Behavioral science consultation to interrogation and debriefing operations: Ethical considerations. In C. H. Kennedy & T. J. Williams (Eds.), *Ethical practice in operational psychology: Military and national intelligence applications* (pp. 51–68). Washington, DC: American Psychological Association.

Dunlap, S. L., Holloway, I. W., Pickering, C. E., Tzen, M., Goldbach, J. T., & Castro, C. A. (2021). Support for transgender military service from active duty United States military personnel. *Sexuality Research and Social Policy, 18,* 137–143.

Fein, R. A., Lehner, P., & Vossekuil, B. (2006). *Educing information, interrogation: Science and art, foundations for the future.* Washington, DC: National Defense Intelligence College.

Galvin, M. (Producer/Director). (2008). *Interrogate this: Psychologists take on terror* [Motion picture]. (Available from MG Productions, 1112 Boylston St., #163, Boston, MA 02215)

Gelles, M. G., & Palarea, R. (2011). Ethics in crisis negotiation: A law enforcement and public safety perspective. In C. H. Kennedy & T. J. Williams (Eds.), *Ethical practice in operational psychology: Military and national intelligence applications* (pp. 107–123). Washington, DC: American Psychological Association.

Glassman, L. H., Mackintosh, M.-A., Talkovsky, A., Wells, S. Y., Walter, K. H., Wickramasinghe, I., et al. (2019). Quality of life following treatment for PTSD: Comparison of videoconferencing and in-person modalities. *Journal of Telemedicine and Telecare, 25*(2), 123–127.

Glynn, L. H., Chen, J. A., Dawson, T. C., Gelman, H., & Zeliadt, S. B. (2021). Bringing chronic-pain care to rural veterans: A telehealth pilot program description. *Psychological Services, 18*(3), 310–318.

Greene, C. H., & Banks, L. M. (2009). Ethical guideline evolution in psychological support to interrogation operations. *Consulting Psychology Journal: Practice and Research, 61,* 25–32.

Gros, D. F., Yoder, M., Tuerk, P. W., Lozano, B. E., & Acierno, R. (2011). Exposure therapy for PTSD delivered to veterans via telehealth: Predictors of treatment completion and outcome and comparison to treatment delivered in person. *Behavior Therapy, 42,* 276–283.

Hoyt, G. B. (2006). Integrated mental health within operational units: Opportunities and challenges. *Military Psychology, 18,* 309–320.

Hoyt, T. (2013). Limits to confidentiality in U.S. Army treatment settings. *Military Psychology, 25*(1), 46–56.

Johnson, W. B. (1995). Perennial ethical quandaries in military psychology: Toward American Psychological Association–Department of Defense collaboration. *Professional Psychology: Research and Practice, 26,* 281–287.

Johnson, W. B. (2008). Top ethical challenges for military clinical psychologists. *Military Psychology, 20,* 49–62.

Johnson, W. B. (2011). "I've got this friend": Multiple roles, informed consent, and friendship in the military. In W. B. Johnson & G. P. Koocher (Eds.), *Ethical conundrums, quandaries, and predicaments in mental health care practice* (pp. 175–182). New York: Oxford University Press.

Johnson, W. B. (2013). Mixed-agency dilemmas in military psychology. In B. A. Moore & J. E. Barnett (Eds.), *Military psychologists' desk reference* (pp. 112–116). New York: Oxford University Press.

Johnson, W. B., Bertschinger, M., Snell, A. K., & Wilson, A. (2014). Secondary trauma and ethical obligations for military psychologists: Preserving compassion and competence in the crucible of combat. *Psychological Services, 11*(1), 68–74.

Johnson, W. B., Grasso, I., & Maslowski, K. (2010). Conflicts between ethics and law for military mental health providers. *Military Medicine, 175,* 548–553.

Johnson, W. B., Johnson, S. J., Sullivan, G. R., Bongar, B., Miller, L., & Sammons, M. T. (2011). Psychology *in extremis*: Preventing problems of professional competence in dangerous practice settings. *Professional Psychology: Research and Practice, 42,* 94–104.

Johnson, W. B., & Kennedy, C. H. (2010). Preparing psychologists for high-risk jobs: Key ethical considerations for military clinical supervisors. *Professional Psychology: Research and Practice, 41,* 298–304.

Johnson, W. B., Ralph, J., & Johnson, S. J. (2005). Managing multiple roles in embedded environments: The case of aircraft carrier psychology. *Professional Psychology: Research and Practice, 36,* 73–81.

Johnson, W. B., Rosenstein, J. E., Buhrke, R. A., & Haldeman, D. C. (2015). After "Don't ask don't tell": Competent care of lesbian, gay and bisexual military personnel during the DoD policy transition. *Professional Psychology: Research and Practice, 46*(2), 107–115.

Johnson, W. B., & Wilson, K. (1993). The military internship: A retrospective analysis. *Professional Psychology: Research and Practice, 24,* 312–318.

Kennedy, C. H. (2009). You want me to do what?: The case of the unlawful order. *Navy Psychologist, 2,* 9–10.

Kennedy, C. H. (2011). Establishing rapport with an "enemy combatant": Cultural competence in Guantanamo Bay. In W. B. Johnson & G. P. Koocher (Eds.), *Ethical conundrums, quandaries, and predicaments in mental health practice: A casebook from the files of experts* (pp. 183–188). New York: Oxford University Press.

Kennedy, C. H. (2012). Institutional ethical conflicts with illustrations from police and military psychology. In S. Knapp & L. VandeCreek (Eds.), *APA handbook of ethics in psychology: Vol. 1. Moral foundations and common themes* (pp. 123–144). Washington, DC: American Psychological Association.

Kennedy, C. H. (2020). *Military stress reactions: Rethinking trauma and PTSD.* New York: Guilford Press.

Kennedy, C. H., Boake, C., & Moore, J. L. (2010). A history and introduction to military neuropsychology. In C. H. Kennedy & J. L. Moore (Eds.), *Military neuropsychology* (pp. 1–28). New York: Springer.

Kennedy, C. H., & Johnson, W. B. (2009). Mixed agency in military psychology: Applying the American Psychological Association's Ethics Code. *Psychological Services, 6,* 22–31.

Kennedy, C. H., Jones, D. E., & Arita, A. A. (2007). Multicultural experiences of U.S. military psychologists: Current trends and training target areas. *Psychological Services, 4,* 158–167.

Kennedy, C. H., & Malone, R. C. (2009). Integration of women into the modern military. In S. M. Freeman, B. A. Moore, & A. Freeman (Eds.), *Living and surviving in harm's way: A psychological treatment handbook for pre- and post-deployment of military personnel* (pp. 67–81). New York: Routledge.

Kennedy, C. H., Malone, R. C., & Franks, M. J. (2009). Provision of mental health services at the detention hospital in Guantanamo Bay. *Psychological Services, 6*, 1–10.

Kennedy, C. H., & Williams, T. J. (2011a). *Ethical practice in operational psychology: Military and national intelligence applications.* Washington, DC: American Psychological Association.

Kennedy, C. H., & Williams, T. J. (2011b). Operational psychology ethics: Addressing evolving dilemmas. In C. H. Kennedy & T. J. Williams (Eds.), *Ethical practice in operational psychology: Military and national intelligence applications* (pp. 3–27). Washington, DC: American Psychological Association.

Kennedy, C. H., & Zillmer, E. A. (2006). *Military psychology: Clinical and operational applications.* New York: Guilford Press.

Kennedy, K., Borum, R., & Fein, R. (2011). Ethical considerations in psychological consultation to counterintelligence and counterterrorism activities. In C. H. Kennedy & T. J. Williams (Eds.), *Ethical practice in operational psychology: Military and national intelligence applications* (pp. 69–83). Washington, DC: American Psychological Association.

Kitchener, R. F., & Kitchener, K. S. (2012). Ethical foundations of psychology. In S. J. Knapp, M. C. Gottlieb, M. M. Handelsman, & L. D. VandeCreek (Eds.), *APA handbook of ethics in psychology: Vol. 1. Moral foundations and common themes* (pp. 3–42). Washington, DC: American Psychological Association.

Koocher, G. P. (2009). Ethics and the invisible psychologist. *Psychological Services, 6*, 97–107.

Laskow, G. B., & Grill, D. J. (2003). The Department of Defense experiment: The psychopharmacology demonstration project. In M. T. Sammons, R. F. Levant, & R. U. Page (Eds.), *Prescriptive authority for psychologists: A history and guide* (pp. 77–101). Washington, DC: American Psychological Association.

Linnerooth, P. J., Mrdjenovich, A. J., & Moore, B. A. (2011). Professional burnout in clinical military psychologists: Recommendations before, during, and after deployment. *Professional Psychology: Research and Practice, 42*(1), 87–93.

Loftus, E. F. (2011). Intelligence gathering post-9/11. *American Psychologist, 66*, 532–541.

Maltzman, S. (2011). An organizational self-care model: Practical suggestions for development and implementation. *The Counseling Psychologist, 39*, 303–319.

McCauley, M., Hughes, J. H., & Liebling-Kalifani, H. (2008). Ethical considerations for military clinical psychologists: A review of selected literature. *Military Psychology, 20*, 7–20.

McCutcheon, J. L. (2011). Ethical issues in policy psychology: Challenges and decision-making models to resolve ethical dilemmas. In J. Kitaeff (Ed.), *Handbook of police psychology* (pp. 89–108). New York: Routledge.

Mullins, W. C., & McMains, M. J. (2011). The role of psychologist as a member of a crisis negotiation team. In J. Kitaeff (Ed.), *Handbook of police psychology* (pp. 345–361). New York: Routledge.

Nagy, T. F. (2012). Competence. In S. J. Knapp, M. C. Gottlieb, M. M. Handelsman, & L. D. VandeCreek (Eds.), *APA handbook of ethics in psychology: Vol. 1. Moral foundations and common themes* (pp. 147–174). Washington, DC: American Psychological Association.

National Immigration Forum. (2017). *For love of country: New Americans serving in our Armed Forces.* Washington, DC: Author. Retrieved September 10, 2020, from *http://immigrationforum.org/wp-content/uploads/2017/11/FOR-THE-LOVE-OF-COUNTRY-DIGITAL.pdf.*

Picano, J., Williams, T. J., Roland, R., & Long, C. (2011). Operational psychologists in support of assessment and selection: Ethical considerations. In C. H. Kennedy & T. J. Williams (Eds.), *Ethical practice in operational psychology* (pp. 29–49). Washington, DC: American Psychological Association.

Pierce, B. S., Perrin, P. B., Tyler, C. M., McKee, G. B., & Watson, J. D. (2021). The COVID-19 telepsychology revolution: A national study of pandemic-based changes in U.S. mental health care delivery. *American Psychologist, 76*(1), 14–25.

Ragusea, A. S. (2012). The more things change, the more they stay the same: Ethical issues in the provision of telehealth. In S. J. Knapp, M. C. Gottlieb, M. M. Handelsmann, & L. D. VandeCreek (Eds.), *APA handbook of ethics in psychology: Vol. 2. Practice, teaching, and research* (pp. 183–198). Washington, DC: American Psychological Association.

Ralph, J. A., & Sammons, M. T. (2006). Future directions of military psychology. In C. H. Kennedy & E. A. Zillmer (Eds.), *Military psychology: Clinical and operational applications* (pp. 371–386). New York: Guilford Press.

Reger, M. A., Etherage, J. R., Reger, G. M., & Gahm, G. A. (2008). Civilian psychologists in an Army culture: The ethical challenge of cultural competence. *Military Psychology, 20,* 21–35.

Schank, J. A., Helbok, C. M., Haldeman, D. C., & Gallardo, M. E. (2010). Challenges and benefits of ethical small-community practice. *Professional Psychology: Research and Practice, 41,* 502–510.

Schendel, C., & Kennedy, C. H. (2020). Consultation within the military setting. In C. A. Falender & E. P. Shafranske (Eds.), *Consultation in health service psychology: Advancing professional practice—a competency-based approach* (pp. 301–318). Washington, DC: American Psychological Association.

Shumate, S., & Borum, R. (2006). Psychological support to defense counterintelligence operations. *Military Psychology, 18,* 283–296.

Soldz, S. (2008). Healers or interrogators: Psychology and the United States torture regime. *Psychoanalytic Dialogues, 18,* 592–613.

Sommers-Flanagan, R. (2012). Boundaries, multiple roles, and the professional relationship. In S. J. Knapp, M. C. Gottlieb, M. M. Handelsmann, & L. D. VandeCreek (Eds.), *APA handbook of ethics in psychology: Vol. 1, Moral foundations and common themes* (pp. 241–277). Washington, DC: American Psychological Association.

Staal, M. A. (2019). Behavioral science consultation to military interrogations. In M. A. Staal & S. C. Harvey (Eds.), *Operational psychology: A new field to support national security and public safety* (pp. 241–260). Santa Barbara, CA: Praeger.

Staal, M. A., & King, R. E. (2000). Managing a multiple relationship environment: The ethics of military psychology. *Professional Psychology, Research and Practice, 31,* 698–705.

Staal, M. A., & Stephenson, J. A. (2006). Operational psychology: An emerging subdiscipline. *Military Psychology, 18,* 269–282.

Stone, A. M. (2008). Dual agency for VA clinicians: Defining an evolving ethical question. *Military Psychology, 20,* 37–48.

Tobin, J. (2005). The challenges and ethical dilemmas of a military medical officer serving with a peacekeeping operation in regard to the medical care of the local population. *Journal of Medical Ethics, 31,* 571–574.

Toye, R., & Smith, M. (2011). Behavioral health issues and detained individuals. In M. K. Lenhart (Ed.), *Combat and operational behavioral health* (pp. 645–656). Fort Detrick, MD: Borden Institute.

Tuerk, P. W., Yoder, M., Ruggiero, K. J., Gros, D. R., & Acierno, R. (2010). A pilot study of prolonged exposure therapy for posttraumatic stress disorder delivered via telehealth technology. *Journal of Traumatic Stress, 23,* 116–123.

Vaughan, C. A., Farmer, C. M., Breslau, J., & Burnette, C. (2015). *Evaluation of the Operational Stress Control and Readiness (OSCAR) Program.* Santa Monica, CA: RAND Corporation. Downloaded on September 7, 2020 from *www.rand.org/pubs/research_reports/RR562.html.*

Wood, D. W., Koffman, R. L., & Arita, A. A. (2003). Psychiatric medevacs during a 6–month aircraft carrier battle group deployment to the Persian Gulf: A Navy force health protection preliminary report. *Military Medicine, 168,* 43–47.

Young, J., Harvey, S., & Staal, M. A. (2011). Ethical considerations in the conduct of security clearance evaluations. In C. H. Kennedy & T. J. Williams (Eds.), *Ethical practice in operational psychology: Military and national intelligence applications* (pp. 51–68). Washington, DC: American Psychological Association.

Index

Note. f, t, or n after a page number indicates a figure, a table, or a note.

Index

Note. f, t, or n after a page number indicates a figure, a table, or a note.

441